Oxford Core Texts

CLINICAL DERMATOLOGY
ENDOCRINOLOGY
PAEDIATRICS
NEUROLOGY

ENDOCRINOLOGY

Andrew Levy

*Consultant Senior Lecturer
in Medicine and Endocrinology,
Bristol Royal Infirmary*

and

Stafford L. Lightman

*Professor of Medicine and
Head of Department,
Bristol Royal Infirmary*

Oxford   New York   Tokyo

Oxford University Press

1997

Oxford University Press, Great Clarendon Street, Oxford OX2 6DP

Oxford   New York
Athens   Auckland   Bangkok   Bogota   Bombay   Buenos Aires
Calcutta   Cape Town   Dar es Salaam   Delhi   Florence   Hong Kong
Istanbul   Karachi   Kuala Lumpur   Madras   Madrid   Melbourne
Mexico City   Nairobi   Paris   Singapore   Taipei   Tokyo   Toronto
and associated companies in
Berlin   Ibadan

Oxford is a trade mark of Oxford University Press

Published in the United States
by Oxford University Press Inc., New York

© Andrew Levy and Stafford L. Lightman, 1997

A catalogue record for this book is available from the British Library

Library of Congress Cataloging in Publication Data
(Data available)

ISBN 0 19 262766 X

Typeset by
EXPO Holdings, Malaysia

Printed in Hong Kong

To Ainslie, Rebecca, Hannah, and Daniel.

Contents

Preface   ix

Acknowledgements   x

Abbreviations   xi

Introduction   1

1 The hypothalamus   13

2 The pituitary gland   25

3 The thyroid gland   57

4 The adrenal glands   83

5 The ovary   103

6 The menstrual cycle   117

7 Fertility   133

8 Pregnancy   143

9 Contraception   155

10 Hirsutism   163

11 The breast   175

12 The testis   185

13 Erectile dysfunction   199

14 Puberty   211

15 Short and tall stature   225

16 Food and energy   239

17 Diabetes mellitus   253

18 Hyperlipidaemia   285

19 Calcium metabolism and bone   299

20 Water and salt   323

21 Endocrine hypertension   337

22 Endocrine neoplasia   345

23 Endocrine prophylaxis   363

24 Endocrine function tests   369

25 Examination hints   379

Index   385

Preface

For a medical undergraduate, the goal of becoming a superb clinician, a brilliant communicator, an astute administrator, and an innovative researcher while sustaining a family and social life of unsurpassed quality and tranquility, may seem entirely practical. In reality, there is scarcely time to meet just a few of these objectives, and the shrewd clinician has to find an appropriate compromise between depth and breadth of knowledge in each field. This is no easy task, as medicine is an ever-changing science, with new diagnostic methods and treatment modalities trailing only a little way behind a fast increasing body of information. Fortunately, within each medical subspeciality there is a definable body of knowledge of fairly modest proportion, that constitutes almost everything that almost everyone needs to know. It is this core that is being increasingly exploited to rationalize medical training so that clinicians have time to develop as free-thinking, caring individuals who are able to manage their patients, the health service, and their own lives as effectively as possible.

The object of this book is to describe the core knowledge of endocrinology in an entertaining, concise, and memorable fashion. In so doing, many rare endocrine disorders that even in a specialized clinic constitute a small fraction of the work, are reduced to a passing mention that befits their clinical importance, rather than the intrigue with which they are associated. Nevertheless, we hope at the same time to communicate the fascination of endocrinology to those who might wish to explore further. In addition to a systematic approach to endocrinology, a number of common scenarios typically seen on the ward and in the endocrine out-patient department have been highlighted by discussing them from a problem-orientated standpoint. Over 450 multiple choice questions have been included to both reinforce important aspects of the text and to introduce fascinating but relatively unimportant points. Chapters devoted to commonly used endocrine tests, subsections on the most informative aspects of examination, flow diagrams, and 'grey cases', representing common presentation of endocrine disease, have also been included.

After digesting the contents of this book, the reader should be confident to manage almost all the patients with endocrine problems that he or she will come across during his or her career, as well as having sufficient knowledge to pass any examination hurdles along the way.

Bristol A. L.
January 1997 S. L. L.

Acknowledgements

We would like to thank Dr Julian Kabala for the radiographs, Dr Ed Sheffield for pathology specimens, Gill Bennerson and Judy Furber for fundal photographs and visual fields, and Gary James and others in the Medical Illustration Department at the Bristol Royal Infirmary. 'The Child Growth Foundation' and Aura Scientific kindly permitted their nine centile growth charts and DEXA scan outputs, respectively, to be reproduced.

Abbreviations

ACE	angiotensin-converting enzyme
ACTH	andrenocorticotrophic hormone
AD	androstenedione
ADH	antidiuretic hormone = vasopressin
AMP	adenosine monophosphate
ANP	atrial natriuretic peptide
AVP	arginine vasopressin
BMD	bone mineral density
BMI	body mass index
bpm	beats per minute
CAH	congenital adrenal hyperplasia
cAMP	cyclic AMP
cGMP	cyclic GMP
CCK-PZ	cholecystokinin–pancreozymin
CHD	coronary heart disease
CRH	corticotrophin-releasing hormone
CRP	C reactive protein
CSF	cerebrospinal fluid
CT	computed tomography
CVA	cerebrovascular accident
DA	dopamine
DEXA	dual energy X-ray absorptiometry
DHEA	dehydroepiandrosterone
DHEAS	dehydroepiandrosterone sulphate
DI	diabetes insipidus
DM	diabetes mellitus
ESR	erythrocyte sedimentation rate
FBC	full blood count
FNAB	fine-needle aspiration biopsy
FSH	follicle-stimulating hormone
FT_4	free T_4
GAP	GTPase activating peptide
GDP	guanosine diphosphate
γGT	Gamma-glutamytranspeptidase
GH	growth hormone
GHRH	growth-hormone-releasing hormone

GMP	guanosine monophosphate
GnRH	gonadotrophin-releasing hormone
GTP	guanosine triphosphate
hCG	human chorionic gonadotrophin
HDL	high density lipoprotein
5-HIAA	5-hydroxyindoleacetic acid
HMG CoA	3-hydroxy-3-methylglutaryl CoA
HRT	hormone replacement therapy
5HT	5-hydroxytryptamine
IDDM	insulin-dependent diabetes mellitus
IGF	insulin-like growth factor
IGFBP	insulin-like growth factor binding protein
im	intramuscular(ly)
iv	intravenous(ly)
LDL	low density lipoprotein
LH	luteinizing hormone
LHRH	luteinizing hormone-releasing hormone (now GnRH)
LINAC	linear accelerator
Lp(a)	lipoprotein little a
LPL	lipoprotein lipase
MAB	maximum androgen blockade
MEN	multiple endocrine neoplasia
MHC	major histocompatibility complex
MIBG	meta-iodobenzylguanidine
MIH	Müllerian inhibiting hormone
MR(I)	magnetic resonance (imaging)
MSH	melanocyte-stimulating hormone
NCAM	neural cell adhesion molecule
NIDDM	non-insulin-dependent diabetes mellitus
$1,25(OH)_2D$	1,25-dihydroxycholecalciferol
OT	oxytocin
PCOD	polycystic ovarian disease
PMS	pre-menstrual syndrome
PNMT	phenylethanolamine N-methyl transferase
PRL	prolactin
PTH	parathyroid hormone
PTHrp	PTH-related peptide
PTU	propylthiouracil
RDS	respiratory distress syndrome
SD	standard deviation
SHBG	sex hormone binding globulin
SHRT	sex hormone replacement therapy
SIADH	syndrome of inappropriate vasopressin secretion

SLE	systemic lupus erythematosus
T_3	tri-iodothyronine
T_4	thyroxine
TRH	thyrotrophin-releasing hormone
TSH	thyrotrophin = thyroid-stimulating hormone
U & E	urea and electrolytes
VIP	vasoactive intestinal polypeptide
VLDL	very low density lipoprotein
VMA	vanillylmandelic acid

Introduction

- General introduction
- What is endocrinology?
- Hormone synthesis
- Hormone storage and release
- Hormone transport
- Hormone actions
- Hormone targeting
- Hormone feedback effects
- Hormone measurement

General introduction

The three extracellular communication systems that allow specialized cells and tissues in an intact organism to function in an integrated fashion are the nervous system, the immune system, and the endocrine system. The nervous system channels two-way information between the central nervous system and periphery. It is specific and fast, but expensive in terms of energy and hardware, easily damaged, and difficult to repair when it fails. The immune system, which provides protection from infection, recognizes foreign protein as a result of immune surveillance, and mediates its effects through a series of specialized cells and soluble proteins, such as antibodies and cytokines—the secretions of activated lymphocytes. The endocrine system exploits hard-wired neurochemical signals from higher brain centres that are transduced by the hypothalamus to hormonal signals. These signalling peptides are released into the portal bloodstream that runs from the hypothalamus to the pituitary gland, where they lead to the controlled release of further peptide signals that are transported in blood to influence distant endocrine glands and other tissues. The endocrine system also encompasses a number of local sensor mechanisms that detect and respond to ambient conditions. Examples are the parathyroid glands, which rapidly increase secretion of parathyroid hormone as plasma calcium levels fall, and the pancreas, which secretes insulin in response to rising glucose levels. With advances in hormone assays and imaging, the diagnosis and management of many endocrine problems are now straightforward.

What is endocrinology?

Endocrinology, as originally defined, is the study of the physiological system in which the activity of distant organs is influenced by chemical substances secreted into the bloodstream. In addition to the dedicated endocrine organs (such as the pituitary, thyroid, and adrenal glands) this definition also includes endocrine organs that have other important functions, such as the gonads and kidneys, and multifunctional tissues whose endocrine activity is not immediately apparent, such as vascular endothelium, the skin, brain, and peripheral fat. In recent years, the importance of local hormonal effects, either on the cell that released the hormone or on adjacent cells, has also been appreciated. Hormones are responsible for controlling body fluid and electrolyte balance, blood pressure, heart rate, acid–base balance, bone mass, muscle and fat mass, cell growth, cell death, development, mental state, and body temperature. In fact all major body systems have a significant endocrine control input.

Hormone synthesis

There are three major categories of hormones: steroids, amines, and peptide or peptide derivative.

- Peptide hormones are coded by genes, transcribed to messenger RNA, translated into protein, and in many cases further modified (e.g. by cleavage or glycosylation) to give the final hormonal product. Insulin, for instance, is translated from mature messenger RNA to give the peptide pro-insulin, then cleaved to give equal amounts of mature insulin and 'C peptide'. Although hormones themselves may be coded for by a single gene, many other genes have to work correctly to ensure that a hormone will function appropriately. These include the genes for proteases that cleave the protein product to the final form, binding proteins that carry the hormone in the blood, receptor proteins that allow cells to respond to the signal, and the many 'second messenger' components within cells that deliver the signal to the appropriate site.
- Steroid hormones, such as cortisol, aldosterone, oestradiol, and testosterone, are made from the precursor cholesterol (or in the case of vitamin D synthesis in the skin, 7-dehydrocholesterol) by the sequential action of a series of enzymes.
- Amines, such as adrenaline and noradrenaline, are also made through the concerted action of a series of enzymes, with tyrosine as the precursor.

Hormone storage and release

With the exception of the thyroid, which contains enough stored hormone in the form of thyroglobulin to last for 2 weeks, most endocrine glands store relatively little pre-formed hormone. Stores of insulin in the pancreas and testosterone in the testes, for example, are enough for a few hours only. Hormone release is often *pulsatile* and in many cases the amplitude and sometimes qualitative response to the hormone depends on this pattern. The stimulatory effect of hypothalamic gonadotrophin-releasing hormone (GnRH) on the pituitary, for example, becomes profoundly inhibitory if GnRH is delivered as a continuous infusion, rather than a series of short pulses. In addition to pulsatility, hormone release is characterized by *biorhythmicity*. Fluctuation in hormone release may occur on a minute-to-minute basis, leading to rapid changes in the concentration of hormone in the blood if its half-life is short.

Secretion of hormones also varies on an hourly, daily (circadian or diurnal), and sometimes monthly basis, often in response to environmental factors. These patterns are further complicated by seasonal variations and by changes confined to different stage of life, such as puberty, pregnancy, or suckling.

Hormone transport

Many hormones are transported in the blood in dynamic equilibrium between protein-bound and free forms, with the small proportion of unbound hormone available to act at the target site. Some proteins have relatively specific binding capacities (such as sex hormone binding globulin) and others, such as albumin, are more general in their binding capacity. Although confusion can still arise if total hormone levels (bound + free) are measured in patients with unrecognized abnormalities of plasma proteins, many modern biochemical assays, although not infallible, take account of this by correcting for protein binding.

Hormone actions

A single hormone may have a number of different actions. Somatostatin, for example, is released from the hypothalamus into the hypothalamo-pituitary portal system and inhibits growth hormone release from the pituitary. It also inhibits release of thyroid-stimulating hormone from the pituitary, and when released from other sites, exerts inhibitory effects on almost all endocrine and exocrine secretions from the pancreas and gastrointestinal tract.

Equally, multiple hormones may be involved in a single action. The control of blood glucose, for example, is directly influenced by insulin, glucagon, growth hormone, somatostatin, cortisol, adrenaline, and noradrenaline.

Hormone targeting

Because hormones are present in the blood at such low levels, their actions are directed to specific sites by a number of mechanisms:

High-affinity receptors

Target tissues often express high-affinity receptors either on the cell surface, within the cytoplasm, or on the nuclear membrane. It is now appreciated that in addition to 'their own' high-affinity receptors, some hormones may also interact with other receptors at lower affinity, perhaps at subsidiary binding sites, producing an integrated and more divergent cascade of intra- and extracellular signals than was previously anticipated.

Portal circulations

Hormone can be contained within a restricted circulation. For example, the hypothalamo-pituitary portal system delivers high levels of hypothalamic-releasing hormone to the pituitary, and the portal blood supply from the gut delivers pancreatic insulin directly to the liver.

Paracrine effects

Local diffusion delivers high concentrations of hormone to adjacent cells and tissue, or even to the cell that originated the hormone. Testosterone synthesized by the Leydig cells of the testes, for example, provide the adjacent seminiferous tubules with high levels of hormone required to promote spermatogenesis. This is called a *paracrine* effect.

Autocrine effects

Hormone released from cells that are then influenced by the same hormone (often observed with growth factors), is called an *autocrine* effect.

Intracrine effects

Hormone can be synthesized from precursors *in situ* within a cell. The formation of dihydrotestosterone (a potent androgen) from pre-androgens within cells of the prostate that subsequently respond to it themselves is sometimes called an *intracrine* effect (see p.353).

Second messengers

Superficially, hormone binding to high-affinity receptors on a cell surface may appear to be the ultimate in targeting. However, at the cellular and molecular level the signal still has to be delivered to the appropriate machinery within the cell, often via a variety of effectors such as cyclic adenosine monophosphate (cAMP), inositol trisphosphate, Ca^{2+}, cyclic guanosine monophosphate (cGMP), and arachidonic acid. The so-called second messenger systems that carry the signal from the cell surface not only interact with each other, but also allow the signal to be amplified or attenuated, according to physiological circumstances.

- Some receptors, such as those for growth factors and insulin, are directly coupled to *tyrosine kinases*. These are proteins that direct the phosphorylation and hence activation of other proteins.
- Amines and neurotransmitters interact with *ligand-gated ion channels*. These are cell surface receptors that, when coupled to their ligand, allow ions to flow into or out of the cell.
- Many peptide hormones, neurotransmitters, and prostaglandins interact with *G protein-coupled receptors*. These transduce peptidergic, muscarinic, dopaminergic, serotoninergic, and adrenergic signals, and are the most abundant group of membrane receptors.

    G proteins consist of a complex of three proteins, an α-, β- and γ-subunit. They are called 'G' proteins because in their activated state they bind guanosine triphosphate (GTP). The duration of activation is limited by the time taken for the G protein to hydrolyse GTP to guanosine diphosphate (GDP), which it binds in the inactive state. Because hydrolysis of GTP to GDP is an enzymatic reaction, G proteins are also called *GTPases*.

    G protein-coupled receptors also interact with the inositol phospholipid second messenger pathway.

Hormone feedback effects

An almost universal feature of the endocrine system is feedback control. Whether the effects are inhibitory, as they usually are, or stimulatory, the presence of these

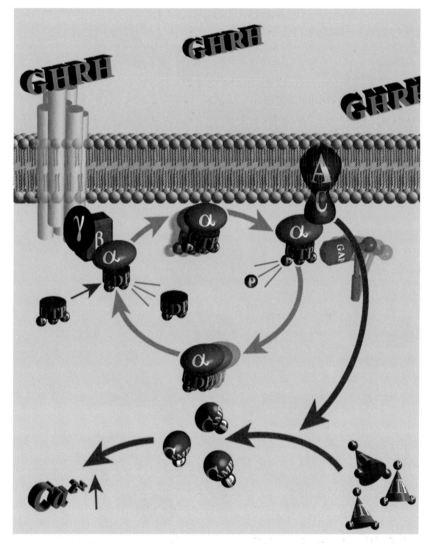

In the activated GTP-bound state, the α-subunit of the GTPase dissociates from the β- and γ-subunits and stimulates adenylyl cyclase to use ATP as a substrate for cyclic AMP production. Cyclic AMP activates cyclic AMP-dependent protein kinases, increases calcium ion level, and mediates a large number of cellular activities, such as stimulating hormone secretion, growth, and division. The weak, intrinsic GTPase activity of the α-subunit, potentiated by the action of GTPase activating peptides (GAPs), hydrolyses GTP and terminates the response.

elegant regulatory mechanisms makes it necessary when assessing endocrine function, to measure the levels of stimulatory hormone and end-organ hormone secretion simultaneously.

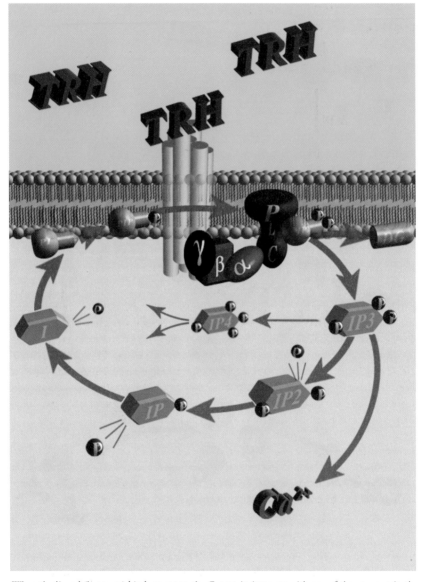

When the ligand (hormone) binds receptor, the G protein interacts with one of the enzymes in the phospholipase C group (PLC). Phospholipase C cleaves a membrane phospholipid 'phosphatidylinositol bisphosphonate (PIP2)' into diacylglycerol (DG) and inositol trisphosphate (IP3), both of which have signalling functions. IP3 causes an increase in intracellular calcium ion levels which, in turn, modulates the activity of protein kinases regulated by calcium-binding regulatory proteins such as calmodulin. IP3 is rapidly dephosphorylated to inositol bisphosphate (IP2), inositol phosphate (IP), and then to free inositol (I), before being reincorporated into the lipid membrane as phosphatidylinositol (PI), then phosphorylated back to PIP2.

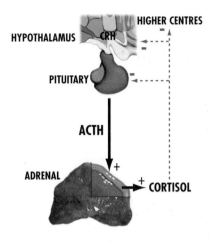

A typical example of *long-loop feedback* is shown above. In this example, corticotrophin-releasing hormone (CRH) from the hypothalamus is released into the portal blood system that connects the hypothalamus to the anterior lobe of the pituitary. The CRH acts on pituitary corticotrophs to stimulate the production and secretion of adrenocorticotrophic hormone (ACTH). ACTH stimulates production of cortisol from the adrenal cortex and the cortisol 'feeds back' to inhibit pituitary ACTH production, hypothalamic CRH production, and also the activity of higher brain centres that influence the hypothalamus. A similar 'long-loop' pattern of feedback control is evident in gonadal and thyroid regulation.

Short-loop feedback is said to occur when the local actions of a hormone inhibit its own release (demonstrated for a number of pituitary hormones), and *ultrashort-loop feedback* occurs when the release of a hypothalamic peptide is inhibited by the peptide itself, immediately after release from the same source (shown for somatostatin and growth hormone-releasing hormone).

Hormone measurement

There have been dramatic technological developments in analytical methods for measuring hormones over the past decade. Instead of slow, labour-intensive and operator-dependent radioimmunoassays, in which hormone in the test sample was displaced from binding a specific antibody by a defined amount of radiolabelled hormone, many routine hormone assays are now carried out in rapid chemiluminescent, immunometric assays by automated systems. Results are produced within minutes rather than days and individual samples rather than batches can be analysed economically. One of the most familiar examples of this kind of new

Examples of the practical significance of understanding mechanisms of hormone action

Mechanism	Example	Explanation
Receptor mutations	Laron dwarfism. A form of inherited dwarfism	Dwarfism with high growth hormone (GH) levels. The GH receptor is abnormal.
Anti-receptor antibodies	Graves' disease. A cause of hyperthyroidism (see page 62)	An autoimmune condition in which thyroid stimulating hormone (TSH) receptor antibodies are produced. Paradoxically, their effect is stimulatory.
Defects in hormone synthesis	Congenital adrenal hyperplasia. A cause of hirsutism & virilism (see page 94)	A group of abnormalities of the adrenal cortical enzymes involved in synthesis of cortisol, aldosterone and other hormones from cholesterol.
Second messenger mutation	Acromegaly: excessive pituitary growth hormone secretion (see page 38)	An activating mutation of a component of the second messenger system is thought to be responsible for 40% of cases of acromegaly.
Paracrine effects	Male fertility (see page 188)	Spermatogenesis is dependent on high levels of androgens diffusing from adjacent leydig cells.
Autocrine effects	Prostatic carcinoma. Hormone synthesis within tumour cells (see page 353)	Formation of 'tumour growth-promoting' androgens within prostatic tumour cells from circulating adrenal pre-androgens, make androgen receptor blockers an intuitive addition to treatments that prevent testicular androgen synthesis.
'Long loop feedback'	Adrenal failure (see page 89)	In primary adrenal failure, cortisol levels & feedback inhibition falls, so pituitary ACTH levels rise. In secondary failure (ie. Pituitary disease), ACTH levels are low.
Hormone transport	Mistaken diagnosis of endocrine overactivity (see page 76)	Oestrogen stimulates production of hormone binding proteins by the liver. In normal women taking 'the pill', *total*, but not *free* thyroid hormones are often raised.
Pulsatility of hormone release	Misleading blood results	Single measurement of hormones with short half lives that are released in pulses (such as growth hormone & ACTH) are notoriously unrepresentative of mean levels.
New laboratory technology	Management of endocrine disease	Rapid diagnosis facilitates management. The finding of a high prolactin level in a patient admitted for urgent treatment of visual failure, secures the diagnosis of macroprolactinoma (see page 36), and allows first line management to be oral dopamine agonists rather than neurosurgery.

technology is the solid-phase colorimetric (rather than chemiluminescent) assay of urinary human chorionic gonadotrophin (hCG) available 'over the counter' to detect early pregnancy. Rapid and reliable laboratory backup is central to the diagnosis and management of endocrine problems.

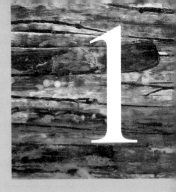

1

The hypothalamus

- Summary
- Introduction
- Key points
- Case histories
- Multiple-choice questions

Summary

Normal function

- In close association with the pituitary gland, the hypothalamus is the principle central regulator and integrator of the endocrine system.
- Vasopressin (formerly known as ADH—antidiuretic hormone) and oxytocin *synthesized* by the hypothalamus are *released* from the terminals of hypothalamic neurones that extend down into the posterior lobe of the pituitary gland.
- The synthesis and release of hormones from the anterior lobe of the pituitary gland is regulated by peptides or amines secreted from the hypothalamus into the hypothalamo-hypophyseal portal system. With the exception of gonadotrophin-releasing hormone (GnRH, formerly LHRH) and dopamine, abnormalities of these systems rarely give rise to clinical conditions.
  - → The secretory response of the pituitary to GnRH is critically dependent on its pulsatile pattern of release.
  - → Hypothalamic dopamine inhibits anterior pituitary prolactin secretion.

Typical pathology

- Hypothalamic underactivity
  - → Hypothalamic underactivity is usually caused by transcranial surgery to remove tumours within the hypothalamus, such as craniopharyngiomas, or pituitary tumours that have grown up into it.
  - → Typical effects are diabetes insipidus, weight gain, and somnolence.
  - → By reducing pulsatile release of GnRH, the hypothalamus is responsible for the amenorrhoea that occurs under conditions of acute stress or low body weight.
  - → If hypothalamic dopamine is prevented from reaching the normal pituitary (usually through compression of the pituitary stalk by an endocrinologically inactive pituitary adenoma) and the pituitary gland is still functioning, hyperprolactinaemia will result.
- → Hypothalamic overactivity
  This is not a clinical entity.

Typical clinical scenario

- A patient with amenorrhoea, who exercises excessively and considers herself 'fit', but is underweight for her height, and has 'hypothalamic amenorrhoea'.
- A panhypopituitary patient, following transcranial, subfrontal surgery to remove a craniopharyngioma, who is somnolent and gaining weight, despite claiming to eat no more than usual.

Table 1.1
Clinically significant hypothalamic hormone dysfunction

Vasopressin Diabetes insipidus	• Vasopressin released from the neural lobe is made in no fewer than 4 discrete locations in the hypothalamus. Localized hypothalamic damage is therefore less likely to cause diabetes insipidus than a diffuse problem such as cranial sarcoidosis or autoimmune destruction. The exception is the formation of craniopharyngiomas which although not strictly of hypothalamic origin, often appear in that location.
• For the same reason, when traumatic diabetes insipidus does occur, for example, following subfrontal surgery, recovery may occur within a few days, although it sometimes takes as long as a year or two—if it occurs at all.
• The release of vasopressin into the bloodsteam does not necessarily depend on the presence of an intact posterior pituitary. It can reach the bloodstream from the remaining pituitary stalk
Dopamine Hyperprolactinaemia	• Compression of the lower part of the median eminence or the pituitary stalk reduces the flow of dopamine from the hypothalamus and disinhibits prolactin release from the pituitary gland.
• Therefore the association of a pituitary mass with hyperprolactinaemia (typically with levels of between 1000 and 3000mu/l) does not invariably indicate the presence of a prolactinoma, as a non-secreting adenoma might cause hyperprolactinaemia by 'pituitary stalk compression'
GnRH (LHRH) Amenorrhoea & infertility	• Hypogonadotrophic hypogonadism is ovarian or testicular failure due to lack of FSH and LH. Lack of pulsatile GnRH release turns off pituitary gonadotrophin (FSH and LH) release
• Kallmann's syndrome, failure of GnRH production by the hypothalamus, is the most common cause of isolated hypogonadotrophic hypogonadism. In this syndrome, during embryogenesis, GnRH-secreting neurones do not migrate backwards from the forebrain to the anterior hypothalamus, and olfactory pathways also fail to connect up. Patients with Kallmann's syndrome do not enter puberty spontaneously and are usually anosmic. Blood tests show low testosterone or oestrogen, in association with a low FSH and LH. Patients rarely volunteer the fact that they have no sense of smell—you need to ask

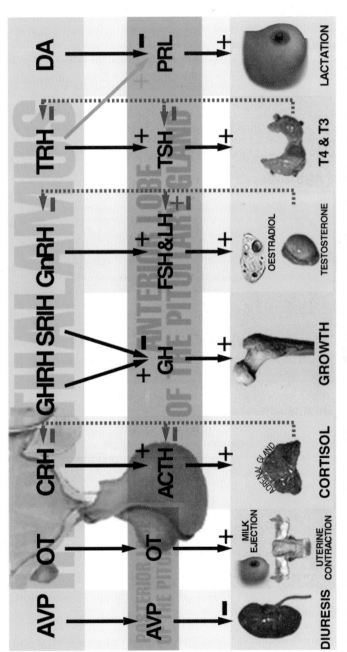

Fig. 1.1 Relationship between the hypothalamus and the anterior pituitary. Hormones are released from the hypothalamo–pituitary portal system to influence anterior pituitary hormone release: corticotrophin-releasing hormone (CRH) stimulates adrenocorticotrophic hormone (ACTH) release; growth-hormone-releasing hormone (GHRH) stimulates and somatostatin (SRIH) inhibits growth hormone (GH) release; gonadotrophin-releasing hormone (GnRH, formerly known as LHRH) stimulates follicle-stimulating hormone (FSH) and luteinizing hormone (LH) release; thyrotropin-releasing hormone (TRH) stimulates thyrotropin (TSH) and to some extent prolactin (PRL) release; and dopamine (DA) inhibits PRL release. Vasopressin (AVP) and oxytocin (OT), synthesized in the hypothalamus, are delivered to the posterior pituitary via neurosecretory nerve terminals, and are released from there in response to appropriate stimuli.

Introduction

The hypothalamus consists of two small, forward-pointing wedges of tissue, barely 15 mm in length, separated by the slit-like third ventricle and joined anteriorly by the lamina terminalis, a thin sheet of tissue that crosses the midline (see p. 326). The superior surface of the hypothalamus is impaled by the fornix, a thick-fibre bundle carrying inhibitory afferents from the hippocampus. The

Table 1.2
Craniopharyngiomas

These are benign, often cystic tumours that usually arise between the pituitary and hypothalamus

They are derived from embryonal squamous cell rests

They are most commonly diagnosed in children but may occur at any age

Because of their position, 80–90 per cent of patients have visual symptoms at presentation

Disturbance of hypothalamic function (either primary or following surgical treatment) is also common

Craniopharyngiomas are a common management problem in the adult endocrine clinic

Table 1.3
Hypothalamic insufficiency

Causes	Effects
Common	Common
Subfrontal surgery	Transient diabetes insipidus
	Hyperphagia and weight gain
Less Common	
Kallmann's syndrome	Less Common
Craniopharyngiomas	Permanent diabetes insipidus
	Somnolence and behaviour changes
Rare	
Autoimmune destruction	Rare
Cranial sarcoidosis	Aggression
Other granulomatous conditions	Impairment of thirst sensation

inferior surface of the hypothalamus is marked anteriorly by the optic chiasm, and bounded laterally by the optic tracts as they diverge from the chiasm on their way to the midbrain. Immediately behind the chiasm the hypothalamus is pulled down into a squat cone—'the median eminence'—at the tip of which, about 1 cm below the optic chiasm, is attached the pituitary gland.

Pituitary secretion is controlled by hypothalamic hormones released into the hypothalamo-hypophyseal portal system (Fig. 1.1) and by feedback effects of secretions from peripheral target organs. If the gonads—(primary hypogonadism), adrenal glands (Addison's disease), or thyroid fail, feedback inhibition at the hypothalamus and pituitary is reduced, and circulating levels of follicle-stimulating hormone (FSH) and luteinizing hormone (LH), ACTH or TSH, respectively, increase.

Key points

- The hypothalamus controls pituitary function.
- The menstrual cycle is controlled by pulsatile release of hypothalamic GnRH.
- The hypothalamus mediates amenorrhoea secondary to emotional stress or being under-weight.
- Except for gonadal axis function, primary hypothalamic failure leading to pituitary hormone deficiency is rare.
- The hypothalamus is typically damaged by tumours, or surgery to remove tumours that arise beneath it. Transcranial surgery to resect craniopharyngiomas is the most common cause.
- Typical features of hypothalamic damage are weight gain, diabetes insipidus, and somnolence.

The case histories in this book—almost all of them real-life examples—are typical of the kind of presentation of endocrine conditions seen in the specialist clinic. There are no set protocols for investigation or management of endocrine disease, and many variations on each theme. Thus the outlines of management are suggestions only, and have been chosen more to provide a flavour of endocrinology in practice, than firm guidelines.

'My patient's menstrual periods have never been heavy and they have now stopped altogether, please advise'

History

A 24-year-old secretary was referred to clinic complaining that her menstrual periods had stopped. Her menarche occurred at the age of 12 and from that time on her periods had been regular but fairly light. During the previous 18 months, she estimated that she had had between 6 and 8 periods—each lasting a day or two only—and for the past 6 months she had had no periods at all. Otherwise, the patient claimed to be completely fit and well. She attended a fitness class four nights a week after work, ate 'wholesome food', and smoked five cigarettes daily. She denied dyspareunia (discomfort on intercourse) or galactorrhoea (milk discharge) and was happy without fertility or periods for the time being, provided she could be reassured that nothing was wrong.

Examination

On examination she was slim and well dressed. Her height was 5'6" (1.68 m), weight 9 st 2 lb (58.1 kg fully dressed), and blood pressure 114/78 mmHg.

Investigations

The only investigation carried out was measurement of FSH, LH, and prolactin, all three of which were at the lower end of their normal ranges, and thyroid function tests, which were normal.

Management

The patient was told that a normal, physiological mechanism turns off menstruation when body weight is low, or during periods of stress or strenuous exercise, in order to protect women from pregnancy under unfavourable circumstances. Low oestrogen levels for any length of time, however, are now known to predispose to osteoporosis and cardiovascular disease (as well as dyspareunia) and normalization of sex hormone levels is recommended. The suggestion that the patient should put on a little weight and stop smoking was unfortunately (but not unexpectedly) met with considerable scepticism and indignation. She was prescribed low-dose sex hormone replacement therapy, and reassured that there was no reason to suspect that her fertility would be impaired in the long run.

Explanation

For many years it has been fashionable for women in Western society to be fairly slender. In many women, once the body mass index (BMI) is more than about 10 per cent below the ideal, pulsatile GnRH release from the hypothalamus diminishes and, in turn, secretion of FSH and LH from the pituitary is reduced. Ovarian follicular development is arrested and consequently oestrogen levels fall. Without oestrogen, the endometrium fails to proliferate and menstrual cycles stop. Vaginal lubrication is also oestrogen dependent—hence the discomfort on intercourse. In this patient, it is likely that excessive exercise and smoking contributed further to reduced circulating oestrogen.

The normal gonadotrophins (FSH and LH) exclude premature ovarian failure (premature menopause), and the normal prolactin excluded amenorrhoea secondary to hyperprolactinaemia.

Multiple-choice questions

1. Hypothalamic failure can cause:
   a. Hypothyroidism;
   b. Pubertal failure;
   c. Failure to enter and progress through labour;
   d. Hypoprolactinaemia;
   e. Diabetes insipidus.

2. The hypothalamus is intimately involved in the regulation of:
   a. Thirst;
   b. Food intake;
   c. Mood;
   d. Pituitary hormone secretion;
   e. Adrenal cortical aldosterone production.

3. Craniopharyngiomas:
   a. Are derived from hypothalamic tissue;
   b. Can rapidly increase in size after remaining static for some time;
   c. Are not sensitive to radiotherapy;
   d. Can secrete prolactin;
   e. Occur in children.

Answers

1. Hypothalamic failure can cause:
   a. Hypothyroidism   T

   It is true, but destruction of the hypothalamus causing hypopituitarism is very rare except after surgery. If circulating thyroid hormone levels are found to be low, in association with a low TSH, think of pituitary disease, rather than a problem 'higher' up.

   b. Pubertal failure   T

   Kallmann's syndrome has an incidence in men of 1/7500 (it is much more common than Cushing's disease or acromegaly). The inheritance can be autosomal dominant, autosomal recessive, or X-linked. About 15 per cent of patients are not anosmic.

   c. Failure to enter and progress through labour   F

   Although oxytocin secretion might be low, the onset of labour is not mediated by oxytocin, neither, somewhat surprisingly, does the absence of oxytocin seem to affect progression through labour.

   d. Hypoprolactinaemia   F

   Changes in prolactin resulting directly from hypothalamic failure are not well described. If anything, one would expect the reduction in hypothalamic dopamine reaching the pituitary to result in *hyper*prolactinaemia.

   e. Diabetes insipidus   T

   The hypothalamus makes the vasopressin that is released from the posterior lobe of the pituitary gland in response to an increase in plasma osmolality and hypotension.

2. The hypothalamus is intimately involved in the regulation of:
   a. Thirst   T

   The complex processes giving rise to the sensation of 'thirst' are hypothalamic in origin. Consequently, the sinister association of diabetes insipidus with impaired thirst sensation is well described.

   b. Food intake   T

   Hypothalamic mechanisms that control satiety are often damaged by transcranial pituitary surgery. The subtle hyperphagia that follows can produce obesity that is difficult to control and often more distressing for the patient than other aspects of hypothalamic damage, such as diabetes insipidus. None of the classic hypothalamic hormones appear to be directly responsible for appetite, although a number of hypothalamic peptides (such as 'neuropeptide Y') have been implicated. The hypothalamus may be one of the principal sites of feedback control of hunger by peptide hormones released from adipose tissue. This is currently an area of intensive research and great commercial excitement.

   c. Mood   T

   There are often subtle mood changes after hypothalamic damage. More severe changes in mood or personality can be one of the after-effects of the underlying disease, or surgery. However, significant changes are fairly unusual.

d. Pituitary hormone secretion   T

Although this is true, in clinical practice, primary hypothalamic problems are rare in comparison with pituitary disease. The blood–brain barrier does not prevent feedback inhibition on hypothalamic neurones by circulating hormones. However, with the exception of gonadal hormones, feedback inhibition is more marked, and more clinically relevant, at the level of the pituitary.

e. Adrenal cortical aldosterone production   F

Pituitary failure (of whatever cause), leaves the renin–angiotensin–aldosterone mechanism unscathed, as ACTH is of only minor importance in this pathway.

3. Craniopharyngiomas:

a. Are derived from hypothalamic tissue   F

They are derived from the remnants of Rathke's pouch—the epithelial evagination of the stomodeum that carries anterior pituitary precursor cells rostrally. As they may appear at any location along the embryonal craniopharyngeal canal, they can be intrasellar or extrasellar. Most are extrasellar, and the incidence of visual symptoms at presentation is high (80–90 per cent). About 50 per cent are calcified—a characteristic finding on computed tomography (CT) (but not magnetic resonance imaging (MRI) examination. In addition to presenting with the classical features of hypothalamic damage (diabetes insipidus, weight gain, and somnolence), they also occasionally present with headaches, loss of short-term memory, growth failure, premature puberty, or hydrocephalus.

b. Can rapidly increase in size after remaining static for some time   T

Craniopharyngiomas often consist of a collection of small cysts containing dark-brown, oily liquid. These can increase rapidly in size after remaining almost unchanged for years. Although benign, in as much as they do not metastasize, the mortality and morbidity from craniopharyngiomas are high, particularly in children under 5 years old.

c. Are not sensitive to radiotherapy   F

Radiotherapy can be useful in prevention of rapid enlargement of cysts.

d. Can secrete prolactin   F

They do not secrete pituitary hormones, but they may, however, lead to hyperprolactinaemia by compressing the pituitary stalk. This reduces the flow of hypothalamic dopamine (which inhibits prolactin release) to the anterior pituitary.

e. Occur in children   T

They are diagnosed in childhood as well as adulthood. Their management remains a major problem in the adult endocrinology clinic.

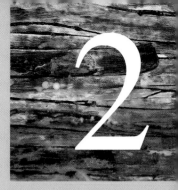

2

The pituitary gland

- Summary
- Introduction
- Pituitary tumours
- Hypopituitarism
- Key points
- Case histories
- Multiple-choice questions

Summary

Normal function

- The anterior lobe of the pituitary gland synthesizes and releases prolactin, growth hormone (GH), thyrotrophin (TSH), adrenocorticotrophin (ACTH, containing the subunit MSH), follicle-stimulating hormone (FSH), and luteinizing hormone (LH).
- Hypothalamic vasopressin and oxytocin are *released* from the posterior lobe.
- Pituitary hormone secretion amplifies and modulates instructions passed down from the hypothalamus.
- Hormone release is modulated by feedback signals from peripheral endocrine organs.

Typical pathology

- Pituitary underactivity (hypopituitarism)
  - → Compression of the normal pituitary by an adjacent pituitary adenoma.
  - → This more commonly results from trans-sphenoidal surgery to resect a pituitary tumour, or from external beam radiotherapy to treat pituitary adenomas that could not (as is usually the case) be completely resected.
- Pituitary overactivity
  - → This is almost always related to the formation of hormone-secreting adenomas. Prolactinomas causing hyperprolactinaemia are the most common. Acromegaly (GH) and Cushing's disease (ACTH) are less frequently seen, and TSH-secreting adenomas are extremely rare.
  - → The exception to the above is hyperprolactinaemia caused by an endocrinologically inactive (i.e. non-hormone-secreting) pituitary adenoma compressing the pituitary stalk and preventing hypothalamic dopamine (prolactin release inhibitor) from reaching pituitary prolactin-secreting cells.
- Other effects of pituitary pathology
  - → Pituitary tumours extending beyond the fossa (macroadenomas) can compress related structures such as the optic chiasm. Assessment of visual fields is central to the management of pituitary tumours.

'Typical clinical scenario'

- A 45-year-old man with acromegaly who, 4 years previously, had a trans-sphenoidal resection of the pituitary tumour, followed by external beam radiotherapy to the pituitary region. He is now taking pituitary hormone replacement therapy (hydrocortisone and thyroxine orally and testosterone by intramascular depot injection: see p. 24).

Introduction

The anterior lobe of the pituitary gland amplifies and modulates instructions passed down from the hypothalamus. It synthesizes and releases prolactin, growth hormone (GH), thyrotrophin (TSH), adrenocorticotrophic hormone (ACTH), follicle-stimulating hormone (FSH), and luteinizing hormone (LH). The hypothalamic hormones vasopressin and oxytocin are *released* from the posterior lobe.

The most common clinical disorders of the pituitary are adenoma formation and hypopituitarism. The latter most often follows the treatment of pituitary tumours. Hormone-secreting adenomas usually present as a result of the hormonal syndrome they cause, while non-secreting pituitary adenomas often come to light because they disturb the function of the adjacent normal pituitary, or compress related structures such as the optic chiasm. They are often treated by surgical excision ± external beam radiotherapy and/or drugs, such as dopamine agonists for prolactinomas or somatostatin (growth hormone release-*inhibiting* hormone) analogues for GH-secreting adenomas.

In hypopituitarism, so-called 'pituitary hormone replacement therapy' is for the most part replacement of peripheral endocrine organ hormone production, i.e. cortisol, thyroxine, and oestradiol or androgens (rather than replacement of pituitary hormones themselves). However, if fertility is required in either sex, true pituitary hormone replacement with intramuscular gonadotrophin injections (FSH and LH) is required, but only as an aid to conception.

Structure

The human pituitary has only two lobes, the anterior lobe and the posterior lobe.

Table 2.1
Pituitary development and anatomy

Very early in embryogenesis, cells destined to form the anterior lobe of the pituitary gland migrate rostrally above an outpouching of the roof of the primitive buccal cavity known as Rathke's pouch. At the same time a downgrowth from the floor of the third ventricle of the brain forms the posterior lobe of the pituitary. After only 7 weeks of gestation the primitive pituitary cells are isolated by the completion of the floor of the sella turcica ('Turkish saddle', after its shape), and by the end of gestation the pituitary has developed into a complex and highly ordered structure that has the highest blood flow (per unit weight) of any tissue in the body. The pituitary averages 13 mm wide by 9 mm anteroposteriorally and 6 mm high, but is considerably bigger during pregnancy. It is largely surrounded by the sphenoid bone and covered by a sheet of dura (the diaphragma sellae) through which the pituitary stalk passes. Anteriorly lies the sphenoid sinus and to either side the cavernous sinuses containing the carotid arteries and the third, fourth, and the upper two divisions of the fifth cranial nerves. Above the pituitary lies the optic chiasm and posteriorly, the brain stem, with the lower border of the pituitary usually lying parallel to the junction of the upper third and lower two-thirds of the pons.

THE ANTERIOR PITUITARY consists principally of 5 cells types:- somatotrophs, which produce growth hormone (GH) 50%, lactotrophs (or mammotrophs), which produce prolactin (PRL) 10 - 25% (up to 70% when lactating), corticotrophs, which produce adrenocorticotrophic hormone (ACTH - which contains melanocyte stimulating hormone (MSH)) 15%, thyrotrophs, which produce thyrotrophin (TSH) 5 - 10% and gonadotrophs, which produce follicle stimulating and luteinizing hormone (FSH & LH) 10%.

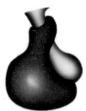

THE POSTERIOR OR NEURAL LOBE consists of a framework of cells similar to the glial cells of the brain (so-called pituicytes), interspersed with the terminals of hypothalamic neurosecretory neurons. Vasopressin and oxytocin, synthesized in the hypothalamus, are stored in and released from the posterior pituitary. The exact function of the pituitary gland in this respect remains uncertain, as controlled release of these hormones can be maintained after total hypophysectomy (pituitary excision), provided the hypothalamus remains undamaged.

Fig. 2.1 The anterior pituitary.

Table 2.2
Immunocytochemistry

Immunocytochemistry is a technique that provides a sensitive and clinically highly relevant classification of pituitary adenomas by hormone content of tumour cells. Tumour sections are incubated with antibodies raised against specific human pituitary hormones in rabbits. A second universal antibody, raised against rabbit antibodies in another species (such as goat), is then applied. The second antibody is chemically linked to a molecule such as biotin, or an enzyme such as 'peroxidase' that can be detected at very low concentrations with a further reaction. As the latter results in a densely coloured product, cells containing specific hormones, in which the colour develops, can be easily identified under the light microscope.

Pituitary tumours

Pituitary tumours can be completely silent and benign, or cause one or more of the symptoms described in Table 2.3.

General investigations

Hormonal

If the patient is phenotypically cushingoid (i.e. shows the physical signs of excessive circulating cortisol, such as central obesity, thin skin, and easy bruising) or acromegalic (i.e. signs of excessive GH effects, such as coarse features, sweating, and enlarged hands), the diagnosis should be confirmed biochemically. If a patient with a pituitary adenoma appears normal, surgery should always be

Table 2.3
Presenting symptoms of pituitary tumours

COMPRESSION OF RELATED STRUCTURES	INAPPROPRIATE HORMONE SECRETION	COMPRESSION OF THE REMAINING PITUITARY
Visual pathway Visual symptoms are typical but almost always limited to vague descriptions of 'fuzzy all over', or 'difficulty reading'. Examine particularly the upper outer fields. Bitemporal hemianopia is the classical defect, but remember that ANY visual defect can occur. **Pituitary stalk** Pituitary stalk compression can lead to hyperprolactinaemia by preventing dopamine reaching the normal pituitary, even though the tumour itself might be 'non-functioning'. **Hypothalamus** Diabetes insipidus caused by compression of the hypothalamus by pituitary tumour (rather than the surgery or radiotherapy used to treat it) is very unusual.	Prolactin-secreting adenomas are the most common symptomatic type of pituitary adenoma (the exact incidence is unknown) Somatotroph adenomas, secreting GH give rise to acromegaly (incidence approx 3 per million.year). Corticotroph adenomas give rise to Cushing's disease (incidence < 1 per million.year). Gonadotrophin and thyrotrophin-producing tumours are very rare.	Any pituitary hormones may be affected either singly or together. Secondary hormone deficiencies, caused by pituitary disease, are usually less dramatic than those caused by primary endocrine gland failure, and may appear relatively slowly. If 3 or more pituitary hormones are deficient, there is a very high chance that GH (deficiency of which is troublesome to diagnose in adulthood) will also be deficient.

preceded by a prolactin measurement to prevent inappropriate surgical treatment of a prolactinoma, as these tumours rarely produce phenotypic changes and are best managed medically, with dopamine agonists such as bromocriptine.

Thyroid function should also be assessed as hypothyroidism itself can very occasionally cause symptomatic pituitary enlargement (i.e. visual field restriction). The 'space occupying' signs resolve once euthyroidism (normal thyroid function) has been restored (see answer to multiple-choice question 4a).

As hydrocortisone cover is routinely used perioperatively, no preoperative *dynamic* tests of pituitary function are usually necessary.

Visual fields

Formal visual field testing (Fig. 2.3) using a Goldmann perimeter or a computerized system (Humphrey Allergan) is important in all cases of pituitary macroadenomas as the presence and rate of change of visual field defects can profoundly affect patient management. If inappropriate hormone secretion is not a problem and visual field testing excludes the presence or progression of visual field defects, treatment, particularly in the elderly, can be limited to pituitary hormone replacement therapy alone.

Table 2.4
Anterior pituitary cell types

	Function	Pattern of release	Notes
Lactotroph	Lactotrophs produce prolactin (PRL), which is essential for lactation. PRL also depresses gonadotrophin (FSH & LH) release & consequently gonadal steroid (ie. oestradiol & androgen) production. This protects nursing mothers from further pregnancy, at least for the first few months after giving birth.	PRL is a stress hormone. Anxiety (about having blood taken, for example) may result in spuriously high levels. PRL also rises during suckling, sleep & after a Grand Mal fit. Nevertheless, a single sample is usually representative of mean circulating levels. PRL release is blocked by hypothalamic dopamine.	High oestrogen levels during pregnancy stimulate lactotrophs to produce PRL. This prepares the breast for lactation. During pregnancy, increased vascularity and an increase in the number & size of lactotrophs doubles pituitary size. This accounts for the susceptibility of the pituitary to infarction following a post-partum haemorrhage (Sheehan's syndrome)
Somatotroph 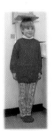	Somatotrophs produce growth hormone (GH). GH acts directly and indirectly (via insulin-like growth factors, 'IGFs') to stimulate linear growth. The metabolic effects tend to counteract those of insulin. The physiological functions of GH in adulthood are not clear, although lack of GH after pituitary surgery does appear to 'adversely' affect body composition.	GH is released in short pulses, mostly during the night. In normal adults, GH levels are low during the day. Glucose ingestion blocks GH secretion. Single blood samples can be misleading. GHRH stimulates GH release, and somatostatin blocks it.	To detect excessive production of GH, mean blood levels, an IGF-1 measurement, failure of oral glucose to adequately suppress GH and a paradoxical GH secretory response to TRH are used. The diagnosis of GH deficiency is much less certain. In children, auxological data (ie. growth rate) is used: in adults, GH secretion in response to insulin-induced hypoglycaemia. Many of the effects of GH are mediated by the IGFs.
Thyrotroph	Thyrotrophs produce thyrotrophin (TSH). This hormone has a unique β subunit and an α subunit identical to the α subunit of FSH, LH & chorionic gonadotrophin. TSH stimulates the synthesis and release of thyroid hormones.	Circulating TSH levels are essentially steady. A single sample is representative of thyrotroph function. Hypothalamic TRH released into the portal blood, stimulates TSH (& at high levels, PRL) release. Thyroid hormones feed back to inhibit TRH and TSH release.	After correction of primary thyrotoxicosis, suppressed thyrotroph function (and TSH levels) often takes several weeks or even months to recover.
Corticotroph	Corticotrophs produce ACTH, which stimulates adrenal glucocorticoid production. MSH, the hormone responsible for skin pigmentation, is a subunit of ACTH.	Pulsatile release of ACTH overlies a pronounced circadian rhythm (high at 6am, low at 10pm). Corticotrophs respond dramatically & rapidly to stress of any kind - including venesection. Hypothalamic CRH stimulates ACTH release. Cortisol feed back inhibits CRH and ACTH release.	ACTH in whole blood is labile. Samples have to be collected onto ice and separated reasonably quickly. Measurement of ACTH is only of use clinically in the differential diagnosis of cortisol hypersecretion.
Gonadotroph	Gonadotrophs produce the glycopeptide hormones follicle-stimulating hormone (FSH) and luteinizing hormone (LH). Biological specificity is conferred by the β subunit. The α subunit is identical to that of TSH and chorionic gonadotrophin (hCG)	The release of both FSH & LH is pulsatile. The FSH pulse length is 3-4h. If the phase of the menstrual cycle is taken into account, a single sample is reasonably representative. LH pulse length is only 60 mins, & levels change dramatically during the menstrual cycle. Thus single LH samples may be misleading. Feedback effects of gonadal hormones at the pituitary and hypothalamus can be inhibitory or stimulatory	FSH stimulates ovarian follicle development, and oestradiol synthesis by the granulosa cells that surround them. LH stimulates ovarian theca cells to produce androgens. These are converted to oestrogens by the granulosa. The LH surge triggers ovulation. Subsequently, LH contributes to corpus luteum formation. Pituitary FSH & LH are not necessary to sustain pregnancy. In the male, LH stimulates androgen production by the testes, and FSH, the initiation of spermatogenesis.

Table 2.5
Less common presenting features

Headaches

Pituitary apoplexy. Haemorrhage into the pituitary and subarachnoid space

Cranial nerve palsies

Temporal lobe epilepsy

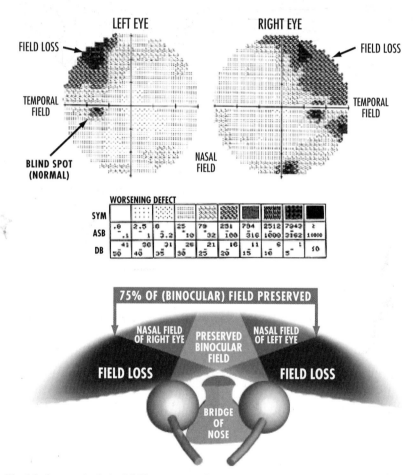

Fig. 2.2 Computerized visual field testing provides accurate, quantitative information about visual field loss. The field data for each eye are presented graphically 'as seen by the patient'. The location of visual loss is shown by the position of shading, and increasing severity of loss by the intensity of shading. The patient shown has predominantly an upper, quadratic bitemporal defect. The lower panel demonstrates how even a complete bitemporal hemianopia produces relatively subtle field loss when both eyes are open.

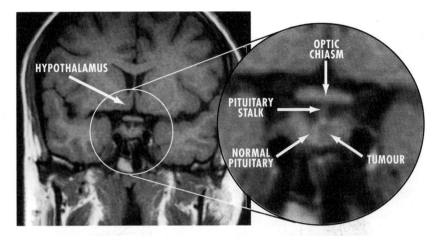

Fig. 2.3 Magnetic resonance images of the brain and pituitary gland in the coronal plane, showing a microadenoma.

Imaging

Magnetic resonance imaging (MRI) has transformed the management of pituitary adenomas, because high-definition soft-tissue images (Fig. 2.4) can be obtained safely at regular intervals, provided the patient can tolerate the claustrophobic and noisy surroundings of the scanner. The sensitivity of detection of *surgically proven* microadenoma approaches 100 per cent with MRI, compared to 50 per cent with computed tomography (CT). However, about 1 in 5 pituitary lesions causing Cushing's disease are too small or diffuse to be identified reliably by either technique.

Plain skull radiography no longer has a place in the diagnosis or management of pituitary adenoma.

Treatment

- Surgery—usually trans-sphenoidal, but occasionally subfrontal or by other routes, reduces excessive hormone secretion and, in the best hands, improves or at least arrests deterioration in visual fields in almost all patients. The peri-operative period is covered with either hydrocortisone or dexamethasone.
- Radiotherapy—fractionated supervoltage radiotherapy consisting of 20–25 treatments over 4–6 weeks, halves the rate of subsequent tumour recurrence, and is often carried out as an adjunct to surgery (Fig. 2.5). However, the ease of follow-up with repeated MR-scanning has made many clinicians think more carefully about the routine use of radiotherapy.
- Drugs—dopamine agonists such as bromocriptine or cabergoline are first treatment for prolactin-secreting pituitary adenomas. Metyrapone is occa

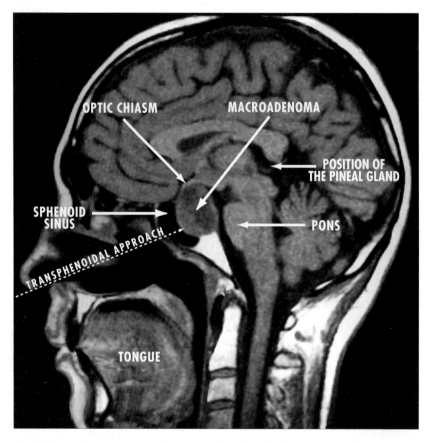

OPTIC CHIASM

MACROADENOMA

POSITION OF
THE PINEAL GLAND

SPHENOID
SINUS

PONS

TRANSPHENOIDAL APPROACH

TONGUE

Fig. 2.4 Magnetic resonance image of the brain and pituitary gland in the sagittal plane, showing an endocrinologically inactive macroadenoma. In this patient the optic chiasm is being lifted and flattened by the tumour compressing it from below. The elegant trans-sphenoidal approach to the pituitary is shown.

ally used in Cushing's disease to lower cortisol prior to pituitary surgery or until pituitary radiotherapy takes effect. Long-acting somatostatin analogues are increasingly used to lower GH secretion in acromegaly.

• Bilateral adrenalectomy cures the biochemical affects of Cushings disease, but stimulates growth and ACTH secretion from remaining corticotroph adenomas cells. This causes skin pigmentation known as Nelson's syndrome and local problems of tumour regrowth.

Outlook

Corticotroph adenomas, the tumours that give rise to Cushing's disease, and large pituitary tumours, particularly in young people, can be troublesome. However, in

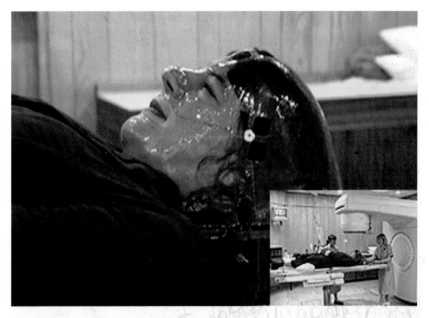

Fig. 2.5 Linear accelerator (LINAC) external-beam radiotherapy for a pituitary tumour. The tailor-made, clear plastic mask holding the patient's head still during the brief procedure shows the targeting marks lined up against the cross-beams of a red laser set into the walls of the radiotherapy room.

the majority of cases the long-term outlook for patients with pituitary adenomas is very good, even though tumours are rarely removed in their entirety.

Specific tumour types

Glycopeptide hormone-secreting adenomas

Pituitary tumours secreting clinically significant amounts of glycopeptide hormones (FSH, LH, or TSH) are very rare. Whenever biochemical hyperthyroidism (i.e. raised F T_4) occurs in the presence of an unsuppressed or frankly elevated TSH, the most common reason is that treatment of primary hypothyroidism has just been started with too high a dose of thyroxine, or, having 'forgotten' to take the thyroxine, the patient is taking a higher dose for a week or two before clinic to try to obscure the fact. In untreated patients, however, the rare TSH-secreting pituitary tumour must be excluded. As a cause of premature puberty or postmenopausal bleeding, gonadotrophin-secreting pituitary tumours should be at the very bottom of a very complete list of differential diagnoses.

Prolactin-secreting adenomas

Table 2.6
Prolactinomas

Microprolactinomas	Macroprolactinomas
Are <10 mm in diameter by definition and confined by a normal pituitary fossa	Are > 10 mm in diameter by definition and spread beyond and/or distort the pituitary fossa
They do not become macroprolactinomas	More commonly diagnosed than microprolactinomas in men and often large at presentation
Typical presenting features are amenorrhoea and/or galactorrhoea	Surgery is very rarely curative
Diagnosis in males is unusual, at least in part because the clinical signs are less obvious	Prolactin levels usually exceed 5000 mU/l
Fewer than 1 in 10 resolve spontaneously	There is a rough association between tumour size and prolactin production. Thus a large tumour with a prolactin of <2500 mU/l is much more likely
Prolactin levels usually vary from 1000 to 4000 mU/l	to be an inactive adenoma compressing the pituitary stalk than a prolactinoma

Treatment of prolactinomas

Dopamine agonists such as bromocriptine restore prolactin to normal in the majority of patients and visual field defects rapidly return to normal in at least 75 per cent. It is first-line treatment for prolactinomas. Unfortunately, nausea, lethargy and nasal stuffiness sometimes limit the dose of bromocriptine or prevent its use altogether. Other dopamine agonists such as cabergoline, pergolide, or quinagolide can be tried, but may produce similar effects

Side-effects of bromocriptine can be reduced by starting at low doses, taking the tablets after food, taking the main dose in the evening, and sometimes by using the tablets vaginally

Although there is no evidence of teratogenicity, most clinicians stop bromocriptine when pregnancy is diagnosed. Macroprolactinomas may increase in size during pregnancy, but symptomatic enlargement is fairly unusual (<16 per cent). If it does occur, bromocriptine can be reinstituted

Hypoprolactinaemia

No attempt is made to diagnose prolactin deficiency as no specific problems arise apart from potential difficulty with initiation and maintenance of breast feeding in females. Curiously, although pharmacological doses of oxytocin are widely used to accelerate labour, oxytocin deficiency appears to have no effect on spontaneous parturition.

Growth hormone-secreting adenomas

[handwritten: Inhibited by use of somato Statin.]

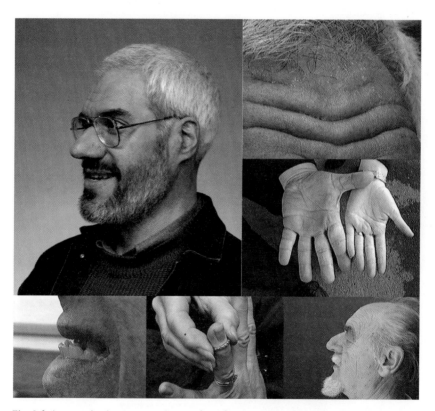

Fig. 2.6 Acromegaly, showing typical coarse facial features and prognathism (forward movement of the jaw). Other features are carpal tunnel syndrome, growth of the extremities, increased sweating (in some patients), weight gain and muscle weakness with widespread osteoarthritis, which together produce a characteristic stooped posture. Characteristically, the spouses are disturbed by the patients' loud snoring—often interrupted by episodes of obstructive sleep apnoea.

[handwritten: Prolactin ↓ by use of dopamine agonists]

Table 2.7
Acromegaly

Diagnosis of acromegaly	Treatment of acromegaly
The diagnosis based on continuing somatic changes, usually accompanied by sweating and headaches, is usually obvious, and easily confirmed by GH estimation	Primary treatment is transphenoidal adenomectomy
A GH series (samples every 10 min for 1 h, or every 30 min for 4 h + IGF-I estimation) confirms the diagnosis	Radiotherapy reduces GH by 15–20 per cent per annum
In borderline cases, failure of a 75 g glucose load to suppress GH to <2 mU/l or a paradoxical GH secretory response to 100 μg of TRH iv ($\geq$ 150 per cent baseline) can be useful	Long-acting somatostatin analogues are increasingly used and may, in future, become first-line agents, although side-effects such as headaches, abdominal cramps, and gallstones may be limiting
	Bromocriptine modestly lowers GH in some patients
	Most patients are helped but not cured by treatment (i.e. mean GH level remains $\geq$ 5 mU/l)

Adrenocorticotrophic hormone-secreting adenomas

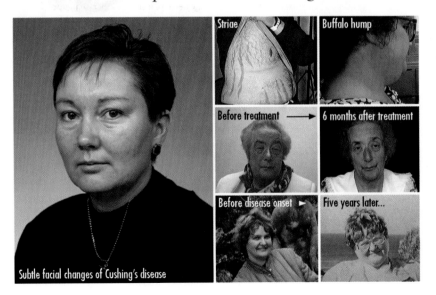

Fig. 2.7 A patient with Cushing's disease, showing the characteristic rounded (moon) face. Typical features are central obesity (with relatively thin arms and legs caused by muscle wasting), deposition of fat over the upper back (a buffalo hump), hirsutism (excessive hair growth, often over the whole body), and thin skin with a tendency to bruise easily. The appearance of violaceous striae is a further manifestation of weakening of skin structure, and an increase in appetite and psychiatric disturbance are also frequently observed.

Table 2.8
Diagnostic steps in suspected Cushing's syndrome (hypercortisolaemia)

1. Is there excessive circulating cortisol?	2. What is the source of the cortisol?
2 × 24 h urinary free cortisol estimation (with creatinine to ensure completeness of collection). A level of > 275 nmol/24 h warrants further investigation	Iatrogenic? Glucocorticoid treatment is by far the most common cause of Cushing's syndrome. Check with the patient before you get this far!
Overnight dexamethasone suppression test. Measure serum cortisol at 8 or 9 a.m. following a 1 mg dose of dexamethasone taken at home the previous evening at 11 p.m. Failure of cortisol to suppress to less than 138 nM warrants further investigation	Measure ACTH level. Undetectable levels suggest an adrenal tumour. Moderately raised levels (40–180 pg/ml) with an ACTH secretory response to CRH (100 μg iv) suggests Cushing's disease, and high levels (> 200 pg/ml) suggest ectopic ACTH production
	High-dose dexamethasone suppression test (2 mg qds orally for 48 h) *Any* suppression of circulating cortisol suggests pituitary, rather than adrenal disease

Although the above appears 'cut and dried', diagnosing the cause of Cushing's syndrome, and treating it effectively when it has been diagnosed, can be notoriously difficult. A number of different tests have to be applied and sometimes repeated, as Cushing's disease can fluctuate in intensity. In some cases, sampling of the venous outflow of the pituitary (petrosal sinus samples) both left and right side, under basal conditions and after CRH stimulation needs to be undertaken to identify the pituitary as the source of excessive ACTH secretion—ie Cushings *disease* other than Cushing's *syndrome.*

Hypopituitarism

Table 2.9
Causes of hypopituitarism

Common	
Surgical hypophysectomy	An adenoma with a fibrous texture at the back of the fossa may be particularly difficult to remove without damaging or resecting some of the adjacent normal pituitary
Compression by tumour	Large pituitary adenomas can disturb the function of adjacent normal pituitary tissue by compression, ischaemia, or by diverting portal blood from the hypothalamus
Pituitary radiotherapy	Radiotherapy reduces anterior pituitary hormone synthesis by about 10 per cent per year. Long-term follow-up is required even if no deficiencies are present at the outset
Relatively rare	
Sheehan's syndrome	Postpartum pituitary infarction (Sheehan's syndrome) occurs when the highly vascular pituitary of a pregnant woman is suddenly rendered ischaemic by hypotension at delivery
'Empty sellar' syndrome	Pituitary tissue is absent on MR or CT scanning without prior surgery or radiotherapy. It is assumed that the pituitary has been destroyed by CSF pressure or an immune process
Idiopathic (in childhood)	Children have normal body proportions but are markedly growth retarded and tend to be overweight for height. For unknown reasons, hypothyroidism in these patients is rare

Table 2.10
Diagnosis and management of hypopituitarism

Hormone	Diagnosis of deficiency	Treatment
TSH → Thyroxine	Measure TSH and free T_4 The free T_4 will be below the normal range $(10–23 \text{ pmol/l})$, usually with a TSH towards the bottom of, or just below the normal range	The average replacement dose of thyroxine is about 100 μg/day The half-life of T_4 is almost 1 week. If a tablet is forgotten one day, the patient can take double the next. The aim is to keep free T_4 within the normal range as TSH will remain low in these circumstances irrespective of circulating thyroid hormone levels
ACTH → Cortisol	Synacthen test If ACTH levels are inadequate for more than a few days, the adrenal cortex (with the exception of the zona glomerulosa) rapidly atrophies. A single iv dose of exogenous ACTH (250 μg Synacthen® (syn ACTHen)) will then produce an inadequate cortisol response (i.e. failing to exceed 495 nmol/l after 1 h)	The dose of hydrocortisone should be kept to a minimum, typically 15–30 mg/day, unless the patient is under stress. An attempt is made to mimic the normal cortisol diurnal variation by giving 10–15 mg orally in the morning, and 5–10 mg in the early afternoon—sometimes as 5 mg at lunchtime, and 5 mg between 3 and 5 p.m. Circulating cortisol levels are usually very low between 6 p.m. and 6 a.m., therefore, the 'evening' dose of cortisol should ideally be taken at about 4 p.m.

continued next page

Hormone	Diagnosis of deficiency	Treatment
LH and FSH	The diagnosis is made symptomatically in females, and by measuring testosterone in males	*Fertility not required*
Oestradiol	In women, amenorrhoea, with other signs of low levels of circulating oestrogen, such as vaginal dryness leading to dyspareunia (painful intercourse) —are cardinal signs. FSH, LH, and oestradiol are often at the low end of the normal range or below	In women, cyclical oral or transcutaneous oestrogen/progesterone replacement
Testosterone		In men, an oily mixture of androgens is given by injection every few weeks. Transcutaneous patches are also available. Testosterone depots can be inserted subcutaneously every few months. Even in men for whom potency is not an issue, testosterone levels of <3 nmol/l (normal range 10–35 nmol/l) are associated with osteoporosis, and should probably be treated.
	In men, low androgen levels lead to loss of libido, lethargy, and impotence. The latter is not a frequent complaint, perhaps because of embarrassment and partly through loss of libido	*Fertility required*
		In women, FSH/LH replacement by daily IM injection, with additional hCG to mimic the LH surge and induce ovulation at the appropriate time. Further progesterone treatment is sometimes given to support the early pregnancy
		In men, as sperm maturation is a slow process, daily FSH and LH injections are required for many months before fertile sperm appear

continued below

Hormone	Diagnosis of deficiency	Treatment
Vasopressin	Symptomatic polyuria. A formal water deprivation test is occasionally required	Vasopressin is most easily given as a nasal aerosol of DDAVP, 1–2 puffs 1–3 times daily. It can also be given as a tablet (200 mg 1–3 times daily). Patients usually arrive at a suitable dose themselves but should be warned that water intoxication can occur
Urine concentration	Usually, the symptoms of polyuria, thirst, and polydypsia are obvious, but if the condition is mild, the mental state of the patient uncertain, or the symptoms inconsistent, a water deprivation test is useful. Look for a decrease in volume and increase in osmolality of urine passed at hourly intervals during the test. Remember to weigh the patient *before and after* they have passed urine each time, to check that they have not taken a surreptitious drink and to identify excessive fluid loss	Advising the patient to leave treatment off for half a day a week to allow for a diuresis to re-establish normal osmotic balance and thirst, is a useful precaution to prevent water overload
		There is no easy way of knowing whether diabetes insipidus (DI) has resolved spontaneously, as it sometimes does after surgery, except to stop treatment and see what happens. The patient may have to bear with what appears to be mild polyuria for a while

continued next page

Hormone	Diagnosis of deficiency	Treatment
Growth hormone	In children, the diagnosis is made on the basis of short stature and slow growth velocity. The GH secretory response to insulin-induced hypoglycaemia is also used but is less reliable	In hypopituitary children with growth potential, GH is routinely replaced with daily subcutaneous injections of biosynthetic GH
Growth	In children in response to hypoglycaemia (glucose <2.2 mmol/l), a GH of <15 is said to be deficient, levels of 17–20 are borderline and over 20, probably normal. Slow growth velocity with a dramatic response to GH treatment is a more reliable sign	There are many anecdotes about the remarkable physical and psychological benefits of replacing GH in GH-deficient adults. As yet, there is little objective evidence of a significant long-term advantage for GH-deficient patients
	The formal diagnosis of GH deficiency is not routinely made in adult patients. When a diagnosis is required, a GH response to hypoglycaemia of <3 mU/l probably indicates deficiency, although this is a matter of ongoing debate	The reason for increased cardiovascular mortality in panhypopituitary patients even when thyroid, gonadal, and adrenal-cortical hormones have been replaced, remains to be explained
		GH is not routinely replaced in adult patients

Table 2.11
Typical anterior pituitary hormone replacement regimen

Male		Female	
Thyroxine	100–125 μg daily	Thyroxine	100–125 μg daily
Hydrocortisone	15 mg a.m. and 5 mg p.m.	Hydrocortisone	15 mg a.m. and 5 mg p.m.
Sustanon®	250 mg every 3 weeks	Oestrogen/ progestogen	Prempak-C® or equivalent

Key points

- Pituitary tumours can secrete hormones inappropriately and/or compress surrounding structures, such as the remaining normal pituitary and the optic chiasm.
- Dopamine agonists, such as bromocriptine or cabergoline are first-line treatment for prolactinomas.
- Compression of the pituitary stalk by a non-secreting pituitary adenoma can cause hyperprolactinaemia.
- A synacthen test is used to diagnose secondary hypoadrenalism. Deprived of ACTH stimulation, cortisol-producing cells of the adrenal rapidly atrophy, and a bolus of exogenous ACTH (Synacthen®) fails to produce an adequate cortisol response.
- Pituitary hormone replacement consists of hydrocortisone, thyroxine, and sex hormones, with vasopressin in the form of DDAVP, if the patient has diabetes insipidus.

'My patient's optician suspects a pituitary tumour, please see and advise'

History

The 58-year-old patient, previously completely well, had recently had a road traffic accident involving a mutual exchange of paintwork between the left side of her car and the right side of a bus. Looking back, she realized that she had had trouble focusing on magazines and newspapers for some months. Her optician confirmed that the prescription of her current spectacles was appropriate but had identified another problem and asked her to see her GP.

Examination

The only abnormality was the suggestion of a field loss in the upper temporal quadrant of her left eye on confrontation.

Investigations

Her gonadotrophins (FSH and LH), free T_4 (FT_4), and TSH were quoted as within their normal ranges. A random cortisol was 340 nmol/l (normal range 150–800 nmol/l); prolactin was 1800 mU/l (normal range $\leq$ 800). Computerized visual field analysis (see p. 32) confirmed the presence of upper quadrantic bitemporal loss, worse on the left than the right. Subsequently, an MRI of her pituitary fossa showed a large pituitary adenoma, 2 cm in anteroposterior and lateral diameter and 1.8 cm high, in contact with the optic chiasm (see Fig. 2.4).

Management

She had a trans-sphenoidal hypophysectomy to decompress her optic chiasm, followed by radiotherapy to the remaining tumour, entailing 25 daily treatments over a 5-week period. Postoperatively, her cortisol rose from 130 nmol/l to 430 nmol/l following a 250 μg dose of intramuscular Synacthen® (normal should reach 495 nmol/l), and the hydrocortisone that had been used to cover the perioperative period was therefore continued in the long term. The patient was advised to increase the dose temporarily during episodes of illness or severe stress. She declined sex hormone replacement therapy, but was started on thyroxine, as both her FT_4 and TSH were low.

Explanation

The diagnosis is an endocrinologically inactive pituitary adenoma. Visual changes are often so gradual in onset that the patient does not realize a problem exists until a considerable deficit has developed. If a tumour of this size (a large marble) had been a prolactinoma, it would have been expected to give rise to a circulating prolactin level exceeding 5000 mU/l. The modest elevation of prolactin was due to compression of the pituitary stalk blocking hypothalamic dopamine (prolactin release inhibiting hormone) from reaching the normal pituitary. The low postoperative FT_4 and TSH indicate secondary hypothyroidism (i.e. due to primary failure).

After a short period without ACTH stimulation, the adrenal cortex (with the exception of the cells producing aldosterone) atrophies. Under these circumstances a single exogenous pulse of ACTH fails to produce a satisfactory increase in circulating cortisol, as it did here.

Finally, although the FSH and LH were in the 'normal range', the levels were much lower than would be expected for a postmenopausal woman, indicating that even before surgery the patient had a degree of pituitary failure. Sex hormone replacement therapy was offered to the patient for its cardioprotective effects, and to prevent further bone mineral loss. Anxiety about breast cancer led her to decline treatment.

'My patient fell and hit his head: a skull X-ray showed an enlarged pituitary fossa'

History

To create that 'extra bit of sparkle', the cleaning lady decided to polish the shower tray. The 68-year-old owner of the house discovered the slippery effects of this rather spectacularly, and was dazed for a few minutes after hitting his occiput. He did not seek help until that evening, however, when he vomited. Nothing untoward was found on examination in casualty and he was sent home with a head injury chart. The pituitary fossa abnormality did not come to light until the skull radiograph was reviewed by a radiologist the following morning, and the GP was informed. The patient himself had not noted any change in his vision and felt well. On direct questioning he stated that his sexual function was normal, with no change in libido or potency.

Examination

The patient had no phenotypic characteristics of acromegaly or Cushing's disease. Careful examination of his vision by confrontation did not reveal any field deficits.

Investigations

A prolactin estimation was 640 m U/l (normal range < 800); TSH was 1.5 m U/l (normal range 0.3–6); FT$_4$, 12.6 pmol/l (normal range 10–23); and testosterone, 11 nmol/l (normal range 10–35). Computerized perimetry (i.e. visual field measurement) was normal. An MR scan of his pituitary fossa confirmed the presence of a macroadenoma.

Management

The diagnosis is an endocrinologically inactive adenoma. As the visual fields were full, the patient was followed up with repeat visual field tests at intervals of 6–18 months, with further baseline pituitary hormone measurements to identify hypopituitarism when, or if, it occurred. The only indication for surgery in this patient would be the development of visual impairment or other evidence of compression of surrounding structures.

Explanation

The differential diagnosis from the skull radiograph and hormone tests was either a non-functioning pituitary adenoma (a so-called incidentaloma) or the empty sella syndrome. Occult non-functioning pituitary adenomas are very common. As their natural history is to grow extremely slowly, they are unlikely to cause any problems. The most significant complication of these tumours is compression of the optic chiasm (followed by compression of the normal pituitary gland, causing hypopituitarism). In the empty sella syndrome, a fold of dura appears to herniate into the pituitary fossa and on MR or CT scanning the sella is seen to be CSF-filled. This condition may have a primarily mechanical aetiology from transmitted CSF pressure or may follow infarction of an occult pituitary adenoma. Frequently, pituitary function remains intact, although different combinations of pituitary hormone hyposecretion may also occur.

A macroprolactinoma is excluded by the normal prolactin estimation.

Multiple-choice questions

1. In pituitary disease:
   a. The intermediate lobe of the pituitary is rarely involved;
   b. First-line treatment for macroprolactinomas is trans-sphenoidal surgery;
   c. Adrenal hormone replacement therapy consists of both glucocorticoids and mineralocorticoids;
   d. Acute stress in a panhypopituitary patient necessitates treatment with catecholamines;
   e. A raised prolactin in association with a pituitary tumour indicates a prolactinoma.

2. The following are causes of hyperprolactinaemia:
   a. Pregnancy;
   b. Stress or anxiety;
   c. Treatment with dopamine agonists;
   d. Pituitary stalk compression;
   e. Breast manipulation.

3. In pituitary hormone replacement:
   a. A low FT_4 with a high TSH indicates anterior pituitary failure;
   b. Hydrocortisone for adrenal cortical replacement should be taken in divided doses;
   c. Testosterone is best given parenterally;
   d. Testosterone injections are required to restore spermatogenesis;

e. Restoration of male and female fertility requires daily treatment with gonadotrophin tablets.

4. The pituitary is situated close to:
   a. The optic tract;
   b. The carotid arteries;
   c. The pineal;
   d. The median eminence;
   e. The fourth cranial nerve.

5. Pituitary hormones:
   a. The actions of GH are mediated entirely through hepatic IGF-I production;
   b. To more closely approximate normal physiology, thyroid hormone replacement should ideally consist of both T_4 and T_3;
   c. Antidopaminergic drugs are used to stimulate lactation in women who deliver twins;
   d. In untreated panhypopituitarism, the patient is usually lethargic and pigmented;
   e. Can all be administered orally.

6. The following are useful clinical signs of Cushing's syndrome (hypercortisolaemia):
   a. Weight gain;
   b. Easy bruising;
   c. Difficulty standing from squatting;
   d. Mental changes;
   e. Osteoporotic fracture in a young obese patient.

7. The following are useful treatments in pituitary disease:
   a. Transcranial, subfrontal surgery for microadenomas;
   b. Bromocriptine for endocrinologically inactive adenomas;
   c. Carbimazole (reducing from 30 mg initially to 5 mg maintenance) for macroprolactinomas;
   d. External-beam radiotherapy (LINAC) for slow-growing, endocrinologically inactive adenomas;
   e. Aldosterone (i.e. mineralocorticoid) replacement in complete anterior pituitary failure.

8. The following are typical:
   a. Symptoms of mania (disorganized mental overactivity) following hypothalamic damage;
   b. SIADH (syndrome of inappropriate vasopressin secretion) following pituitary damage;
   c. Menorrhagia (heavy menstrual periods) in association with weight loss;
   d. Oliguria in cranial (central) diabetes insipidus;
   e. Carpal tunnel syndrome in Cushing's disease.

Answers

1. In pituitary disease:
   a. The intermediate lobe of the pituitary is rarely involved   T

   The intermediate lobe is not present in man. However, in many mammals it is a distinct cell layer composed almost entirely of corticotrophs (cells producing hormones of the ACTH family) that, unlike anterior- lobe corticotrophs, express D2 dopaminergic receptors. When these dopaminergic receptors are stimulated, intermediate lobe hormone secretion is inhibited. If (very rarely) in a case of Cushing's disease, D2 agonists such as bromocriptine are found to reduce ACTH, it has been suggested that the tumour may have originated from cells of the 'intermediate lobe type'.

   b. First-line treatment for macroprolactinomas is trans-sphenoidal surgery   F

   First-line treatment for prolactin-secreting pituitary tumours is bromocriptine or another dopamine agonist. A surgical cure for macroprolactinomas is unusual, even if the tumour is accessible, while dopamine agonists are usually remarkably successful in both shrinking the tumour and reducing prolactin secretion. Most specialist centres also treat microprolactinomas with dopamine agonists as their first-line therapy.

   c. Adrenal hormone replacement therapy consists of both glucocorticoids and mineralocorticoids   F

   Although *primary* adrenal failure will need treatment with both glucocorticoids and mineralocorticoids, adrenal failure secondary to pituitary disease does not, as adrenal aldosterone production is not controlled by pituitary ACTH, but by the renin–angiotensin system (see p. 87).

   d. Acute stress in a panhypopituitary patient necessitates treatment with catecholamines   F

   The adrenal medulla seems to be fairly redundant. Although the capacity of the body to produce circulating adrenaline is abolished, the sympathetic nervous system (which uses noradrenaline) remains intact.

   e. A raised prolactin in association with a pituitary tumour indicates a prolactinoma   F

   Not necessarily. A non-secreting tumour might 'compress the pituitary stalk' and prevent dopamine from inhibiting prolactin secretion from the normal prolactin-secreting cells in the adjacent pituitary tissue.

2. The following are causes of hyperprolactinaemia:
   a. Pregnancy   T

   Lactation during pregnancy is thought to be prevented by high circulating levels of oestrogens and progesterone.

   b. Stress or anxiety   T

   If a patient is unduly anxious about venesection, this alone can cause significant hyperprolactinaemia; so can a grand mal convulsion—a fact that has been exploited to differentiate true from pseudo fits.

   c. Treatment with dopamine agonists   F
      It is treatment with dopamine *antagonists*, such as the phenothiazines and domperidone, that cause hyperprolactinaemia.

   d. Pituitary stalk compression   T
      By blocking hypothalamic dopamine from reaching the anterior pituitary.

   e. Breast manipulation   T
      This is the wet-nurse phenomenon. A woman who keeps checking to see whether galactorrhoea is still present by attempting to express milk, will stimulate prolactin and oxytocin production and perpetuate the neuro-endocrine reflex. Other causes of hyperprolactinaemia commonly seen in the endocrine clinic are prolactinomas, exogenous oestrogen therapy and, sometimes, primary hypothyroidism.

3. In pituitary hormone replacement:

   a. A low FT_4 with a high TSH indicates anterior pituitary failure   F
      In pituitary failure, as distinct from primary hypothyroidism, TSH will not be elevated. The TSH might be 'within the normal range', but would be inappropriately low in the presence of a subnormal T_4.

   b. Hydrocortisone for adrenal cortical replacement should be taken in divided doses   T
      The biological half-life of oral hydrocortisone is quite short (about 3–4 hours). If a single dose is taken when the patient gets up in the morning, very little remains by lunchtime. As circulating cortisol levels in normal people are very low by about 6 p.m., the 'evening' dose of hydro-cortisone should be taken as early as 4 p.m. and if patients feel exhausted at midday, it may be worth splitting the dose into three—for example, 10–15 mg at 7 a.m. 5 mg at lunchtime, and a further 5 mg at 4 p.m. The dose is generally kept as low as possible, but should, of course, be increased, typically to 3 or 4 times the normal daily dose for 2 or 3 days if the patient develops a fever or undergoes a major period of stress. A dose taken too late in the evening may cause insomnia.

   c. Testosterone is best given parenterally   T
      Testosterone tablets (Restandol®) are not well absorbed and do not usually return androgen levels to the normal range. Scrotal patches (at-tached to the shaved scrotum, because the skin is thin and absorbant as well as being rich in 5α-reductase which converts testosterone to the more active dihydrotestosterone as it passes through) are expensive and less effective than injections. Newer delivery systems (Andropatch®) allow androgens to be absorbed effectively across normal skin. Injections of a mixture of testosterone esters (Sustanon®) work well, given as 100 mg every 2 weeks, or 250 mg every 3 weeks. Testosterone implants are also available.

   d. Testosterone injections are required to restore spermatogenesis   F
      High endogenous levels of testosterone made by the Leydig cells of the testis are required for spermatogenesis. Exogenous testosterone merely

turns off gonadotrophins (FSH and LH) and reduces the sperm count. The corresponding situation in women would be to use oestrogens and progestogens—components of the contraceptive pill.

e. Restoration of male and female fertility requires daily treatment with gonadotrophin tablets   F

Unfortunately, FSH and LH have to be given by daily injection. A course of injections lasting 6–9 months is usually required before fertile sperm are evident, as spermatogenesis (from beginning to end) takes many months. It is also sensible to offer to cryopreserve semen after treatment so that another course of treatment is not obligatory should the patient want to have further children at a later date. In women, daily injections of FSH (±LH) are used to induce follicular development. An injection of LH (as chorionic gonadotrophin, which has similar effects) is given to induce ovulation, and increasingly, progestogens are then given orally for the first trimester to 'support the developing pregnancy'.

4. The pituitary is situated close to:

a. The optic tract   T

The optic tract starts immediately behind the chiasm, and the optic nerve ends immediately in front of it. The position of the chiasm and the direction of growth of pituitary tumours is variable, so any kind of visual field loss can occur. Occasionally, even a physiologically enlarged pituitary can impinge on the optic chiasm and affect vision. This may occur very rarely in prolonged, primary hypothyroidism, where the fall in circulating thyroid hormones reduces feedback inhibition of hypothalamic TRH production and pituitary TSH production. The TRH stimulates thyrotrophs (and lactotrophs), both of which increase in size and activity.

b. The carotid arteries   T

Neurosurgeons make every effort to stick to the midline. If they deviate to one side, or the carotid deviates towards the midline and is punctured, the vessel may have to be tied off in the neck.

c. The pineal   F

The pineal gland is a neurosecretory gland, about 5 mm × 7 mm in size that lies in the midline against the superior colliculi at the back of the midbrain (see Fig. 2.4). The function of the pineal is not well established in man, but in lower vertebrates the pineal is light sensitive and, in some rodents, pinealectomy enhances gonadal axis activity and can modestly advance puberty. The pineal produces a number of biologically active peptides, including melatonin, the secretion of which is high at night and low during the day. If the sympathetic nerve input to the pineal is cut, pineal rhythms persist but are no longer 'entrained' to (i.e. follow) light and dark. Oral melatonin supplements are reputed to reduce the effect of jet lag. The association of pineal tumours (pinealomas) with premature puberty is almost certainly due to hypothalamic damage rather than a direct effect of changes in pineal secretory activity.

    d. The median eminence   T
       This is the inverted cone of hypothalamus that merges inferiorally with the pituitary stalk.

    e. The fourth cranial nerve   T
       The fourth, fifth, and sixth cranial nerves run in the cavernous sinuses, either side of the pituitary fossa. Infiltration of the cavernous sinuses and cranial nerve palsies are unusual, but do occur. The factors that determine the direction of expansion of pituitary adenomas are unknown at present.

5. Pituitary hormones:

    a. The actions of GH are mediated entirely through hepatic IGF-I production   F
       Growth of cartilage *in vivo* is GH dependent, but adding GH to cartilage fragments *in vitro* was found to have no effect, implicating that its effects were mediated through another hormonal messenger. An intermediate molecule, 'somatomedin C', now known as IGF-I was identified. In the past it was thought that hepatic production of IGF-I mediated all of the effects of GH. It now seems that GH receptors are widespread and that, in many GH-responsive tissues, IGF-I is synthesized locally and acts in an autocrine or paracrine fashion.

    b. To more closely approximate normal physiology, thyroid hormone replacement should ideally consist of both T_4 and T_3 F
       Exogenous T_4 is de-iodinated to T_3 within the tissues of the body to produce appropriate levels of the more active thyroid hormone T_3. Exogenous T_3 is completely unnecessary.

    c. Antidopaminergic drugs are used to stimulate lactation in women who deliver twins   F
       The relationship between prolaction and lactation is more complex than this. A month or two after delivery, prolactin levels are often completely normal between nursing episodes. In addition, it is prudent to avoid drug treatment in pregnant women and nursing mothers as some (listed at the back of the British National Formulary (BNF)), reach substantial concentrations in breast milk.

    d. In untreated panhypopituitarism, the patient is usually lethargic and pigmented   F
       Lethargy is certainly a feature, as the patient would be hypothyroid (due to lack of TSH) and hypoadrenal (due to lack of ACTH). However, as ACTH has melanin-stimulating hormone effects, the patient would be pale, rather than pigmented. Furthermore, public and axillary hair would be lost as both ACTH (which drives adrenal androgen formation) and GnRH (which stimulates ovarian androgen production) are deficient.

    e. Can all be administered orally   F
       Not quite. Thyroxine, cortisol, and sex hormone replacement therapy for women are certainly active orally. Testosterone is poorly absorbed orally,

but it can (like DDAVP, a vasopressin analogue) be given in tablet form. GH can only be given by subcutaneous injection, and oxytocin (used by obstetricians to accelerate labour) is given by intravenous infusion.

6. The following are useful clinical signs of Cushing's syndrome (hyper-cortisolaemia):

   a. Weight gain   F

   Although weight gain is a consistent feature of Cushing's disease, the sign is not particularly useful as Cushing's disease is very rare (incidence ≤ 1 in 10^6.year), while obesity is very common. It is also worth remembering that in ectopic ACTH production by small-cell lung cancer, progression of the underlying disease can be so rapid that the classical physical appearance of Cushing's syndrome has no time to develop. In these cases the correct diagnosis is suggested by rapidly progressive weakness, hypokalaemia, glucose intolerance, and hypertension.

   b. Easy bruising   T

   The effects of glucocorticoids on the integrity of the skin and blood vessels are very specific. Patients almost always complain that they bruise more easily, and the presence of bruising, particularly if the patient has no idea how they got there, is very useful. Severe bruising at venepuncture sites is also a suggestive sign.

   c. Difficulty standing from squatting   T

   Proximal myopathy is another very useful sign of Cushing's. Obese people, particularly young obese people are not usually weak, as increased muscle strength develops in response to normal movement (the equivalent of weight training). Profound proximal myopathy in Cushing's makes it very hard for them to stand from squatting five times. At home, they may find it difficult to climb stairs, and sometimes even to get up off the floor or carry a kettle full of water. Often, the patient will also complain of an associated 'bad back', not realizing that muscle weakness affecting the spinal muscles can lead to backache.

   d. Mental changes   T

   Subtle mental changes often precede any other symptoms or signs of Cushing's disease. As many as 50% of patients with Cushing's disease are clinically depressed.

   e. Osteoporotic fracture in a young obese patient   T

   High levels of glucocorticoids produce dramatic bone mineral loss. Osteoporotic fractures in young patients are very rare, of course, but the presence of osteopaenia (measured by dual energy X-ray absorptiometry (DEXA) scan) is almost universal in patients with chronic hypercortisolaemia. Put another way, the absence of osteopaenia makes the diagnosis of Cushing's disease less likely.

7. The following are useful treatments in pituitary disease:

   a. Transcranial, subfrontal surgery for microadenomas   F

As microadenomas do not extend beyond the pituitary fossa, they are not accessible from the anterior cranial fossa.

b. Bromocriptine for endocrinologically inactive adenomas   F

Dopamine agonists have been tried in most types of pituitary adenoma. They are remarkably successful in prolactinomas and less effective in somatotroph adenomas (secreting GH), but have no significant effects in inactive adenomas.

c. Carbimazole (reducing from 30 mg initially to 5 mg maintenance) for macroprolactinomas   F

Carbimazole is an antithyroid drug (see p. 67).

d. External-beam radiotherapy (LINAC) for slow-growing, endocrinologically inactive adenomas   T

External-beam radiotherapy remains an extremely successful treatment for many types of pituitary adenomas, including endocrinologically inactive adenomas, usually as an adjunct to surgery. The symptomatic recurrence rate is greatly reduced.

e. Aldosterone (i.e. mineralocorticoid) replacement in complete anterior pituitary failure   F

This is not usually required as aldosterone production by the adrenal cortex, unlike production of cortisol and adrenal androgens, is largely controlled by the renin–angiotensin system, rather than by pituitary ACTH (see p. 87).

8. The following are typical:

a. Symptoms of mania (disorganized mental overactivity) following hypothalamic damage   F

The opposite tends to be the case. Patients tend to be somnolent and lethargic.

b. SIADH (syndrome of inappropriate vasopressin secretion) following pituitary damage   F

Inadequate, rather than excessive vasopressin secretion leading to diabetes insipidus is much more frequent.

c. Menorrhagia (heavy menstrual periods) in association with weight loss   F

'Hypothalamic amenorrhoea' tends to occur.

d. Oliguria in cranial (central) diabetes insipidus   F

Polyuria occurs.

e. Carpal tunnel syndrome in Cushing's disease   F

Carpal tunnel syndrome is much more commonly associated with acromegaly and may be the first sign of the condition to come to medical attention.

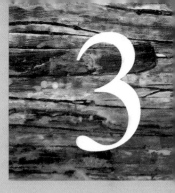

3

The thyroid gland

- Summary

- Introduction

- Overactivity of the thyroid gland

- Underactivity of the thyroid gland

- Thyroid enlargement in a euthyroid patient

- Thyroid carcinoma

- Subacute thyroiditis

- Key points

- Case histories

- Multiple-choice questions

Summary

Normal function

- Production, storage, and secretion of thyroid hormones.
- Calcitonin is produced by the 'C' cells of the thyroid, but has no significant effects on calcium metabolism at physiological concentrations.

Typical pathology

- Thyroid overactivity (hyperthyroidism or thyrotoxicosis) is very common
  - → Usually caused by Graves' disease or toxic multinodular goitre. Treatment is with radioiodine or antithyroid drugs such as carbimazole. *neomerozole*
- Thyroid underactivity (hypothyroidism) is also very common
  - → Usually caused by Hashimoto's (autoimmune) thyroiditis or radioiodine treatment for an overactive thyroid.

'Typical clinical scenario'

- A rather anxious and irritable 23-year-old with Graves' disease. She complains of 'weight loss and sore eyes' and of feeling 'tired but wound up all the time so that she cannot really sleep'.

Introduction

Thyroid disease is a very common problem seen in the endocrine clinic; auto-immune thyroid disease alone is more prevalent than diabetes mellitus. Graves' disease is autoimmune hyperthyroidism (thyrotoxicosis) and Hashimoto's disease, autoimmune hypothyroidism. Reliable, straightforward laboratory investigations such as TSH and free thyroid hormone levels (FT_4 and FT_3), together with treatments for hyperthyroidism and hypothyroidism that are unsurpassed in safety and efficacy, make dealing with these problems for the most part a gratifying experience.

Thyroid tumours, although accounting for only about 1 per cent of all invasive carcinomas, are the most common of all endocrine malignancies with an annual incidence of about 36/million. Most tend to be relatively benign in behaviour, with 75 per cent of thyroid tumour sufferers dying from other conditions.

Thyroiditis, inflammation of the thyroid (other than that caused by Hashimoto's disease) is relatively rare.

Overactivity of the thyroid gland

Biochemically, hyperthyroidism is characterized by a suppressed TSH with raised free thyroid hormone levels.

Table 3.1
Thyroid anatomy and development

The thyroid is one of the largest endocrine glands. It consists of two lobes about 4 cm in length and 2 cm in thickness, joined by an isthmus that crosses the midline just below the cricoid cartilage. It is bound to the trachea by loose connective tissue. The blood flow to the normal thyroid exceeds that to the kidneys and in hyperthyroidism is often so great that it can be heard with a stethoscope as a thyroid bruit

The thyroid gland originates early in fetal development as an epithelial proliferation at a point in the developing foregut that becomes the back of the tongue. It migrates downwards from there as a bilobed diverticulum, trailing behind it the thyroglossal duct, remnants of which may persist into adult life. It begins to function at the end of the first trimester.

Table 3.2
Thyroid hormone production and actions

Iodine is present in sea-food, iodized salt, and meat and vegetables, the latter depending on the amount in their food or the soil that they grew in, respectively. Iodine is actively transported into the thyroid gland (trapped) and rapidly oxidized by thyroid peroxidase to form a series of iodinated proteins, principally thyroglobulin, in a reaction that is stimulated by TSH and inhibited by many antithyroid drugs. Thyroglobulin, the principle component of the colloid within thyroid follicles is hydrolysed by proteases and cleaved by peptidases to yield mono- and di-iodothyronine. These are coupled together to form the active thyroid hormones tri-iodothyronine (T_3) and tetra-iodothyronine (thyroxine or T_4) that are released into the circulation. In blood, T_4 and T_3 are almost entirely bound to thyroid-binding globulin, thyroid-binding pre-albumin, and albumin. The remaining 'free' hormone is available to act on the tissues at the nuclear and mitochondrial level via thyroid hormone receptors to influence growth, differentiation, and energy expenditure

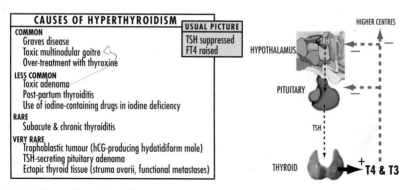

Fig. 3.1 Causes of hyperthyroidism.

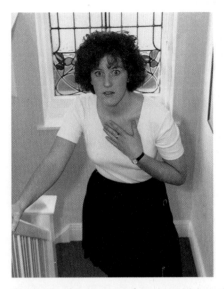

Fig. 3.2 Typical appearance of a patient with hyperthyroidism. Lid retraction is seen, and the patient has had to stop while ascending stairs because of palpitations and proximal myopathy manifesting as pain in the thigh muscles.

Young patients with hyperthyroidism are usually easy to recognize (Fig. 3.2). They tend to wear fewer layers of clothes than other patients and their behaviour may be less rational. There is frequently a history of increased irritability and short attention span, restlessness yet fatigue, proximal muscle weakness (i.e. having to stop and rest while walking upstairs), changes in menstrual pattern (often lighter), moderate increase in frequency of bowel opening, weight loss despite an increase in appetite, and a feeling of heat, sweatiness, and trembling.

Table 3.3
Hyperthyroidism

Symptoms	Incidence (%)	Signs	Incidence (%)
Nervousness, restlessness, and anxiety	99	Tachycardia	100
		Tremor	97
Sweating	91	Thyroid bruit	77
Hypersensitivity and intolerance to heat	89	Eye signs	71
		Atrial fibrillation	10
Palpitations	89	Finger clubbing and pre-tibial myxoedema	Rare
Fatigue	88		
Weight loss	85		

Table 3.4
Epidemiology of Graves' disease

Epidemiology of Graves' disease	
Incidence per annum (female)	~0.5%
Prevalence in females	~1%
Female to male ratio	10:1
Mean age of onset	30–40 years
Pernicious anaemia develops in	3%
Myasthenia gravis develops in	1%

They often appear underweight with warm, moist skin, tachycardia, and a fine tremor of their outstretched hands. Retraction of the upper eyelid leaves a rim of sclera visible above the cornea, and in some patients the eyelid can be shown to lag behind the globe as it turns down (lid lag). A modest goitre (enlarged thyroid) is usually but not always present, and there may be a systolic thyroid bruit. In older patients, the condition may be entirely occult, or present with 'lone atrial fibrillation' (10 per cent of whom turn out to be thyrotoxic), unexplained weight loss, or with worsening angina.

Graves' disease

Graves' disease is the most common cause of hyperthyroidism in patients younger than 40 years. It is characterized by symptoms of hyperthyroidism (see above), infiltrative ophthalmopathy, and a diffuse goitre, in any combination. Infiltrative dermopathy (myxoedema) and finger clubbing (acropachy) are classical but rare associations of Graves' disease. Reduced fertility and an increase in spontaneous early fetal loss are also features of Graves'.

Graves' ophthalmopathy

Graves' eye disease—infiltrative ophthalmopathy (Fig. 3.3)—is distinct from the eye signs of hyperthyroidism (eyelid retraction and 'lid lag'), although both may coexist. Periorbital oedema, soreness, redness, chemosis (watering eyes), and a gritty sensation in the eyes is common (Table 3.5). Infiltration of extraocular muscles and retro-orbital soft tissues with glycosaminoglycans causes proptosis—forward movement of the eyes. Proptosis (>22 mm measured by exophthalmometer (Fig. 3.4) may be entirely unilateral and can even occur in isolation in a clinically and biochemically euthyroid patient. An antibody-dependent mechanism has been suggested but at present the cause of this phenomenon remains unknown. The course of Graves' ophthalmopathy is independent of thyroid status and is independent of treatment of hyperthyroidism, although there is a suggestion that raised levels of TSH may exacerbate the condition.

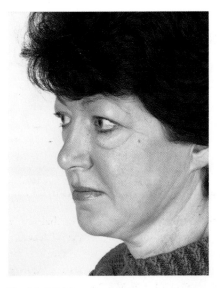

Fig. 3.3 Mild Graves' ophthalmopathy, showing moderate periorbital oedema.

Table 3.5
Characteristics and treatment of Graves' eye disease

Characteristics	Treatment
Lid retraction (the sclera becomes visible above (and below) the cornea)	Mild conjunctival irritation Hypromellose eye drops during the day
Periorbital soft tissue swelling—usually non-pitting and boggy	Simple eye ointment at night
Increased volume of orbital connective tissue, muscles and fat, leading to proptosis—forward movement of globes (>22 mm is 'marked')	Taping the eyes closed at night Chloramphenical ointment
Inability to close the eye (lagophthalmos), which can lead to exposure keratitis	Photophobia
Chemosis (excessive watering of the eye)	Dark glasses or protective shields
Photophobia	
	Diplopia

Tethering of extraocular muscles, particularly the inferior rectus and medial rectus, leading to double vision, particularly on upward gaze (ophthalmoplegia).	Fresnel prisms glued to spectacle lenses
	  Botulinum toxin injections
	  Extraocular muscle surgery

	Severe, progressive ophthalmopathy
	  Prednisolone (120 mg/day)
	  Retro-orbital steroid injections
	  Orbital radiotherapy
	  Tarsorrhaphy or other lid surgery

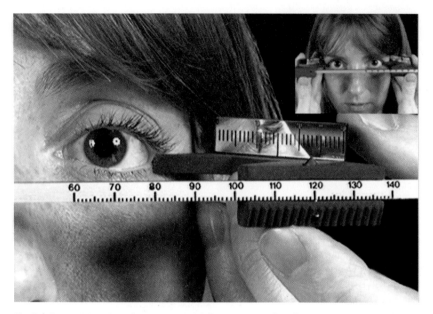

Fig. 3.4 Proptosis is measured using an exophthalmometer. The feet of this small apparatus are rested against the lateral orbital margins formed by the zygomatic bones. Once aligned, by superimposing the blue stud with the reflection of the contralateral one, the position of each cornea can be read off against their reflections on a millimetre scale viewed through a mirror or prism.

Toxic multinodular goitre

This usually develops in older patients ($\geq$ 50 years), some of whom have had non-toxic multinodular goitres for years. In many, no obvious goitre is present. Antithyroid drugs or radioiodine are the treatments of choice.

Toxic adenomas

These are benign, autonomous tumours (i.e. functional in the absence of TSH or stimulating antibody) that usually occur in young middle age and present as a slow-growing, discrete mass that eventually becomes big enough (usually $\geq$ 3 cm in diameter) to cause hyperthyroidism and atrophy of the rest of the thyroid. Radioiodine or surgery are the treatments of choice (see below).

Special cases

T_3 toxicosis

If the patient is clinically thyrotoxic and/or the TSH is suppressed yet the free T_4 is normal, consider isolated elevation of T_3. T_3 toxicosis probably occurs as an early stage of typical hyperthyroidism, and is treated in the same way.

Pregnancy

Features of hyperthyroidism may be masked by similar features of pregnancy. As always, suppressed TSH and elevated *free* thyroid hormone indicates hyperthyroidism. However, a raised *total* T_4 is a normal feature of pregnancy as thyroid-binding globulin is increased in high oestrogen states. Treatment options are more limited during pregnancy (see below), and there is a case for definitive treatment of the condition with radioiodine, 4 months or more before pregnancy is contemplated. As carbimazole and propylthiouracil cross the placenta but maternal thyroid hormones do so only minimally, the dose of antithyroid drugs should be the smallest necessary to control the condition.

Postpartum thyroiditis

During the year after delivery, up to 5 per cent of women develop 'postpartum thyroiditis'. This is a curious condition of unknown aetiology that leads to transient hyperthyroidism in 50 per cent, transient hypothyroidism in 25 per cent, and a biphasic pattern in the remainder. In all but 5 per cent of women (who are rendered permanently hypothyroid), euthyroidism spontaneously returns. The condition tends to recur with subsequent pregnancies.

The first phase of postpartum thyroiditis is characterized by an unregulated discharge of thyroid hormone from the gland and moderate hyperthyroidism. At the same time iodine uptake is greatly depressed (so that antithyroid drugs tend not to work), and the production of thyroid hormone virtually ceases. If the condition persists until stored thyroid hormone is exhausted, hypothyroidism ensues. Subsequently, after a lapse of a few weeks to 9 months, iodine uptake and formation of thyroid hormone resumes. Temporary or permanent treatment with thyroxine may be needed. Hyperthyroidism resulting from postpartum thyroiditis can be distinguished from Graves' disease by reduced or absent uptake of radioactive technetium into the thyroid.

Treatment of hyperthyroidism

Thyroid storm (thyrotoxic crisis)

Thyroid storm is a very rare complication of hyperthyroidism that is typically induced in unrecognized or inadequately treated thyrotoxic patients through an unknown mechanism by stress, such as surgery, toxaemia of pregnancy, parturition, or ketoacidosis. Tremulousness, restlessness, marked pyrexia, and tachycardia are almost invariable. Profuse sweating, nausea, vomiting, abdominal pain, and delirium are followed in untreated patients by apathy, hypotension, coma, and death. Thyroid hormone levels are often not much higher than average thyrotoxic levels and if the condition is suspected, urgent action should be taken even before thyroid function results are available (see Table 3.7). The death rate is about 20 per cent.

Table 3.6
Treatment of hyperthyroidism

Radioiodine	Antithyroid drugs	Notes	Surgery
Highly effective and very safe. The incidence of thyroid cancer after radioiodine is *lower* than that in the general population, and the radiation dose to the gonads is equivalent to that of a barium enema. The dose is calculated to deliver about 5–6 mCi 185–222 mBq of radiation 24 h after treatment There is a cumulative risk of hypothyroidism after treatment, irrespective of the dose used (40–70% or more at 10 years) Carbimazole blocks iodine uptake and is stopped at least 5 days before treatment. It can be resumed 7 days after radioiodine treatment and then gradually withdrawn over the ensuing months *continued below*	Carbimazole A 12–18 month course starting at 40–60 mg as a single daily dose, reducing to a 5–10 mg maintenance dose over a month or two is used in the first instance. A useful alternative for rapid control without necessitating frequent assessment, is to add thyroxine (100 μg daily) to continuous high-dose carbimazole (30 mg/day). The most feared (but very rare) complication is reversible agranulocytosis (incidence ≤1%) usually within the first few weeks of treatment, presenting as sore throat and fever. Treatment must be stopped immediately and antibiotics instituted until granulocytes are restored.	Even mild thyrotoxicosis should be treated to prevent myopathy, osteoporosis, and dysrrhythmias, etc. Postparturm thyroiditis, however, is usually transient and, as iodine uptake is poor, antithyroid drugs are seldom effective. Symptomatic treatment with propranolol may be all that is required	Surgery is not an appropriate treatment for uncomplicated thyrotoxicosis. It is reserved for concurrent cosmetic, malignant, or compressive problems Complications Thyrotoxicosis recurs in ≤18% Hypothyroidism occurs in ≤30% Vocal cord paralysis ≤4% Hypoparathyroidism ≤4%

Radioiodine	Antithyroid drugs	Notes	Surgery
Most of the effect develops within 3–6 months of the dose, which can be repeated if required	Propylthiouracil		
	Propylthiouracil (400–600 mg daily) is reserved for:		
As radioiodine crosses the placenta it is contraindicated in pregnancy	New treatment in pregnancy, as transplacental passage is said to be lower than that of carbimazole		
	Where carbimazole has produced a rash or other side-effect, although there are reports of agranulocytosis recurring after institution of other antithyroid drugs		
	When a particularly rapid antithyroid effect is required, as it also impairs peripheral T_4 to T_3 conversion		
	Note that neither drug significantly alters the course of the disease and that if the condition has not spontaneously regressed during treatment, it will re-emerge. Some clinicians now use these drugs in the long term		

Table 3.7
Special situations

Thyroid storm	Pregnancy	Skin complications

Supportive
Digoxin and diuretics
Paracetamol, cooling fans, and wet packs
 	
Antithyroid
Propylthiouracil:
  300–400 mg by nasogastric tube
    every 4 h
Iodine: sodium ipodate (Biloptin)
  1 g/24 h orally
  or saturated KI solution, 5 drops
    6 hourly orally
  or sodium iodide 250 mg/6 h
Dexamethasone:
  2 mg orally 6 hourly inhibits
    hormone release
  and peripheral conversion of T_4 to T_3
 	
Together these measures usually
  normalize T_3 within 24–48 h
	Propylthiouracil (PTU) is the treatment of
	choice. The lowest possible dose should be
	used (usually $\leq$200 mg/day). Very little PTU is
	found in breast milk, but it is probably best to
	advise mothers not to nurse their babies at all
		Pretibial myxoedema responds poorly to
		treatment, and attempts at surgical excision are
		usually counterproductive
		Steroid creams and occlusive dressings are
		occasionally beneficial

Underactivity of the thyroid gland

Biochemically, primary hypothyroidism is characterized by a raised TSH and a low FT_4.

Many grossly hypothyroid patients are too lethargic to complain of anything. If they did, it would be of weight gain, constipation, dry skin and hair, aching muscles, husky voice, intolerance of the cold, and disturbance of the menstrual cycle. They are facially rather pale and puffy on examination, with non-pitting periorbital oedema, thin scalp hair, and thinning of the outer third of the eyebrows (Fig. 3.5). They are usually obese and tend to move and think slowly. Hypercholesterolaemia (due to reduced lipoprotein lipase activity) is often present and mild hyperprolactinaemia (owing to the raised thyrotrophin-releasing hormone levels) occasionally occurs. Hypothyroidism is sometimes associated with hypertension, and there may be normocytic or macrocytic anaemia. The characteristically slowed tendon reflexes are a result of increased muscular relaxation time, rather than slowing of neuronal conduction velocity.

Hashimoto's thyroiditis

Hashimoto's thyroiditis, although occasionally a cause of transient hyperthyroidism, is the most common cause of permanent hypothyroidism. There is often a family history of the condition and of other autoimmune conditions such

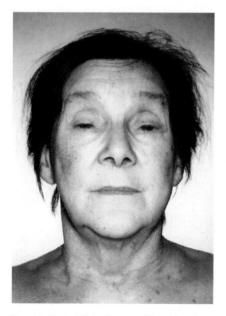

Fig. 3.5 Typical facial features of thyroid underactivity.

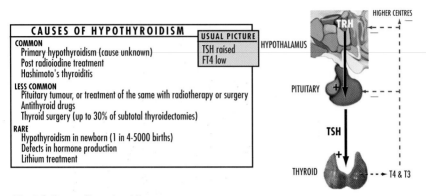

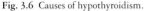

Fig. 3.6 Causes of hypothyroidism.

as pernicious anaemia, diabetes mellitus, and vitiligo. The condition usually presents in the 30–50-year age range, affects females more than males, and is often associated with fairly high titres of antimicrosomal (formerly antiperoxidase) antithyroid autoantibodies. There is no specific treatment for the condition other than replacement of thyroid hormone.

Thyroid enlargement in a euthyroid patient (euthyroid goitre)

A number of different factors, some speculative, are responsible for simple non-toxic goitre. The condition has a 9 : 1 female to male sex ratio and is particularly prevalent during adolescence and pregnancy. Suppression of TSH with thyroxine treatment is occasionally successful in making the goitre regress slightly. Clinically, the problem is usually cosmetic.

A goitre may also accompany many thyroid conditions that have euthyroid phases in addition to increased and impaired thyroid function. Occasionally, a family history of euthyroid goitre suggests an inherited defect in thyroid hormone production that is compensated for by an increase in thyroid size. Rarely, these goitres may cause respiratory symptoms and require further investigation, and surgery or radioiodine treatment to shrink the gland.

Thyroid carcinoma

Although thyroid carcinomas (Table 3.9) are the most common of all endocrine malignancies, they account for fewer than 1 per cent of all invasive carcinomas. Their behaviour tends to be benign, with about 75 per cent of patients dying from other causes. Thyroid tumours are generally treated by total thyroidectomy, or thyroid lobectomy for small, papillary lesions. Thyroid cancer in a thyrotoxic or hypothyroid patient is rare.

Table 3.8
Features and treatment of hypothyroidism

Features			Treatment
Symptoms and signs	Frequency (%)	Diagnostic weight	
Dry skin	60–100	3	• The treatment of hypothyroidism is thyroxine. The dose is adjusted at intervals until (with the exception of secondary hypothyroidism, i.e. pituitary disease) the TSH lies within the normal range. In pituitary disease free T_4 should be normalized
Cold intolerance	60–95	4	
Hoarseness of the voice	50–75	5	
Weight gain	50–75	1	• In elderly patients, or patients with ischaemic heart disease, treatment should be started at a low dose (i.e. 25 μg daily) and increased cautiously, at intervals of a few weeks
Constipation	35–65	2	
			• Once an appropriate replacement dose has been identified, it can be continued without further testing in the long term
Slow movements	70–90	11	
Coarse skin and hair	70–100	7	• In myxoedema coma, iv T_3 (500 μg then 100 μg daily) is given with full (particularly ventilatory) supportive care. Hydrocortisone (100 mg iv daily) is used to cover the possibility of concurrent adrenal failure. The outlook is poor
Periorbital puffiness	40–90	4	
Slow reflexes	50	15	

Diagnostic weight is a measure of the specificity of the symptom or sign, i.e. how good it is at distinguishing hypothyroidism from other conditions—the higher the number, the better it is

Table 3.9
Thyroid carcinoma

Papillary	Follicular	Anaplastic	Medullary
Epidemiology	Epidemiology	Epidemiology	Epidemiology
50–70% of total	10–15% of total	10% of total	1–2% of total
2.5:1 female/male ratio	2.5:1 female/male ratio	Slight female/male preponderance	Slight female/male preponderance
50% occur before the age of 40	>50% occur after the age of 40	Most occur in patients older than 50 years	Associated with parathyroid hyperplasia and phaeochromocytoma in MEN 2a and MEN 2b
Slowest growing of all thyroid cancers	Haematogenous rather than lymphatic spread to bone, lung, and liver	Presentation	Familial cases (20%) often present before 40 years.
90% survival at 20 years: even if local lymph nodes are involved at presentation, only 1% die of the disease	44–86% 5-year survival	Typically presents as rapid, painful enlargement of a mass that has often been present in the thyroid for years	Sporadic cases usually occur in older patients
Prognosis worse in patients older than 50 years with distant metastases and a primary tumour >4 cm in diameter at diagnosis		Outcome	Tumour markers
		Invasion of adjacent structures leads to hoarseness, stridor, and dysphagia. The prognosis is poor	As these arise from parafollicular (C) cells of the thyroid, basal calcitonin is increased in 33–66%

continued below

Papillary	Follicular	Anaplastic	Medullary
Treatment After thyroid lobectomy for a <2 cm lesion in patients aged 20–40 years, thyroxine is given long term to suppress TSH. Follow-up is by physical examination only			**Pentagastrin or calcium infusions elicit an exaggerated calcitonin secretory response** In the familial type, identification of the *RET* oncogene confirms that the phenotype will develop
If the lesion is >2 cm across, total thyroidectomy is followed by an ablative dose of radioiodine			**Treatment** Total thyroidectomy during the pre-malignant phase of C-cell hyperplasia is curative.
Tumour marker A thyroglobulin level of ≤ 2 ng/ml on T_4 is highly indicative of a disease-free state			
A radioiodine scan can be useful to identify metastases			

About 5 per cent of apparently solitary thyroid nodules represent tumours. Diagnosis of the nature of thyroid nodules depends on careful histological exam- ination of cells and tissue fragments obtained by fine-needle aspiration biopsy. This can be carried out in the clinic without an anaesthetic.

Ultrasound scanning is useful to differentiate solid from cystic lesions. Radioiodine uptake scans can be used to differentiate a functioning ('warm or hot') from a non-functioning ('cold') nodule. The order of investigation of a solitary thyroid nodule depends on the preferences of the clinician involved and the available services. Increasingly, fine-needle aspiration is being used in the clinic as a rapid, and in many cases definitive, investigation. A typical flow chart of investigations is given in Fig. 3.7.

Subacute thyroiditis

With the exception of postpartum thyroiditis (and Hashimoto's) these conditions are probably quite rare. Mild cases of subacute thyroiditis (also known as granulo- matous, giant cell, or de Quervain's thyroiditis) might well be mistaken for pharyngitis unless the presence of tenderness localized to the thyroid itself is recognized. Patients often complain of fever and lassitude with pain radiating to the jaw, ear, or occiput that can be exacerbated by turning the head or swallow- ing. Pain may be completely absent, however, and the presenting features limited to nervousness or palpitations. The condition often takes some months to resolve and may be treated with non-steroidal anti-inflammatory drugs or simple anal- gesics such as aspirin or paracetamol, or, if the severity of symptoms warrants it, prednisolone (40 mg daily) until it resolves.

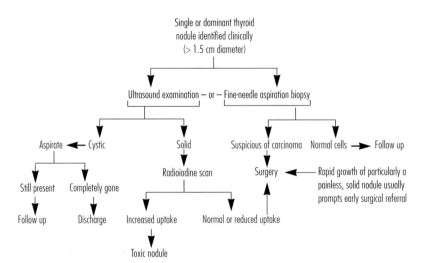

Fig. 3.7 Investigation of thyroid carcinoma. Note that the order of investigation depends on the clinician and on the available resources.

Explanation

Oestrogens, in this case a component of the contraceptive pill, increase hepatic output of thyroid hormone-binding globulin. Thus the *total* T_4 result from the laboratory, while correct, was misleadingly high. The normal TSH gave the game away and, soon after the carbimazole was stopped, a free T_4 and repeat TSH were found to be normal. Patients who are pregnant will tend to have high total T_4 levels, for exactly the same reason.

'My patient has a thyroid nodule please advise'

History

The patient was a completely fit and well 44-year-old male who had a medical examination for insurance purposes and was found to have a thyroid nodule. He had no personal or family history of thyroid or autoimmune disease and had not received external radiotherapy to the neck at any time in the past.

Examination

The only abnormality was a thyroid nodule, 1 cm in diameter in the left lobe of the thyroid gland.

Management

About 40 per cent of people over the age of 40, have one or more thyroid nodules palpable on careful examination. The risk of malignancy if the nodule is less than 1.5 cm in diameter is low, and in many centres, no action would be taken, other than follow-up at intervals to see if it is changing in size. An alternative approach would be to do a fine-needle aspiration biopsy (FNAB) under ultrasound control.

Notes

In nodules this size, FNAB should not necessarily be considered 'a safer option' than observing. There is a 15 per cent chance that the FNAB will be non-diagnostic, and of these, about 14 per cent turn out to be malignant. In patients with a history of neck irradiation or who were exposed to the fallout from the Chernobyl nuclear disaster as young children, however, the risk of malignancy is many times greater and tissue diagnosis should not be delayed.

Multiple-choice questions

1. In thyroid disease:
    a. An anxious young woman is found to have a raised total T_4. Her TSH was found to be within the normal range. The raised total T_4 indicates that she is thyrotoxic.
    b. A patient with primary hypothyroidism has a raised TSH despite being prescribed 200 μg of thyroxine daily. The patient is clearly thyroxine resistant and should have the dose increased further in accordance with her requests.
    c. Two months after carbimazole treatment was started for a toxic nodular goitre, a patient's free T_4 is now low–normal but her TSH remains suppressed. The dose should be increased.
    d. A patient on intensive care is found to have a suppressed FT_4 and TSH. Hypothyroidism is contributing to the clinical problem, and replacement therapy should be started.
    e. Three months after starting replacement therapy for primary hypo-thyroidism, the TSH is normal but the patient still complains of tiredness and aching muscles. The dose should not be increased further as the TSH is within the normal range.

2. The following are useful treatments for hyperthyroidism:
    a. Lugol's iodine;
    b. Carbimazole;
    c. Propranolol;
    d. Glucocorticoids such as dexamethasone and prednisolone;
    e. Amiodarone.

3. In an untreated patient, the following make hyperthyroidism very unlikely:
    a. Constipation;
    b. A TSH in the normal range;
    c. A low free T_4;
    d. Intolerance of the cold;
    e. A suppressed TSH with a low free T_3 and free T_4.

4. The following are characteristic of hypothyroidism:
    a. Hypercholesterolaemia;
    b. Osteoporosis;
    c. Slowed neuronal conductivity leading to delayed ankle reflexes;
    d. Confusion and mental slowness;
    e. Sweating.

Answers

1. In thyroid disease:
    a. An anxious young woman is found to have a raised total T_4. Her TSH was found to be within the normal range. The raised total T_4 indicates that she is thyrotoxic

F

Hepatic production of thyroid-binding globulin and therefore total T_4 (but not free T_4) is increased by oestrogens. She is taking the contraceptive pill.

b. A patient with primary hypothyroidism has a raised TSH despite being prescribed 200 μg of thyroxine daily. The patient is clearly thyroxine resistant and should have the dose increased further in accordance with her requests   F

A thyroxine requirement in excess of 150 μg daily is unusual. The average requirement is 112 ± 19 μg/day. The most likely cause is failure to take the medication as prescribed.

c. Two months after carbimazole treatment was started for a toxic nodular goitre, a patient's free T_4 is now low–normal but her TSH remains suppressed. The dose should be increased   F

After prolonged suppression, the return of normal TSH secretion by the pituitary can be markedly delayed. It may take 3 months or more for levels to return to normal.

d. A patient on intensive care is found to have a suppressed FT_4 and TSH. Hypothyroidism is contributing to the clinical problem, and replacement therapy should be started   F

Probably not. In many types of stress, from fasting to infection, central down-regulation of the thyroid axis occurs. This is called the 'sick euthyroid syndrome'. The pathogenesis remains uncertain, but treatment with thyroxine is not indicated.

e. Three months after starting replacement therapy for primary hypo-thyroidism, the TSH is normal but the patient still complains of tiredness and aching muscles. The dose should not be increased further as the TSH is within the normal range   T

It often takes much longer for stiff muscles and lethargy to disappear than for the FT_4 and TSH to be normalized. The patient should be warned about this at the outset, and may need further reassurance at intervals.

2. The following are useful treatments for hyperthyroidism:
  a. Lugol's iodine   T

The thyroid is the only tissue that takes up significant amounts of iodine. Physiological amounts of iodine produce a short-lived increase in thyroxine formation that rapidly returns to normal or even subnormal levels. For reasons that are unclear, a pharmacological dose of iodine (i.e. iodine in potassium iodide solution (Lugol's iodine)) promptly but temporarily inhibits hormone release and blocks peripheral de-iodination. It is still used in 'thyroid storm' and during the preparation of thyrotoxic patients for surgery. Iodine deficiency, of course, reduces the ability of the thyroid to make hormones, and in areas of endemic deficiency, goitres (so-called Derbyshire neck) are prevalent.

  b. Carbimazole   T

Iodine is transported into the gland (trapped), bound to iodotyrosine (organified), synthesized into thyroxine (T_4) and tri-iodothyronine (T_3), and stored in large amounts. Most antithyroid drugs in common use, of which carbimazole is one, work by reducing the amount of iodine available for thyroid hormone synthesis. Methimazole, the active metabolite of the pro-drug carbimazole, is used in the United States.

c. Propranolol   T

This may be all that is required in postpartum thyroiditis, where the condition is likely to be self-limiting and characterized by failure of iodine uptake (and therefore failure of carbimazole or propylthiouracil effect). Propranolol, while not treating the primary problem, does reduce deiodination of T_4 to the more active T_3, and therefore reduces the activity of circulating thyroid hormones.

d. Glucocorticoids such as dexamethasone and prednisolone   T

Dexamethasone has a number of useful effects in thyroid storm, including inhibition of conversion of T_4 to T_3 in the periphery (usually 2 mg every 6 hours). Prednisolone is also used in severe, progressive Graves' ophthalmopathy, but should only be used under the supervision of an ophthalmologist.

e. Amiodarone   F

This can have almost any effect on thyroid status, the most usual being induction or exacerbation of hyperthyroidism. As its name suggests, it contains a lot of iodine, and abnormal thyroid function tests can occur without evidence of clinical disease. Patients taking lithium as an antipsychotic also occasionally develop overt hypothyroidism and, in the past, lithium has been used as a treatment for hyperthyroidism. If hypothyroidism does develop during lithium therapy, treatment with thyroxine does not reverse its antipsychotic effects.

3. In an untreated patient, the following make hyperthyroidism very unlikely:

a. Constipation   F

Diarrhoea, or at least, relatively loose stools is more common, but by no means invariable.

b. A TSH in the normal range   T

This might, however, occur in a thyrotroph adenoma of the pituitary, but these are extremely rare.

c. A low free T_4 T

A low FT_4 level indicates hypothyroidism.

d. Intolerance of the cold   F

Many, particularly elderly patients complain of this. It is possible to be thyrotoxic without any symptoms at all.

e. A suppressed TSH with a low free T_3 and free T_4 T

This would suggest secondary hypothyroidism in a patient who, for example, might have had pituitary surgery and radiotherapy for a pituitary adenoma.

4. The following are characteristic of hypothyroidism:

   a. Hypercholesterolaemia   T

   Thyroid function should always be checked in a patient with hyperlipidaemia.

   b. Osteoporosis   F

   This is more characteristic of hyperthyroidism.

   c. Slowed neuronal conductivity leading to delayed ankle reflexes   F

   Slowed ankle reflexes do occur, but the predominant effect is a myopathy, with very little change in nerve conduction velocities. This sign is highly specific for hypothyroidism, easy to elicit, and hence extremely useful.

   d. Confusion and mental slowness   T

   This is one of the more disturbing features of the condition that may take months to improve, even after circulating thyroid hormone levels are returned to normal.

   e. Sweating   F

   This is of course a characteristic of hyperthyroidism, rather than hypothyroidism.

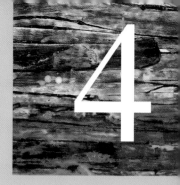

4

The adrenal glands

- Summary

- Introduction

- The adrenal medulla

- The adrenal cortex

- Key points

- Case history

- Multiple-choice questions

Summary

Normal function

- The medulla synthesizes adrenaline and noradrenaline.
- The cortex produces cortisol, pre-androgens, and aldosterone.

Typical pathology

- Adrenal underactivity (unusual or rare)
  - → Primary failure (Addison's disease) leads to a syndrome resulting from low cortisol and aldosterone, with pigmentation from secondary elevation of pituitary ACTH.
  - → Secondary failure (i.e. hypopituitarism) reduces cortisol production but leaves aldosterone unchanged (as it is regulated by the renin–angiotensin pathway). As ACTH is low, pigmentation does not occur.
  - → Failure of the adrenal medulla is not a clinical entity.
  - → Inherited enzyme defects can lead to impaired cortisol (± aldosterone) synthesis and excessive pre-androgen production (congenital adrenal hyperplasia).
- Adrenal overactivity (rare or very rare)
  - → Excessive ACTH stimulation resulting from pituitary or other ACTH-secreting tumours: Cushings *disease* or Cushings *syndrome* respectively
  - → Adrenal medullary tumours can secrete adrenaline and/or noradrenaline (phaeochromocytoma).
  - → Tumours of the adrenal cortex can secrete aldosterone (Conn's syndrome), cortisol (Cushing's syndrome), or androgens (causing virilization in women).

'Typical clinical scenario'

- A 54-year-old man with secondary adrenal cortical failure following pituitary surgery and radiotherapy. He is taking thyroxine and sex hormones in addition to hydrocortisone.

Introduction

The adrenal cortex is the site of production of cortisol, aldosterone, and pre-androgens such as dehydroepiandrosterone (DHEA), dehydroepiandrosterone sulphate (DHEAS), and androstenedione (AD). The adrenal medulla produces catecholamines. Disorders of the adrenal medulla, such as phaeochromocytoma formation, are very rare. Although minor variations in adrenal function are

Table 4.1
Adrenal anatomy and development

The adrenals consist of a gland within a gland. The cortex is derived from a proliferation of mesenchymal cells that line the coelomic cavity adjacent to the urogenital ridge. At 8 weeks' gestation the mesenchymal cell mass of the primitive adrenal cortex is invaded by neuroectodermal cells that form the medulla. In adults, the cortex constitutes 90% of the weight of the adrenal glands. The adrenals lie at the upper poles of the kidneys and are usually surrounded by a layer of fat that facilitates their identification by MR scanning. Each adrenal gland measures approximately $1 \times 3 \times 5$ cm, but may vary in size depending on the physiological circumstance: if one is removed, for example, the other undergoes compensatory hypertrophy

Table 4.2
Adrenal cortical hormone function

Mineralocorticoid	Glucocorticoid	Androgens
Aldosterone has major effects on extracellular fluid volume and potassium homeostasis. It acts on specific receptors in the distal convoluted tubule of the kidney to decrease sodium and increase potassium excretion. Water passively follows sodium ion excretion	Cortisol diffuses into its target cells, combines with receptor protein in the cytoplasm, and is transported to the nucleus where it modifies gene expression and hence protein synthesis. It has many effects on metabolism including stimulation of hepatic glucose synthesis, breakdown of protein in muscle, skin, and bone, an anti-inflammatory effect, and enhancement of lipid mobilization. Cortisol protects us from stress-induced hypotension, shock, and death by mechanisms that are not understood	The pre-androgens, dehydroepiandrosterone (DHEA), dehydroepiandrosterone sulphate (DHEAS), and androstenedione exert most of their androgenic effect following conversion in peripheral adipose tissue to testosterone. In women, androgens are responsible for the normal pattern of female secondary sexual hair. Excess androgen action leads to hirsutism, amenorrhoea, acne, and eventually virilization

implicated in a number of fairly common problems, such as hirsutism and acne, the presentation of primary adrenal problems is uncommon.

Atrial natriuretic peptide (Table 20.1) is another modulator of aldosterone release.

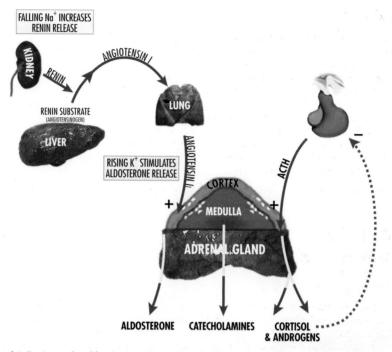

Fig. 4.1 Renin, produced by the juxtaglomerular cells of the renal cortex, is the rate-limiting enzyme for the conversion of circulating angiotensinogen to angiotensinogen I. It is increased by a fall in renal perfusion (standing up, dehydration, renal artery stenosis, etc.), by a decrease in plasma sodium, and by renal sympathetic nerve activity. Angiotensin I is rapidly converted into angiotensin II by angiotensin-converting enzyme (found predominantly in the lungs). ACTH from the anterior pituitary stimulates adrenal production of cortisol and androgens such as androstenedione, DHEA, and DHEAS. Feedback control is via cortisol. Pituitary failure has no effect on aldosterone production.

The adrenal medulla

Underactivity

There is no clinical syndrome associated with adrenal medullary failure. Neither adrenaline nor noradrenaline needs to be replaced following bilateral adrenal failure or removal.

Overactivity

Tumours of the catecholamine-producing cells of the adrenal medulla, 'phaeochromocytomas' (Fig. 4.2), are the only significant cause of adrenal medullary overactivity. The prevalence of these tumours identified at autopsy (1:1000) suggests that their behaviour is generally benign and that most remain

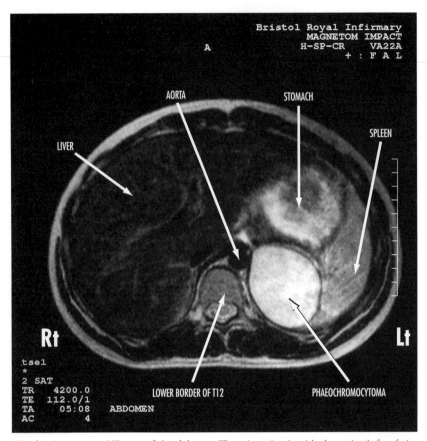

Fig. 4.2 A transverse MR scan of the abdomen. The orientation is with the patient's feet facing towards the observer. The liver, spleen, and stomach are seen, along with a mass above the left kidney—a phaeochromocytoma.

occult. In fact, about 50 per cent of phaeochromocytomas identified at post-mortem were not associated with hypertension during life. Those that are recognized (and on average it takes around 4 years to do so) are usually identified in middle age as the cause of sustained or paroxysmal hypertension and other symptoms associated with sudden, inappropriate, and excessive secretion of adrenaline, noradrenaline, or both, such as headaches, palpitations, sweating, and anxiety (Table 4.3).

Phaeochromocytomas are usually single and benign. In adults, approximately 10 per cent are malignant, 10 per cent are bilateral, 10 per cent are extra-adrenal, and 10 per cent are familial. In children, 20 per cent are bilateral, 30 per cent are extra-adrenal at diagnosis, and over 50 per cent of unifocal tumours initially considered to be benign, ultimately prove to be multifocal and/or malignant.

Table 4.3
Symptoms and diagnosis of phaeochromocytoma

Typical symptoms	Diagnosis
Headache: abrupt in onset, severe, throbbing, generalized; 5 min to 2 h	24 h urinary excretion of adrenaline, noradrenaline, or their metabolic products (metanephrines, normetanephrines, or vanillylmandelic acid (VMA), one of the main urinary metabolites of catecholamines)
Sweating: continuous or paroxysmal, sometimes truncal, with dry periphery	
Palpitations: sometimes intense; may be slow	
Weight loss	
Chest pain: may occur at the height of the attack	CT or MR imaging of the adrenals, sympathetic chain, or elsewhere
Pallor or flushing	
Episodic anxiety	Scintigraphy with MIBG (meta-iodobenzylguanidine)
Hypotension and shock	

Phaeochromocytomas are associated with the multiple endocrine neoplasia syndrome type 2a and 2b (see p. 354).

The adrenal cortex

Underactivity

This can be primary (Addison's disease), or secondary, due to insufficient circulating ACTH (Table 4.4).

Addison's disease

Primary adrenal insufficiency, Addison's disease, seems to be much rarer in clinical practice that incidence figures would suggest. The condition is weakly associated with other causes of autoimmune glandular hypofunction, such as diabetes mellitus, primary gonadal failure, autoimmune thyroid failure, vitiligo, and pernicious anaemia. The strongest association is with hypoparathyroidism, in which there is an 11 per cent prevalence of anti-adrenal antibodies—an antibody rarely evident in other autoimmune diseases.

Addison's disease causes weakness, weight loss, vomiting, pigmentation, and postural hypotension. The symptoms often appear gradually over months and may be hard to spot. Classical biochemical abnormalities of high potassium and low sodium are late features that may not appear until the patient is in crisis. Even then, hyponatraemia may be masked by dehydration.

As soon as an Addisonian crisis is suspected, intravenous saline replacement should be given together with glucocorticoids. Once the condition of the patient is stable, hydrocortisone (glucocorticoid replacement) can be withheld for 36 hours to allow a Synacthen test to be carried out, and restarted pending the results.

Table 4.4
Causes and diagnosis of adrenal cortex underactivity

Primary adrenal failure	Secondary adrenal failure	Diagnosis of adrenal underactivity
The whole cortex is destroyed. Therefore both glucocorticoid and *mineralocorticoid* production is affected. ACTH levels and plasma renin activity are high, cortisol (and aldosterone) levels are low	The zona glomerulosa is not affected by ACTH deficiency. Therefore only glucocorticoid production is affected. Both ACTH and cortisol levels are low. Aldosterone production is normal	The Synacthen test This tests the ability of adrenal cortical cortisol production to respond to ACTH
Major causes Autoimmune atrophy 80% Tuberculosis 20%	Major causes Pituitary adenoma Craniopharyngioma	In primary adrenal failure, cortisol levels fail to reach 495 nmol/l 30 min and 1 h after an im bolus of ACTH (250 μg)
Causes that should be clear from the history Drugs (ketoconazole, metyrapone, etc.) Irradiation Adrenalectomy	Causes that should be clear from the history Pituitary surgery Pituitary radiotherapy Glucocorticoid-induced atrophy	In secondary adrenal cortical failure (i.e. failure of ACTH production by the pituitary), the adrenal cortex rapidly atrophies and the same criteria apply. Note that a false positive (abnormal) test will result if the patient is taking a glucocorticoid at the time.
Rare causes Haemorrhage (i.e. meningococcal sepsis) Replacement by tumour or lymphoma Replacement by amyloid or sarcoidosis Congenital enzyme deficiency	Rare causes Pituitary infarction Primary pituitary failure Hypothalamic sarcoidosis Metastatic tumour in the hypothalamus	ACTH level Once adrenal cortical underactivity has been diagnosed with the synacthen test, a single measurement of ACTH will distinguish primary adrenal failure (high ACTH) from secondary adrenal failure (low ACTH)

Table 4.5
Primary adrenal insufficiency

Incidence	1:25 000
Female/male ratio	5:4
Mean age of diagnosis	41 years
Proportion of cases diagnosed between the third to fifth decade	66%
Death rate	1:250 000
Anti-adrenal antibodies	64%

The importance of doubling the dose of hydrocortisone during times of stress should be emphasized to the patient and the message reinforced at intervals.

The most common cause of hypoadrenalcorticalism is iatrogenic. Systemic glucocorticoid treatment inhibits pituitary ACTH secretion and rapidly induces adrenal cortical atrophy. Rapid withdrawal of glucocorticoids does not afford the adrenal cortex sufficient time to recover, and a physical or psychological stress at this time may induce an Addisonian crisis. Prolonged courses of glucocorticoids must be withdrawn slowly.

Overactivity

The causes of overactivity of the adrenal cortex can be divided into intrinsic adrenal cortical problems, such as the formation of hormone-secreting tumours, and extrinsic problems such as excessive production of ACTH in Cushing's disease or the formation of renin-secreting tumours of the kidneys (Table 4.7).

Although almost all causes of adrenal cortical overactivity are rare or very rare, Conn's syndrome and congenital adrenal hyperplasia are probably both more common than is generally recognized. An overnight dexamethasone suppression test (see p. 372) is almost always sufficient to exclude Cushing's syndrome in patients with hirsutism or obesity.

Conn's syndrome

Conn's syndrome, an aldosterone-secreting adenoma of the adrenal cortex causing hypertension and spontaneous hypokalaemic alkalosis, is responsible for less than 1 per cent of cases of hypertension (see p. 340). It typically occurs in symptomatic, young to middle-aged (30–50-year-old) patients with moderate hypertension. It is slightly more common in females than in males. Malignant hypertension is very unusual, and a potassium of 4 mmol/l or more excludes the diagnosis.

Diagnostic tests are designed to demonstrate a suppressed plasma renin activity and an inappropriately elevated aldosterone level despite the presence of hypokalaemia (which would normally suppress it) and normal dietary intake of potassium and sodium. Conn's syndrome is further suggested if potassium

Table 4.6
Adrenal insufficiency

Primary adrenal insufficiency

Common symptoms
Weakness and fatigue	100%
anorexia	100%
Nausea and vomiting	90%

Common signs
Weight loss	100%
Hyperpigmentation	90%
Hypotension	90%

Adrenal crisis
Unexplained symptoms and
signs, such as:
Hypoglycaemia
Fever
Abdominal pain
Hyponatraemia
Hyperkalaemia
Illness with unexpectedly severe:
Nausea
Vomiting
Dehydration
Hypotension
Shock

Maintenance and emergency treatment of adrenal insufficiency
Secondary hypoadrenalcorticalism
Hydrocortisone
15–20 mg on waking and 5–10 mg in the early afternoon or
10–15 mg on waking, 5 mg at midday, and 5 mg at 4 p.m.
Primary hypoadrenalcorticalism
As above, but add
Fludrocortisone 100 μg (50–200 μg) daily

Emergency treatment
Take blood sample for later cortisol estimation, then give 4 mg dexamethasone
iv or im immediately, with saline infusion (1 l/h) to rehydrate

Laboratory features of Addison's disease

Biochemistry
Hyponatraemia, often absent or minimal early on
    20% do not have hyponatraemia at any time
Hyperkalaemia, often mild
    33% do not have hyperkalaemia at any time
Uraemia
Mild acidosis

Haematology
Anaemia—normochromic, normocytic
    May be masked by dehydration
Eosinophilia
Lymphocytosis
Hypoglycaemia

Unusual features
Hypercalcaemia
Pernicious anaemia

Steroid cover
Minor illnesses
    Increase hydrocortisone to two or three times the
    normal daily dose. Dental surgery under a local
    anaesthetic does not require additional cover

Major surgery
    Give 100 mg hydrocortisone iv with induction of
    anaesthetic and repeat 8 hourly for the first 24 h.
    Decrease by 50% per day until the normal
    maintenance dose is reached

Table 4.7
Adrenal overactivity

Primary adrenal overactivity	Secondary adrenal overactivity
Tumours of the adrenal cortex can secrete any of the hormones normally produced by that tissue. Adrenal cortical tumours are highly malignant, in many cases, but fortunately very rare	Adrenal cortical hormone production is normally controlled by pituitary ACTH and via the renin-angiotensin system. Excess production of these hormones causes adrenal hyperstimulation

Intrinsic hormone produced
Glucocorticoids
   Leading to Cushing's syndrome
Androgens or oestrogens
   Leading to virilism in females or
   feminism in males. In children,
   precocious puberty can result
Aldosterone
   Primary hyperaldosteronism, also
   known as Conn's syndrome. Responsible
   for <1% of hypertension
	Extrinsic hormone produced
	ACTH
	   This is responsible for Cushing's
	   disease—pituitary-dependent ACTH
	   excess (a tumour of corticotroph cells)
	ACTH may be produced ectopically,
	   usually by other tumours such as
	   small-cell lung carcinomas
	Renin
	   Renin-secreting tumours of the kidney
	   can lead to secondary hyperaldosteronism

supplements fail to restore potassium levels, and sodium supplements (which directly inhibit renin production) fail to suppress aldosterone. Once good biochemical evidence of primary hyperaldosteronism has been collected, an MR scan of the adrenals is useful to look for a solitary adenoma.

Treatment

Surgical excision of the adenoma. In zona glomerulosa hyperplasia or if the patient is unfit for surgery, spironolactone, an aldosterone antagonist, is a very effective therapy, with amiloride (which inhibits distal tubule sodium transport) as a useful second-line treatment.

Table 4.8
Normal values of aldosterone and plasma renin

	Aldosterone	Plasma renin activity
After remaining recumbent overnight	100–400 pmol/l (3.6–14.5 ng/dl)	1.1–2.7 pmol/ml.h (3.2 ± 1 μg/l.h)
After 30 min in an upright posture	Double the above	2.8–4.5 pmol/ml.h (9.3 ± 4.3 μg/l.h)
Random		0.5–3.1 pmol/ml.h

Congenital adrenal hyperplasia (CAH)

A series of enzymes in the adrenal cortex is responsible for the biosynthesis of cortisol, aldosterone, and pre-androgens from cholesterol (Fig. 4.3). The whole process is driven by pituitary ACTH and subject to feedback inhibition by cortisol at the level of the pituitary gland and hypothalamus.

In CAH, inborn defects in adrenal cortical enzyme function lead to impaired synthesis of cortisol ± aldosterone. The reduction in cortisol decreases feedback inhibition of ACTH production and increased ACTH compensates for defects in cortisol biosynthesis but leads to excessive activity of other pathways, often leading to increased pre-androgen production and virilization in females (Fig. 4.4).

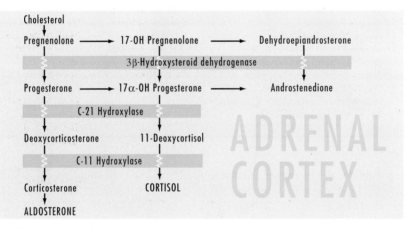

Fig. 4.3 Biosynthesis of adrenal cortical steroid hormones.

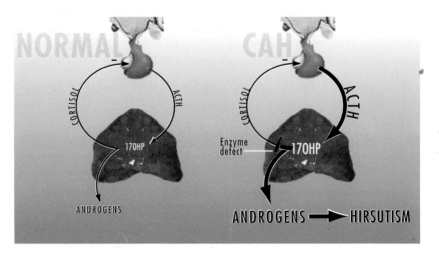

Fig. 4.4 In congenital adrenal hyperplasia, a much higher ACTH drive keeps cortisol within the normal range. The unaffected androgen synthesis pathway is overstimulated.

Table 4.9
Congenital adrenal hyperplasia

Notes	Symptoms and signs	
21-Hydroxylase deficiency (>90%) The full-blown condition affects 1:10 000 births (i.e. at least twice as common as acromegaly) It is the most common cause of ambiguous genitalia The non-classical (i.e. partial) form has an overall incidence of around 1%	Result from excessive androgen production and (in 50% of cases) reduced aldosterone production	
	Neonates	Adults
	Females: mild virilism to complete pseudohermaphroditism Males: sexual precocity, advanced bone age, and loss of final height Salt-wasting crises: hyperkalaemia and hyponatraemia (due to lack of aldosterone)	Females: hirsutes; can be clinically indistinguishable from polycystic ovarian disease Males: no specific symptoms unless salt wasting. Often at least 5 cm below predicted height. Therefore, may be short statured Curiously, the condition can appear to wax and wane markedly
11β-Hydroxylase and 3β-Hydroxysteroid dehydrogenase deficiency Similar to the above, but extremely rare and often associated with hypertension		
	Hypoglycaemia may also occur	

In neonates and young children, impairment of aldosterone synthesis can result in episodes of gross hyperkalaemia, sodium ('salt') wasting, fits, and sometimes death unless the condition is promptly treated. The death rate is higher in males owing to the difficulty and subsequent delay of detecting minor degrees of virilization. Milder variants usually present in childhood or at puberty, and in the adult endocrine clinic, very mild forms of the condition present with hirsutism or acne.

Diagnosis in adults

Congenital adrenal hyperplasia usually presents in females in young adulthood with hirsutism and amenorrhoea or menstrual irregularities (occasionally with mild virilization) that can be clinically almost indistinguishable from the picture seen in polycystic ovarian disease. If hirsutism seems excessive, 17-hydroxyprogesterone is measured in addition to LH, FSH, testosterone, and sex hormone binding globulin. A more definitive diagnosis can be made by observing an excessive increase in 17-hydroxyprogesterone (to >45.4 nM) after an injection of ACTH (Synacthen®, 250 μg).

Treatment

Treatment with glucocorticoids reduces ACTH levels and returns pre-androgen (and 17-hydroxyprogesterone) levels to normal. Mineralocorticoid supplements are also given in salt-wasting forms. The dose of glucocorticoid in children is monitored by measuring growth velocity, skeletal maturation, and 17-hydroxyprogesterone (all three of which increase if the dose is inadequate) at intervals.

Key points

- The primary function of the renin–angiotensin system is to keep the blood volume constant.
- Aldosterone secretion is principally stimulated by:
  - (a) angiotensin II; and
  - (b) an increase in potassium.
- Renin release is principally stimulated by:
  - (a) a fall in renal perfusion pressure;
  - (b) increased sympathetic nervous system activity; and
  - (c) a fall in sodium.
- The symptoms of Addison's disease often appear gradually over many months. Electrolyte changes are late signs.
- Patients with untreated Addison's disease become anorexic, lethargic, and lose weight.
- Emergency treatment of adrenal insufficiency consists of intravenous rehydration with saline and glucocorticoid replacement with dexamethasone.
- The typical replacement dose of glucocorticoids in primary or secondary adrenal cortical failure is 10–15 mg of hydrocortisone in the morning and 5 mg in the early afternoon.

'My patient is tired. Does he have Addison's disease?'

History

A 45-year-old man complained of a 6-month history of increasing tiredness that had now become so severe that it prevented him functioning at work. He had had what he took to be a common cold 7 months previously and was forced to retire to bed for a week. In the past month, he had had two episodes of vomiting and had lost 5 kg in weight over the same time.

Examination

His blood pressure was 110/80 mmHg with no postural drop. There was no buccal pigmentation and a scar from an appendicectomy at the age of 24 was unpigmented. He was untanned.

Investigations

His full blood count, urea, and electrolytes were normal. In particular his Na^+ was 138 mmol/l (normal range (135–153) with a K^+ of 4 mmol/l (normal range 3.7–5.2)) A Synacthen test (250 intramuscular μg of Synacthen®) resulted in an increase in cortisol from 180 nmol/l to 230 nmol/l at 30 min, and to 240 nmol/l at 60 min (normal response ≥495). A random ACTH estimation was 185 ng/l (normal range 5–36 at 9 a.m., <10 at midnight, and ≤76 under conditions of stress). Adrenal autoantibodies were negative. No adrenal calcification was seen on a plain abdominal radiograph.

Management

He was started on hydrocortisone replacement therapy, 10 mg on waking, 5 mg at 1 p.m. and 5 mg at 4 p.m., with fludrocortisone 100 μg daily. The necessity for increasing the dose to 2–4 times basal levels for a few days under conditions of acute mental or physical stress was emphasized to the patient.

Explanation

An inadequate response to Synacthen® identified adrenocortical insufficiency and the raised ACTH confirmed the diagnosis of primary adrenal cortical failure (i.e. Addison's disease). Anti-adrenal autoantibodies are *absent* in almost 40 per cent of autoimmune Addison's disease and a negative test does not detract from the diagnosis. In tuberculous Addison's disease, adrenal calcification is often present and can be seen on plain radiographs.

Addison's disease is rare and the incidence of the condition in patients who are otherwise well, but complain of tiredness is negligible. Scars sustained *after* but not before the onset of Addison's disease tend to pigment. The normal electrolytes in this patient in no way exclude the diagnosis, as the fall in Na^+ and increase in K^+ are usually very mild until the patient is in impending crisis. In secondary adrenal failure (i.e. pituitary failure), electrolyte changes do not occur, as the aldosterone-secreting zona glomerulosa is stimulated by angiotensin II rather than pituitary ACTH.

Multiple-choice questions

1. The adrenal gland:
   a. There are significant clinical interactions between the adrenal cortex and medulla.
   b. In a patient with hypoparathyroidism and new-onset nausea, anorexia, and weight loss, a potassium of 6 mmol/l suggests that primary adrenal cortical failure should be urgently excluded.
   c. A plasma sodium of 140 mM (135–153) in a non-specifically unwell patient excludes adrenal cortical failure.
   d. A random cortisol can be a useful diagnostic aid in adrenal cortical failure.
   e. In full-blown, virilizing forms of congenital adrenal hyperplasia, the Müllerian (female) system involutes.

2. In adrenal metabolism:
   a. Ingestion of large amounts of liquorice produces apparent hyper-aldosteronism;
   b. Bartter's syndrome results from a defect in tubular chloride or potassium transport;
   c. Primary hyperaldosteronism is usually the result of an aldosterone-secreting adenoma of the adrenal cortex (Conn's syndrome);
   d. A markedly depressed 17-hydroxyprogesterone in a hirsute patient suggests congenital adrenal hyperplasia;
   e. Conn's syndrome usually produces severe, uncontrollable hypertension in youth.

3. Phaeochromocytoma:
   a. Normal urinary levels of adrenaline and noradrenaline exclude the diagnosis;
   b. Is associated with papillary thyroid carcinoma;
   c. Phaeochromocytomas and ganglioneuromas (tumours of sympathetic ganglia) are found only in the adrenal medulla and along the extent of the sympathetic chains.
   d. High urinary adrenaline levels suggest an intra-adrenal phaeochromo-cytoma;
   e. Hypertension can be controlled safely with beta-adrenergic blockade.

4. Causes of hypokalaemia include:
   a. Cushing's syndrome;
   b. Bartter's syndrome;
   c. Addison's disease;
   d. Congenital adrenal hyperplasia;
   e. Conn's syndrome.

Answers

1. The adrenal gland:
   a. There are significant clinical interactions between the adrenal cortex and medulla   F

   Phenylethanolamine N-methyl transferase (PNMT), the enzyme that converts noradrenaline to adrenaline in the adrenal medulla, needs high levels of steroids generated by the adrenal cortex to function properly. Clinically, however, the interaction is not significant.

   The 'endocrine gland within an endocrine gland' arrangement of the adrenals is not unique. The calcitonin-secreting 'C' cells are entirely surrounded by the thyroid gland, and the posterior lobe of the pituitary gland is partly (and in some species completely) enveloped by the anterior lobe.

   b. In a patient with hypoparathyroidism and new-onset nausea, anorexia, and weight loss, a potassium of 6 mmol/l suggests that primary adrenal cortical failure should be urgently excluded   T

   The biochemical changes of Addison's disease should not necessarily be relied on, but spontaneous elevation of plasma potassium is a very suggestive sign, and should be followed up with a Synacthen test.

   c. A plasma sodium of 140 mM (135–153) in a non-specifically unwell patient excludes adrenal cortical failure   F

   The biochemical changes of Addison's disease can develop slowly or not at all. Hyponatraemia in particular can be masked by concurrent dehydration, or in secondary adrenal failure (i.e. pituitary failure with low ACTH when the renin–angiotensin–aldosterone axis remains intact) never develop at all.

   d. A random cortisol can be a useful diagnostic aid in adrenal cortical failure   T

   The Synacthen test is 'the test' of course, but if a random cortisol in an ill patient is reported as <50 nmol/l, the diagnosis is very likely, and the Synacthen test results are likely to be <50 nmol/l at time zero, <50 nmol/l at 30 min, and <50 nmol/l at 60 min. The same test results will also be recorded if the patient has been on long-term prednisolone or dexamethasone for another indication!

   e. In full-blown virilizing forms of congenital adrenal hyperplasia, the Müllerian (female) system involutes   F

   Although the adrenals can virilize a female fetus by producing large amounts of pre-androgens, unlike the testes they do not produce Müllerian inhibiting hormone. Hence the uterus and Fallopian tubes persist.

2. In adrenal metabolism:
   a. Ingestion of large amounts of liquorice produces apparent hyperaldosteronism   T

Liquorice and carbenoxolone inhibit the enzyme 11-hydroxysteroid dehydrogenase and therefore allow glucocorticoids to function at mineralocorticoid receptors.

b. Bartter's syndrome results from a defect in tubular chloride or potassium transport   T

Bartter's syndrome is the result of a defect in tubular chloride or potassium transport. It usually presents in childhood as normotensive (or sometimes hypertensive) hypokalaemia with raised aldosterone and renin. The definitive test is to give patients 100 mM chloride per day. If they excrete more than 10 mM, the diagnosis is confirmed. Remember it as a renal potassium chloride leak.

c. Primary hyperaldosteronism is usually the result of an aldosterone-secreting adenoma of the adrenal cortex (Conn's syndrome)   T

Single adrenal adenomas account for 50–90 per cent of primary hyperaldosteronism. The rest are due to bilateral hyperplasia. Together, they account for less than 1 per cent of cases of hypertension, and in neither case is the cause known. An MR scan of the adrenals, which at first sight would seem the most obvious way to distinguish an adenoma from bilateral hyperplasia, may add to the confusion by disclosing non-functioning adrenal nodules that are present in at least 1 per cent of the population as a whole. The diagnostic accuracy of CT and MR in this context are equal, at 70 per cent. Venous sampling has a 95 per cent sensitivity and adrenal iodoscintigraphy, 70 per cent sensitivity.

d. A markedly depressed 17-hydroxyprogesterone in a hirsute patient suggests congenital adrenal hyperplasia   F

The 17-hydroxyprogesterone is characteristically elevated. It is an important branch point of cortisol and pre-androgen metabolism. If cortisol metabolism is blocked, cortisol feedback inhibition diminishes, pituitary ACTH production increases and stimulates adrenal steroid production. Therefore more pre-androgens are produced, as are intermediates such as 17-hydroxyprogesterone. Although severe forms of CAH are often diagnosed clinically at birth, from a day or two after birth (to allow the metabolites to accumulate) neonates can be screened for CAH using blood-spot 17-hydroxyprogesterone.

e. Conn's syndrome usually produces severe, uncontrollable hypertension in youth   F

The hypertension is usually fairly mild. The spontaneous hypokalaemia is a characteristic effect of excessive aldosterone action.

3. Phaeochromocytoma:

a. Normal urinary levels of adrenaline and noradrenaline exclude the diagnosis   F

The absence of raised levels of adrenaline and noradrenaline in the urine certainly help to exclude the diagnosis, but between attacks, 24 h mean levels are often normal. Raised urinary catecholamines are highly suggestive of phaeochromocytoma, but acute and chronic stress, stroke, and sympathomimetic drugs can falsely elevate levels. Extra-adrenal phaeochromocytomas, or paragangliomas, usually secrete noradrenaline exclusively and can occur almost anywhere. Measurement of the noradrenaline/ creatinine ratio in an overnight urine collection may be a more sensitive and specific method to identify phaeochromocytomas.

b. Is associated with papillary thyroid carcinoma   F
Phaeochromocytomas are associated with the multiple endocrine neoplasia syndrome types 2a and 2b. The MEN 2 syndromes are associated with medullary thyroid carcinoma rather than papillary thyroid carcinoma, and in a minority of cases, with hyperparathyroidism. They are also associated with neurofibromatosis (although only 1 per cent of patients with neurofibromatosis have phaeochromocytomas) and in some kindreds with von Hippel–Lindau disease (retinal cerebellar haemangioblastomatosis).

c. Phaeochromocytomas and ganglioneuromas (tumours of sympathetic ganglia) are found only in the adrenal medulla and along the extent of the sympathetic chains   F
These tumours have been described in many locations, including the retroperitoneum, abdomen, mediastinum, skull base, neck, spinal cord, urinary bladder, larynx, orbit, lung, liver, and bone.

d. High urinary adrenaline levels suggest an intra-adrenal phaeochromocytoma   T
The enzyme PNMT (phenylethanolamine N-methyl transferase) in the adrenal converts noradrenaline to adrenaline. Extra-adrenal lesions do not elaborate this enzyme and cannot, therefore, produce adrenaline.

e. Hypertension can be controlled safely with beta-adrenergic blockade   F
Hypertension in phaeochromocytomas can be made catastrophically worse with unopposed beta blockade, as the vasodilator effect of adrenaline is blocked. However, alpha-adrenoreceptor blockers, such as doxazosin, are extremely useful in this context.

4. Causes of hypokalaemia include:

a. Cushing's syndrome   T
Glucocorticoids cause sodium retention and potassium loss. However, in Cushing's disease hypokalaemia is unusual, and its presence in Cushing's syndrome, suggests ectopic ACTH production.

b. Bartter's syndrome   T
Bartter's syndrome is characterized by defective renal tubular chloride and potassium transport.

c. Addison's disease   F
Hyponatraemia and hyperkalaemia are characteristic but often very late manifestations. Hyperkalaemia is more often caused by renal failure, acidosis (such as diabetic ketoacidosis), the use of angiotensin-converting enzyme (ACE) inhibitors or potassium-sparing diuretics, or an artefact caused by haemolysis of the blood sample.

d. Congenital adrenal hyperplasia   F

In salt-losing cases, the salt is sodium, rather than potassium, as aldosterone is low.

e. Conn's syndrome   T

The aldosterone/renin activity ratio (in ng/dl and ng/ml hour, respectively) often exceeds 20 even after the patient is made sodium replete by giving 10 slow-sodium tabs (100 mM) daily for 2 weeks. Failure of plasma aldosterone to suppress to less than 420 pmol/l (15 ng/dl) 2 h after a 25 mg oral dose of captopril (especially if given with 0.3 mg of fludrocortisone) further supports the diagnosis of primary hyperaldosteronism.

In a solitary aldosterone-secreting adenoma, plasma renin activity remains completely suppressed and aldosterone (paradoxically) falls slightly after 3 hours' standing or walking. Under the same circumstances a dramatic rise in aldosterone, presumably in response to a minimal increase in renin, suggests bilateral hyperplasia. As renin is an enzyme, it is expressed as an 'activity', rather than as a concentration.

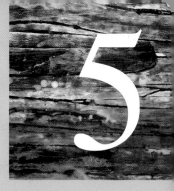

The ovary

- Summary

- Introduction

- Ovarian development

- Ovarian function

- Key points

- Case history

- Multiple-choice questions

Summary

Normal function

- The ovaries are the source of ova and sex hormones from the menarche until the menopause.

Typical pathology

- Disordered menstruation: amenorrhoea or oligomenorrhoea (reduced frequency of menstruation) related to reduced body weight, polycystic ovarian disease, or hyperprolactinaemia.
- Hirsutism (usually related to polycystic ovarian disease).
- Pre-menstrual syndrome ('pre-menstrual tension').
- Ovarian failure
  → Infertility.
  → Oestrogen withdrawal producing vasomotor instability (hot flushes) and vaginal dryness (leading to dyspareunia—painful intercourse) in the short term, and predisposing to heart disease and osteoporosis in the long term.

'Typical clinical scenario'

- A 28-year-old woman with amenorrhoea and mild hirsutism secondary to polycystic ovarian disease.
- A 56-year-old woman, 5 years postmenopause, who is troubled by hot flushes and concerned about osteoporosis, but also worried about the side-effects of sex hormone replacement therapy.

Introduction

A combination of hirsutism, disordered menstruation, and subfertility, usually attributed to polycystic ovarian disease, is one of the most common symptom complexes seen in the endocrine clinic. Osteoporosis resulting from post-menopausal oestrogen deficiency (physiological ovarian failure) is almost universal in the elderly. Most other ovarian problems are either referred directly to gynae-cologists or are very rare, for example precocious puberty secondary to sex hormone production by ovarian tumours.

Ovarian development

In the presence of two complete X chromosomes, the ovaries develop to contain granulosa cells, stromal cells, and ova. Formation of the Fallopian tubes, the uterus, and the upper third of the vagina from the Müllerian ducts is entirely independent of ovarian development. These structures are therefore almost

Table 5.1
Sex differentiation

Genetic sex is determined by the presence of a Y chromosome. Gonadal sex is established by the presence of ovaries or testes, and phenotypic sex (sometimes known as 'delivery room sex' or 'legal sex') is determined by the external genitalia. Gender, the identification of self as male or female, is assigned at about the time that speech develops

Irrespective of genetic sex, the structures that form the gonads and genital apparatus are identical in early embryonic life. Gonadal sex is determined at approximately day 40 of gestation when, depending on the presence or absence of an intact Y chromosome (specifically, expression of the sex-determining region of that chromosome), the undifferentiated gonad becomes either a testis or ovary. The development of phenotypic sex depends on the type of gonad formed

In the male the epididymis, vas deferens, and seminal vesicles are formed from the Wolffian ducts while the Müllerian ducts regress under the influence of 'Müllerian-inhibiting hormone' produced by the fetal testis. In the female (the default sex), the Wolffian ducts regress and the Müllerian ducts form the Fallopian tubes, uterus, and upper part of the vagina

The external genitalia of both sexes develop from the same structures: the genital tubercle becomes either the clitoris or the glans penis; the genital swellings either side become the labia majora or the scrotum; and the urethral fold, the labia minora or penile shaft. In the male fetus, normal development of the prostate and external genitalia is primarily dihydrotestosterone, rather than testosterone, dependent

normal in Turner's syndrome (XO rather than XX genotype) even though the ovaries fail to develop.

Ovarian function

The ovaries produce oestradiol from the granulosa cells that form the developing follicles, androgens from the theca cells that surround them (most of which are aromatized to oestrogens by the granulosa), and progesterone from the corpora lutea that develop after ovulation. The corpus luteum is a temporary endocrine organ that secretes progesterone to prepare the oestradiol-primed endometrium to accept the newly fertilized ovum, and to facilitate establishment of early pregnancy.

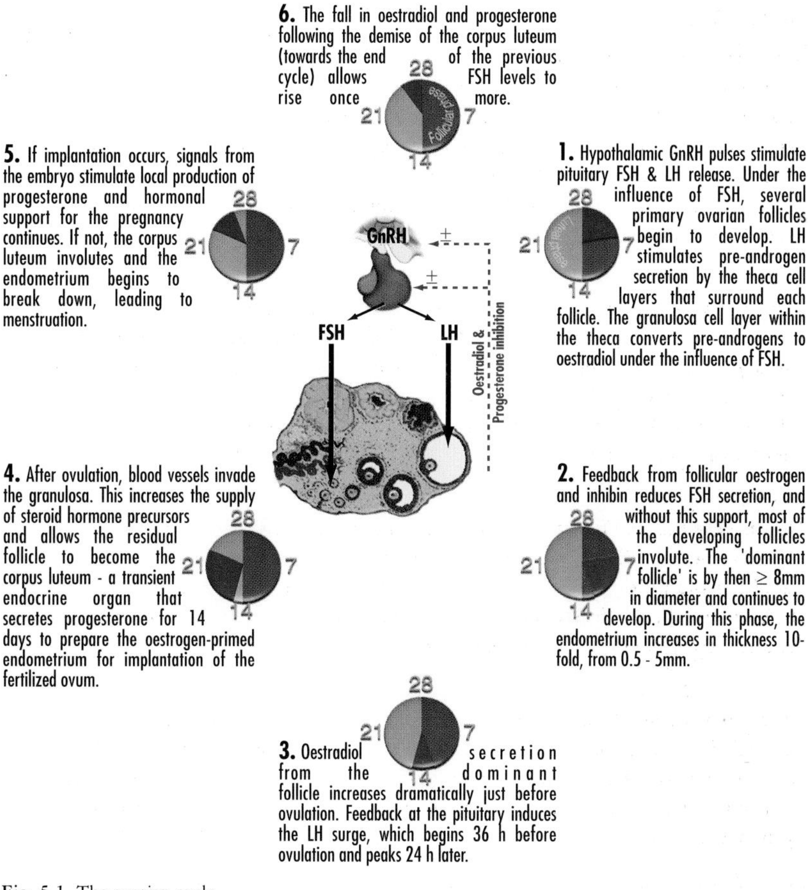

6. The fall in oestradiol and progesterone following the demise of the corpus luteum (towards the end of the previous cycle) allows FSH levels to rise once more.

5. If implantation occurs, signals from the embryo stimulate local production of progesterone and hormonal support for the pregnancy continues. If not, the corpus luteum involutes and the endometrium begins to break down, leading to menstruation.

GnRH

FSH   LH

Oestradiol & Progesterone inhibition

1. Hypothalamic GnRH pulses stimulate pituitary FSH & LH release. Under the influence of FSH, several primary ovarian follicles begin to develop. LH stimulates pre-androgen secretion by the theca cell layers that surround each follicle. The granulosa cell layer within the theca converts pre-androgens to oestradiol under the influence of FSH.

4. After ovulation, blood vessels invade the granulosa. This increases the supply of steroid hormone precursors and allows the residual follicle to become the corpus luteum - a transient endocrine organ that secretes progesterone for 14 days to prepare the oestrogen-primed endometrium for implantation of the fertilized ovum.

2. Feedback from follicular oestrogen and inhibin reduces FSH secretion, and without this support, most of the developing follicles involute. The 'dominant follicle' is by then ≥ 8mm in diameter and continues to develop. During this phase, the endometrium increases in thickness 10-fold, from 0.5 - 5mm.

3. Oestradiol secretion from the dominant follicle increases dramatically just before ovulation. Feedback at the pituitary induces the LH surge, which begins 36 h before ovulation and peaks 24 h later.

Fig. 5.1 The ovarian cycle.

Key points

- Developing ovarian follicles are lined by granulosa cells that synthesize oestrogens from pre-androgens made by the theca cell layers that surround them.
- Raised progesterone levels on days 19–21 of the cycle indicate that ovulation has occurred.
- A withdrawal bleed following 5 days' treatment with 5 mg Provera®, indicates that ovarian oestrogen output is sufficient to cause endometrial proliferation.

Table 5.2
Comparison of oestrogens and progestogens

Oestrogens	Progestogens
Principal effects	**Principal effects**
Development of female secondary sexual characteristics	Induction of secretory activity in the oestrogen-primed endometrium, i.e. prepares it for acceptance of the newly fertilized ovum, and inhibits uterine contractions
Development of the ductal system of the breast	Increases viscosity of cervical mucus
Proliferation of the endometrium	Promotes glandular development of the breast
Thickening of vaginal mucosa	Increases basal body temperature
Thinning of cervical mucus	Makes cervical mucus relatively impenetrable to sperm
Prevention of bone mineral loss	
Prevention of atherosclerosis	
Uses	**Uses**
In conjunction with progestogens in 'the contraceptive pill' or in lower doses as hormone replacement therapy (HRT) to prevent osteoporosis, atherosclerosis, and relieve symptoms of the menopause	Used alone, or in conjunction with oestrogens in 'the contraceptive pill'
Treatment of gonadal failure, and induction and maintenance of secondary sexual characteristics in hypogonadotrophic hypogonadism	Lower doses are used with oestrogens in 'HRT' to prevent endometrial proliferation leading to neoplasia
Preparation of the endometrium before embryo transfer	Used to induced withdrawal bleeding in the diagnosis of amenorrhoea (i.e. identifies evidence of oestrogen priming)

continued below

Oestrogens	Progestogens
Principal side-effects	Principal side-effects
Endometrial proliferation which leads to hyperplasia and in the absence of progesterone to an increased risk of endometrial cancer	Amenorrhoea
Probable slight increase in the risk of breast cancer with long-term use ($\geq$10 years) but may marginally decrease the mortality rate from it	Irregular bleeding or spotting, particularly when used alone
Headaches and induction or exacerbation of migraine	Malaise and depression
Breast tenderness	Weight gain and oedema
Irregular bleeding	Hirsutism
	Acne

Table 5.3
Assessment of ovarian function

Oestrogen status	Progesterone status	Integrated function
Historical data	*Historical data*	*Historical data*
Vaginal lubrication	Basal body temperature	Menstrual cycles
Vaginal dryness, leading to dyspareunia (painful intercourse) suggests that oestrogen levels are low	An increase in basal body temperature (measured on waking, before getting out of bed) by 0.5 °C occurs after ovulation. Asking subfertile patients to keep a temperature diary can be used to predict ovulation, but may also lead to unhealthy preoccupation and anxiety	Completely regular menstrual cycles strongly suggest that gonadotrophins, oestrogens, progesterone, and androgens are adequate, ovulation is occurring, and that the reproductive tract is normal
Clinical signs		
Breast development		Hot flushes
As breast ductal development is oestrogen dependent, normal breast development indicates that oestrogens were present during adolescence	*Clinical signs*	The mechanism responsible for vasomotor instability in ovarian failure has still not been fully elucidated. Strictly speaking a sex hormone withdrawal phenomenon, it is usually synonymous with ovarian failure, but also occurs in men with acute gonadal failure or post-castration (for prostatic cancer)
	Cervical mucus	
	The nature of cervical mucus can be used to assess the oestrogen and progesterone status of the patient. However, obtaining a sample is not practical in endocrinology outpatients	
Tests		
Blood oestradiol level		
These are not particularly useful alone as the 'normal range' is wide, but low levels with raised gonadotrophins strongly suggest primary ovarian failure		

continued below

Oestrogen status	Progesterone status	Integrated function
Provera withdrawal test	*Tests*	*Tests*
Oestrogens cause endometrial proliferation. Progestogens depress oestrogen receptor function. Thus if a short course of progestogen treatment (i.e. medroxyprogesterone acetate (Provera®) 5 mg/day for 5 days) induces a menstrual bleed, the endometrium must previously have been exposed to oestrogens	Blood progesterone level	Ultrasound examination
	An elevated progesterone level measured between days 19 and 21 of the menstrual cycle (i.e. to >30 nmol/l) is a very simple and useful test. It indicates that a corpus luteum is present and therefore that ovulation must have occurred	Transabdominal or transvaginal ultrasound or MR imaging is useful to demonstrate streak ovaries, ovarian tumours, and the presence and size of follicles during ovulation induction. Ovarian imaging can also be used to confirm the diagnosis of polycystic ovarian disease

'My patient complains of secondary amenorrhoea. I have diagnosed premature menopause and told her that there is no treatment that will restore fertility. She has requested a second opinion'

History

A 28-year-old female was referred to clinic with secondary amenorrhoea. Menarche was at the age of 11 years and except for an uneventful, full-term pregnancy at the age of 23, menstrual cycles had been regular from then until 6 months previously, when they stopped. Looking back, she confirmed that sexual intercourse had become uncomfortable, and on two subsequent occasions she had experienced a hot flush.

Examination

Anxious but otherwise normal.

Investigations

FSH was 50 IU/l (normal range 1–9 U/l). No further investigations were carried out.

Management

Unfortunately, the diagnosis made by her GP was accurate, and the patient was told as gently as possible that premature menopause had indeed occurred. Even at a normal age (mean of 51 years) the menopause can be psychologically as well as physically disturbing. It is very tangible reminder of the inevitable processes of ageing, and the perception of permanent loss of fertility can be associated with bereavement reactions. Premature ovarian failure is in many cases much more traumatic. The patient was offered and accepted sex hormone replacement therapy.

Explanation

In this previously fertile young woman, two FSH estimations 6 weeks apart were both high. The discomfort on intercourse and hot flushes were clear evidence of oestrogen withdrawal, and there was little doubt about the diagnosis. However, as the consequences of the diagnosis of ovarian failure are dramatic and permanent, further tests, such as ovarian ultrasound to exclude the presence of follicles, or even ovarian biopsy, are sometimes undertaken. A karyotype was not requested in view of her previous normal pregnancy. Premature ovarian failure can be associated with autoimmune failure of other endocrine glands such as Addison's disease and primary hypothyroidism.

Sex hormone replacement therapy was suggested as a treatment to prevent hot flushes, to prevent osteoporosis, and for its protective effects on the cardiovascular system.

Multiple-choice questions

1. Major targets for oestrogen action are:
   a. Hair follicles;
   b. The endometrium;
   c. The vagina;
   d. Bone;
   e. The breasts.

2. Progesterone:
   a. Is elevated during the first week of the cycle;
   b. Is usually maximal between days 16 and 19 of the cycle;
   c. High levels on day 19 of the cycle indicate that ovulation has occurred;
   d. Makes cervical mucus relatively impermeable to spermatozoa;
   e. Causes proliferation of breast glandular tissue.

3. Oestrogens:
   a. Tend to cause breast tenderness;
   b. Can increase the risk of endometrial cancer;
   c. Increase the risk of breast cancer;
   d. Are made by aromatization of androgens in peripheral fat;
   e. Are absorbed through the skin.

4. Ovaries:
   a. Are present in XXY males;
   b. Are present in completely virilized females with congenital adrenal hyperplasia;
   c. May contain follicles in some patients with Turner's syndrome;
   d. Stop functioning at the time of the menarche;
   e. Contain more ova at birth than they do by menarche.

Answers

1. Major targets for oestrogen action are:
   a. Hair follicles   F
      Androgens are the gonadal steroids that induce vellous follicles to turn into either sebaceous glands or terminal hair follicles. Oestrogens are used in the treatment of hirsutism both for their contraceptive effect (as anti-androgens are by their nature mutagenic) and, secondly, to increase hepatic production of sex hormone binding globulin, thus reducing the levels of free androgens in the blood.
   b. The endometrium   T
      Of course, and the action produced is proliferation. Continuous high oestrogen levels produce amenorrhoea (sometimes with 'spotting' or occasional small bleeds) in the presence of endometrial proliferation. Treatment with medroxyprogesterone acetate (5–10 mg daily for 5 days) will induce a menstrual period under these circumstances—a positive Provera test.
   c. The vagina   T
      Vaginal secretions are oestrogen dependent. Absence of oestrogens leads to poor vaginal lubrication, thinning of the vaginal epithelium, and uncomfortable intercourse (dyspareunia). This is a very useful symptom in the diagnosis of low oestrogen levels.
   d. Bone   T
      One of the most dramatic effects of oestrogen withdrawal is an abrupt increase in bone mineral loss to three times the rate of pre-menopausal loss.
   e. The breasts   T
      The development of breast tissue is largely oestrogen dependent. The 'shield chest' of Turner's syndrome results in part from complete lack of breast development. Histological remains of ovaries ('streak ovaries') are found along the urogenital ridge and as there is no follicular development, oestrogen production is minimal. These patients need early diagnosis followed by treatment with growth hormone, and then oestrogens to take them through puberty at an appropriate age.

2. Progesterone:
   a. Is elevated during the first week of the cycle   F
      The major site of progesterone production in the non-pregnant state is the corpus luteum in the ovary. This is not formed until ovulation has occurred in mid cycle. Therefore progesterone is not elevated until the second half of the cycle.
   b. Is usually maximal between days 16 and 19 of the cycle   F
      Most of the variability in menstrual cycle length is related to variability in the luteal (secretory) or second half of the cycle. Although the peak of progesterone production can occur at slightly different times, days 19 to 21 encompass the most likely time to pick up the progesterone peak from a functional corpus luteum.

c. High levels on day 19 of the cycle indicate that ovulation has occurred T

A corpus luteum must be present, and ovulation must therefore have occurred.

d. Makes cervical mucus relatively impermeable to spermatozoa T

This is one of the principle actions thought to bring about the contraceptive action of the progesterone-only pill.

e. Causes proliferation of breast glandular tissue T

Progesterone and prolactin induce proliferation of breast glandular tissue. High levels of progesterone and oestrogen during pregnancy block lactation until after delivery.

3. Oestrogens:

a. Tend to cause breast tenderness T

This is particularly noticeable in men who experience a sudden increase in the oestrogen/androgen ratio, either when they take drugs with oestrogenic properties, such as digoxin, or anti-androgenic properties such as spironolactone or flutamide. Women taking the contraceptive pill may also notice breast tenderness, as may normal women particularly towards the middle of each menstrual cycle. The return of breast tenderness is a troublesome side-effect of hormone replacement therapy in post-menopausal women.

b. Can increase the risk of endometrial cancer T

Except in women who have had a hysterectomy, continuous unopposed oestrogen treatment (i.e. without progesterone) is now no longer used because of this problem (and others). In polycystic ovarian disease, where endogenous oestrogen levels are chronically raised, endometrial neoplasia is slightly more common, with a peak incidence in young middle age.

c. Increase the risk of breast cancer T

Prolonged treatment, even with the low doses used in sex hormone replacement therapy, do appear to modestly increase the *incidence* but perhaps not the mortality of this disease. Women with a high risk of cardiovascular disease and a low risk of breast cancer should probably be targeted for treatment.

d. Are made by aromatization of androgens in peripheral fat T

Peripheral fat can convert pre-androgens to androgens (testosterone and dihydrotestosterone), and also convert androgens to oestrogen, principally oestrone. The latter is implicated in the metabolic pathways that lead to polycystic ovarian disease.

e. Are absorbed through the skin T

This is exploited as the 'oestrogen patch', a method of administration that circumvents hepatic first-pass metabolism.

4. Ovaries:

a. Are present in XXY males F

Patients with Klinefelter's syndrome have testes.

b. Are present in completely virilized females with congenital adrenal hyperplasia　　　　　　　　　　　　　　　　　　　　T

The excess androgens are derived from the adrenal cortex rather than the gonads. They do have ovaries, and are usually fertile.

c. May contain follicles in some patients with Turner's syndrome　　　T

Depending on the extent of genomic deletion of the second 'X' chromosome and the presence of mosaicism.

d. Stop functioning at the time of the menarche　　　　　　　　　F

The menopause is the time they stop, and the mean age of this has remained 51 years for decades—unlike the menarche, the mean age of which is gradually falling.

e. Contain more ova at birth than they do by menarche　　　　　T

From the time they are fully formed *in utero* (at about 10 weeks), the number of ova progressively declines, so that by birth, there are approximately 10^6, and by the menarche 400 000. At the time of the menopause, only a few remain.

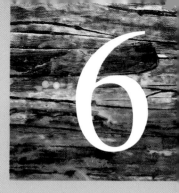

6

The menstrual cycle

- Summary

- Introduction

- Amenorrhoea

- Polycystic ovarian disease

- Other disorders of the menstrual cycle

- Menopause

- Key points

- Case history

- Multiple-choice questions

Summary

Normal function

- The menstrual cycle prepares the endometrium for implantation of the fertilized ovum and restores it to its unproliferated state if implantation does not occur.

Typical pathology

- Oligomenorrhoea or amenorrhoea
  - → Polycystic ovarian disease (one of the most common pathological causes of oligomenorrhoea).
  - → Weight loss, stress, or excessive exercise (≥10 per cent below ideal weight is enough).
  - → Hyperprolactinaemia (usually pituitary microprolactinoma formation).
  - → Premature menopause, Turner's syndrome, and constitutional delay of puberty are less often seen. The distinction between primary and secondary amenorrhoea (no history of menstruation and amenorrhoea following at least 6 months' of normal menstrual cycles, respectively) is not particularly helpful clinically as a number of common problems can cause either.

'Typical clinical scenario'

- A 34-year-old with a 5 month history of amenorrhoea. A raised prolactin (2900 mU/l) was found on testing and a microprolactinoma diagnosed on pituitary MR imaging.

Introduction

Sexual reproduction is the only way that offspring can end up with fewer mutations than their parents. The cost of this evolutionary necessity is the complex and risky process of having to liberate ova into an environment in which they are free to interact with male gametes, yet retain them within the body so that they can be nurtured once fertilized. Unlike cells from a metastasizing neoplasm that are able to embed themselves in previously unmodified tissue, for the fertilized ovum, a unique and evanescent host tissue has to be prepared specially to facilitate implantation (Table 6.1). The endometrium does not remain in a proliferated, 'ovum-ready' state for long, however, and the result is menstruation, an event that would hardly have existed in the past, as fertile females would have been pregnant or lactating almost throughout their reproductive lives.

Typical causes of amenorrhoea are pregnancy, the menopause, polycystic ovarian disease (PCOD, although oligomenorrhoea is more common), hyperprolactinaemia, psychological stress, being underweight for height (≤90 per cent ideal body weight), and Turner's syndrome.

Table 6.1
Endometrial changes during the menstrual cycle

Simultaneous with the decline in corpus luteum function and the falling levels of oestrogen (and progesterone), local production of prostaglandins produces intense vasospasm in the endometrial spiral arterioles. This leads to ischaemic necrosis and endometrial loss in association with the bleeding that marks the first day of the menstrual cycle.

As oestrogen levels start to rise at the fourth or fifth day, rapid oestrogen-induced endometrial growth occurs. Endometrial thickening slows as progesterone levels increase after ovulation, as progesterone decreases the number of oestrogen receptors. The main change in the second half of the cycle is maturational, however, with an increase in the tortuosity of the endometrial glands and spiral arterioles

What is menstruation?

Menstruation is the cyclical loss of blood from the uterus, averaging once every 28 ± 3 days and lasting for 4 ± 2 days. The first menstrual period or 'menarche', occurs at a mean age of 13, approximately 2 years after the beginning of breast development. With the exception of pregnancy and lactation, menstrual cycles then continue until the menopause at the average age of 51.

The menstrual cycle is divided into two phases, the first of which, the follicular or proliferative phase, is a remarkably constant 14 days in length. During this phase, the thickness of the endometrium increases tenfold. The second phase, the luteal or secretory phase, lasts from 10 to 16 days, and is the cause of the variation in menstrual cycle length in normal women.

Amenorrhoea

Amenorrhoea is subdivided into primary amenorrhoea, the absence of menstruation by the age of 16, and secondary amenorrhoea, failure of menstruation for 6 months in a woman who previously had regular menses. The classification is far from absolute, as a number of common conditions can cause either. Pregnancy is the most common cause of amenorrhoea. Even patients who have been amenorrhoeic for years can present with an abdominal mass that turns out to be a gravid uterus.

Clinical evaluation

Amenorrhoea is a common problem, and as such, it is the province of general practitioners, family planning clinics, paediatricians, and gynaecologists as well as endocrinologists. The majority of cases of amenorrhoea seen in adult endocrine clinics are of secondary amenorrhoea, and the cause of most of these is clear from the history alone, sometimes supplemented with the results of baseline pituitary function tests, such as gonadotrophins, sex hormones, sex hormone binding globulin, and prolactin (Fig. 6.1, Table 6.2).

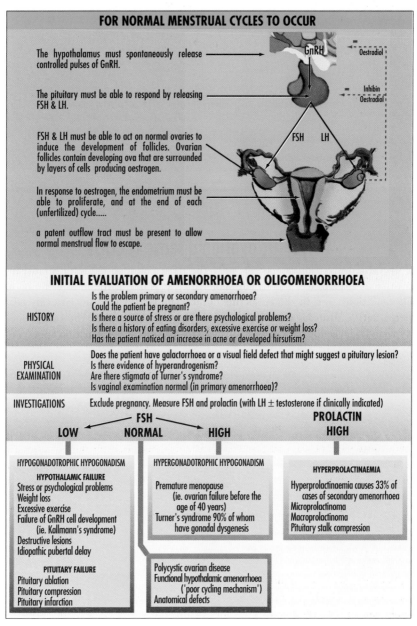

FOR NORMAL MENSTRUAL CYCLES TO OCCUR

The hypothalamus must spontaneously release controlled pulses of GnRH. → GnRH ⟶ Oestradiol

The pituitary must be able to respond by releasing FSH & LH. ← Inhibin Oestradiol

FSH & LH must be able to act on normal ovaries to induce the development of follicles. Ovarian follicles contain developing ova that are surrounded by layers of cells producing oestrogen. FSH LH

In response to oestrogen, the endometrium must be able to proliferate, and at the end of each (unfertilized) cycle.....

a patent outflow tract must be present to allow normal menstrual flow to escape.

INITIAL EVALUATION OF AMENORRHOEA OR OLIGOMENORRHOEA

HISTORY	Is the problem primary or secondary amenorrhoea? Could the patient be pregnant? Is there a source of stress or are there psychological problems? Is there a history of eating disorders, excessive exercise or weight loss? Has the patient noticed an increase in acne or developed hirsutism?
PHYSICAL EXAMINATION	Does the patient have galactorrhoea or a visual field defect that might suggest a pituitary lesion? Is there evidence of hyperandrogenism? Are there stigmata of Turner's syndrome? Is vaginal examination normal (in primary amenorrhoea)?
INVESTIGATIONS	Exclude pregnancy. Measure FSH and prolactin (with LH ± testosterone if clinically indicated)

← **FSH** →

PROLACTIN

LOW   **NORMAL**   **HIGH**   **HIGH**

HYPOGONADOTROPHIC HYPOGONADISM	HYPERGONADOTROPHIC HYPOGONADISM	HYPERPROLACTINAEMIA
HYPOTHALAMIC FAILURE Stress or psychological problems Weight loss Excessive exercise Failure of GnRH cell development (ie. Kallmann's syndrome) Destructive lesions Idiopathic pubertal delay	Premature menopause (ie. ovarian failure before the age of 40 years) Turner's syndrome 90% of whom have gonadal dysgenesis	Hyperprolactinaemia causes 33% of cases of secondary amenorrhoea Microprolactinoma Macroprolactinoma Pituitary stalk compression
PITUITARY FAILURE Pituitary ablation Pituitary compression Pituitary infarction	Polycystic ovarian disease Functional hypothalamic amenorrhoea ('poor cycling mechanism') Anatomical defects	

Fig. 6.1 Causes of amenorrhoea.

Table 6.2
Common causes of amenorrhoea in the general endocrine clinic

1. Polycystic ovarian disease (PCOD)
2. Weight loss to <90% of ideal, i.e. anorexics and slimmers—often coupled to excessive exercise
3. Hyperprolactinaemia (most commonly microprolactinoma formation)
4. Premature menopause (i.e. premature ovarian failure)
5. Hypopituitarism (e.g. postpartum pituitary infarction—Sheehan's syndrome)
6. Idiopathic pubertal delay
7. Anxiety, e.g. exams and other traumatic life events
8. Pregnancy, the most common cause of amenorrhoea but rarely referred for investigation

Polycystic ovarian disease (PCOD)

Polycystic ovarian disease is not only the most common cause of hirsutism, menstrual disturbance, and female subfertility, it is one of the most common of all conditions seen in the endocrine clinic. The factors that initiate this self-perpetuating disorder are still a matter of debate. Whatever the cause, once hyperandrogenaemia has been established, the pattern of perpetuation appears to be as shown in Fig. 6.2.

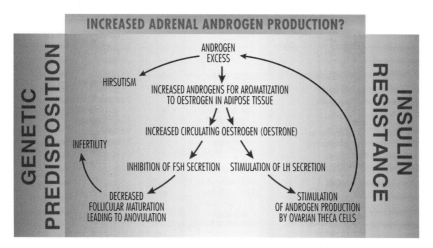

Fig. 6.2 Perpetuation of hyperandrogenaemia.

Table 6.3
Laboratory features of PCOD

LH elevated & FSH suppressed - ie. increased LH/FSH ratio	Gonadotrophins are normal in at least 20% of women with PCOD, but often the LH/FSH ratio is higher than 2 or 3. Although not usually tested, there is an exaggerated release of LH after GnRH stimulation
Hyperinsulinaemia. Tested by observing a raised fasting insulin level	30% of patients who have fewer than 6 menstrual periods per annum & chronic anovulatory cycles have insulin resistance with impaired glucose tolerance or non-insulin dependent diabetes mellitus
Raised circulating androgen and preandrogen levels	Testosterone is usually modestly increased and sex hormone binding globulin is often low
Raised prolactin level (in some patients)	The 15-20% prevalence of hyperprolactinaemia results from the raised circulating oestrogen levels. This finding sometimes brings 'a microprolactinoma' into the differential diagnosis
Provera withdrawal bleed positive	Because PCOD is characterized by chronic anovulation in the presence of oestrogen, progesterone treatment, by acutely reducing oestrogen action at the endometrium, produces a withdrawal bleed.

Table 6.4
Treatment of polycystic ovarian disease

TREATMENT	RATIONALE	BENEFITS		
		AMENORRHOEA	HIRSUTES	INFERTILITY
WEIGHT LOSS	This will reduce peripheral aromatization, & decrease the LH/FSH ratio. It is difficult to achieve but important if other treatments are to be effective	✓	✓	✓
CYCLICAL PROGESTOGEN TREATMENT	Medroxyprogesterone acetate (Provera, 5mg/day for 5-10 days every 28 days) will restore regular menstrual cycles & prevent endometrial hyperplasia that may be associated with neoplasia	✓	✗	✗
CLOMIPHENE CITRATE	50-150mg/day for 5 days from day 2 of the cycle (or at any time if cycles have ceased) blocks oestrogen feedback & increases FSH secretion. 75% of women ovulate on this treatment; the pregnancy rate is 30-50%	✓	✗	✓
COMBINED OESTROGEN AND PROGESTOGEN PILL	All types of combined contraceptive 'pill' lower LH levels. Dianette, a combined 'pill' marketed as a contraceptive, uses the antiandrogen cyproterone as the progestogen.	✓	✓	✗
ANTIANDROGEN TREATMENT	Cyproterone acetate (50-100mg on days 5-15 of the cycle) cannot be used alone as it is not a reliable contraceptive, & would feminize a male foetus. It is therefore prescribed with ethinyloestradiol, 20-50μg on days 5-26 of the cycle.	✓	✓	✗
INJECTIONS OF FSH OR FSH & LH	This directly stimulates ovarian follicle development. It is followed by a dose of LH (hCG) to induce ovulation ± further progesterone treatment to support the corpus luteum	✗	✗	✓
SURGICAL REDUCTION OF OVARIAN STROMA	Not often resorted to, but may be more widely applicable with advances in laparoscopic diathermy	✓	✓	✓

✓, Effective; ✗, counterproductive

Diagnosis

The diagnosis of PCOD is usually made on historical and clinical grounds of chronic oligomenorrhoea and varying degrees of hirsutism. Menarche occurs in most at the normal time, but 5–10 per cent have primary amenorrhoea. Infertility and hirsutism occur in 75 per cent, amenorrhoea in 50 per cent, and obesity is present in 40 per cent of patients. Rarely, virilization can occur. The diagnosis is supported by a single measurement of circulating testosterone, FSH, LH ± sex hormone binding globulin. Other confirmatory tests, such as Provera®-induced withdrawal bleed or transvaginal ultrasound imaging of the ovaries (to show that they are polycystic), does not often change the management.

Treatment

The management of PCOD depends entirely on the patient's symptoms or aspirations. Most treatments that are useful for hirsutism, for example, are contraceptive (Table 6.4).

Other disorders of the menstrual cycle

About 50 per cent of women will seek help for dysmenorrhoea (pain associated with menstrual periods) at some point during their reproductive life. Primary dysmenorrhoea (i.e. in the presence of a structurally normal genital tract), often associated with nausea, diarrhoea, headaches, and emotional disorders, is the result of prostaglandin-induced uterine smooth muscle contractions during the second half of ovulatory cycles. It is usually relieved by preventing ovulation with the contraceptive pill. If, after a reasonable trial, the pain persists, a gynaecological opinion should be sought.

Secondary dysmenorrhoea is cyclical pain in women who have other gynaecological problems, such as endometriosis, pelvic inflammatory disease, or fibroids. Again, the problem is gynaecological rather than endocrinological.

Pre-menstrual syndrome (pre-menstrual 'tension' or 'PMT')

Almost all women experience a variety of symptoms between ovulation and menstruation, such as breast tenderness, abdominal bloating, headache, weight gain, and behavioural changes. Although there is no evidence that the hormonal milieu of women who suffer from pre-menstrual tension is any different from those who do not, there is no doubt that symptoms of pre-menstrual syndrome in some women can be physically and emotionally disabling.

Treatment

Suggesting subtle changes in life style such as an improved diet and increased exercise may be perceived as trivializing a very real problem. The initial treatment, depending on symptoms, is to try analgesics ± oil of evening primrose (Efamast® 40 mg three or four times a day). A more aggressive approach is to prevent ovulation with the contraceptive pill. In exceptional patients, a GnRH superagonist is needed to turn off cyclical gonadotrophin release, along with hormone replacement therapy. Provided the diagnosis is secure, the only certain way of helping is ovariectomy, but even then, symptoms of oestrogen withdrawal and anxiety about atherosclerosis and bone mineral integrity means that some form of hormone replacement will be required.

Abnormal uterine bleeding

In most cases abnormal uterine bleeding is the province of general practitioners, family planning clinics, and gynaecologists rather than endocrinologists. Nevertheless, there are primary endocrine causes of abnormal bleeding, such as hypothyroidism-induced menorrhagia and oligomenorrhoea in mild hyper-prolactinaemia secondary to microprolactinoma. Heavy menstrual loss (in excess of the usual 30 ml over 4–6 days) may also be attributable to structural problems such as fibroids, endometriosis, or uterine polyps, and regular but very light bleeding to thyrotoxicosis, polycystic ovarian disease, or obstructive pathological conditions such as intrauterine adhesions (synechiae) or cervical scarring. Intermenstrual bleeding or spotting between episodes of regular, ovulatory menstruation may be the result of cervical or endometrial lesions requiring gynaecological evaluation and treatment.

Bleeding associated with anovulatory cycles—dysfunctional uterine bleed-ing—is characteristic of cycles at either end of reproductive life. Menstrual loss in dysfunctional bleeding is unpredictable in timing, duration, and amount and, as ovulation does not occur, is usually painless. The most common cause is poly-cystic ovarian disease. Similar 'oestrogen breakthrough bleeding' can occur par-ticularly when unopposed oestrogens are given in the longer term without intermittent progestogen-induced bleeds.

Menopause

The menopause has come to mean the sequence of symptoms and endocrine events leading up to and extending beyond the last menstrual period, rather than, as is strictly the case, the last menstrual period itself. Gradual but progressive loss of ovarian function is often associated with somatic and psychological changes that lead up to 40 per cent of women entering the climacteric to seek medical help.

Cyclical ovarian activity ceases at an average age of 51. Unlike the menarche, the mean age of the menopause has not changed over the years and is completely independent of height, weight, and, if smoking habits are excluded, social class. Cigarette smoking is anti-oestrogenic and the symptoms of the climacteric can often be postponed for a year or two if the habit is stopped.

Symptoms and signs

The pattern of menstruation leading up to the menopause is variable. Often the interval between periods diminishes as the follicular phase of the cycles shorten, but lengthening of the cycle or intermittent bleeding is common. The fall in oestrogen gives rise to hot flushes which usually resolve spontaneously within 2–5 years of the menopause. The fall in oestrogen leads to a decrease in size of reproductive organs and breasts, atrophy of urogenital epithelium and skin, and an increasing risk of cardiovascular disease and osteoporosis. Mean FSH and LH levels gradually rise and an increasing proportion of cycles become anovulatory.

In obese women, aromatization of adrenal androgens may maintain fairly normal oestrogen levels and symptoms of the climacteric may be minimal.

Treatment with sex hormone replacement therapy (SHRT)

The major short-term indication for prescribing SHRT is to alleviate the symptoms of hot flushes and dyspareunia (painful intercourse) as described above. Longer-term benefits include a reduced risk of osteoporosis (amounting to a 50 per cent reduction in subsequent lifetime risk of osteoporotic fracture after 5 years' treatment, even though bone mineral loss resumes after oestrogen with-

Table 6.5
Female sex hormone replacement regimens

Cyclical regimens

Many sex hormone replacement regimens simulate the normal menstrual cycle with combinations of oral or transdermal oestrogen together with a monthly course of progestogen

For women who find continuation of the monthly cycle troublesome, regimens in which a course of progestogen is given only once every 3 months are also available

Continuous regimens

In women who have had a hysterectomy, treatment with progestogens is not required. Continuous oestrogen such as daily oral conjugated oestrogens (0.625 μg), or oestradiol implants or patches are usually used

For women who retain a uterus, newer 'non-bleed' preparations in which oestrogens (oestradiol or conjugated oestrogen) and progestogens (norethisterone or medroxyprogesterone acetate) are given on a daily basis without interruption have recently become available for use from 12 months or more after the last menstrual period

drawal) and a 50 per cent reduction in the incidence of cardiovascular disease. The small increased risk of breast cancer is still being examined.

Key points

- The most common cause of secondary amenorrhoea (amenorrhoea after the establishment of regular cyclical menstruation) is pregnancy, and the second most common, the menopause.
- Raised gonadotrophins (FSH and LH) with a low oestrogen suggests ovarian failure.
- Low gonadotrophins and low oestrogen indicates secondary hypogonadism.
- A single, normal serum prolactin is sufficient to exclude the presence of hyperprolactinaemia.
- Amenorrhoea in the presence of oestrogen and raised testosterone is usually caused by PCOD.

'My patient has pre-menstrual tension. None of my treatments has worked for her'

History

The life of an otherwise fit 36-year-old woman had become increasingly disrupted by mood swings coinciding with the latter part of each menstrual cycle. She described uncontrollable aggressive outbursts, very much against her nature, and had even found herself close to accosting another passenger on the top deck of a bus, completely without provocation. Her symptoms had not been improved by treatment with the combined or the progesterone-only contraceptive pill.

Examination

Normal

Investigations

None

Management

By the time the patient sees an endocrinologist, reassurance, explanation, and evening primrose oil may not be enough. Typically, the combined contraceptive pill is stopped if the patient is on it, or started, if she is not, or a progesterone-only pill or injection substituted. Antidepressants are usually ineffective as are vitamin B_6 supplements, tranquillizers, and aspirin-like drugs. If mood disturbance is severe and clearly related to pre-menstrual syndrome (PMS), a suitable first-line treatment would be continuous ethinyloestradiol with a short course of progesterone to induce a withdrawal bleed (without stopping the oestrogen) every 3 months. If this is ineffective, menstrual periods can be stopped completely with a long-acting GnRH analogue (although this is not a licensed use for these drugs), sometimes with cyclical oestrogen and progesterone added back. If all else fails and the symptoms are incapacitating, hysterectomy has been found to improve some of the symptoms of PMS in about half of the women who are forced to resort to it.

Explanation

Despite intensive research since the term 'pre-menstrual' syndrome was coined in 1931, there remains no overall agreement about the definition, cause, or treatment of the pre-menstrual syndrome. Although almost all doctors believe that PMS exists, careful studies have found no relationship between mood fluctuation and menstrual cycle phase, and 'task performance' or ability to process information does not change during the menstrual cycle. Nevertheless, many women from diverse cultural backgrounds claim to suffer from PMS, and cyclical mood changes have been reported even in women who are generally unaware of PMS. It also seems likely that the feeling of well-being experienced by some pregnant women and post-natal mood swings, are at least to some extent related to hormonal changes. Typical symptoms consist of abdominal bloating and swelling, breast tenderness, changes in appetite, memory changes, altered sex drive, aggression, mood swings and headaches.

Multiple-choice questions

1. Amenorrhoea can be caused by the following:
   a. Moving house;
   b. Kallmann's syndrome (hypothalamic hypogonadotrophic hypogonadism);
   c. Excessive exercise;

    d. Being fashionably slim;

    e. Turner's syndrome.

2. The following laboratory and dynamic tests suggest ovarian failure:

    a. Raised FSH and LH;

    b. Raised circulating GnRH;

    c. Raised progesterone;

    d. Oestrogen levels within normal limits;

    e. A withdrawal bleed after a Provera (progesterone) challenge.

3. The following drugs can produce amenorrhoea:

    a. Phenothiazines;

    b. Ethinyloestradiol;

    c. Goserelin (a GnRH superagonist);

    d. Continuous use of the progesterone-only pill;

    e. Combined, cyclical oestrogen and progestogen contraceptive pill.

4. The following conditions are associated with oligomenorrhoea:

    a. Polycystic ovarian disease;

    b. Thyrotoxicosis;

    c. Hyperprolactinaemia;

    d. Androgen-secreting ovarian neoplasms;

    e. Anorexia nervosa.

5. Polycystic ovarian disease:

    a. Is typically associated with fewer than six menstrual periods per year;

    b. Is characterized by hypoandrogenization;

    c. Is an oestrogen-deficient state;

    d. May be partly or completely reversed by weight gain;

    e. Tends to be associated with a high LH/FSH ratio.

6. The pre-menstrual syndrome (pre-menstrual tension):

    a. Produces characteristic changes in hormone levels and fluid balance;

    b. Is recognized in all societies;

    c. Can be ameliorated by blocking ovulation with the contraceptive pill;

    d. May be bad enough to warrant oophorectomy;

    e. Can cause aggressive outbursts, headaches, and pyrexia.

Answers

1. Amenorrhoea can be caused by the following:

    a. Moving house   T
       Stress, of which this is one, can certainly cause menstrual disturbances.

    b. Kallmann's syndrome (hypothalamic hypogonadotrophic hypo-
       gonadism)   T
       In early fetal life the GnRH neurones (of which there are only about 1000)
       lie at the front of the brain, near the olfactory placode. They migrate back

from there towards the anterior pole of the hypothalamus, following a trail of neural cell adhesion molecules (NCAMs). This 'chemical trail' is absent in Kallmann's syndrome, hence the association of absent GnRH and anosmia in 85 per cent of those with this syndrome. The male to female ratio is 5:1.

c. Excessive exercise   T
Another mechanism to limit fertility at times of stress.

d. Being 'fashionably' slim   T
This is not a flippant or frivolous question. The 'social ideal' is near the level (10 per cent under ideal body weight) at which amenorrhoea occurs. Low oestrogen levels will affect bone mineral accretion and predispose to osteoporosis in later life.

e. Turner's syndrome   T
Turner's syndrome is a form of gonadal dysgenesis marked by short stature, sexual infantilism, streak gonads, and phenotypic changes such as a 'shield chest' and neck webbing. Partial X-chromosome deletions may occur. Preservation of Xq26–28 is required for normal ovarian function, and women who have only a short arm deletion may be fertile.

2. The following laboratory and dynamic tests suggest ovarian failure:
   a. Raised FSH and LH   T
   This is exactly what happens in the menopause.

   b. Raised circulating GnRH   F
   GnRH would probably be raised but it is undetectable peripherally, and it is not possible to sample hypothalamo-hypophyseal portal blood in humans.

   c. Raised progesterone   F
   In ovarian failure there is no follicular development, and therefore no corpora lutea—the main source of progesterone.

   d. Oestrogen levels within normal limits   F
   Granulosa cells surrounding ovarian follicles make oestrogen by aromatizing androgens. In ovarian failure, there are no developing follicles, and oestrogen levels tend to be very low.

   e. A withdrawal bleed after a Provera (progesterone) challenge   F
   Provera® rapidly down-regulates oestrogen receptors in the endometrium. If the endometrium has been exposed to oestrogens and is in a proliferated state, a withdrawal bleed results. Thus a withdrawal bleed distinguishes polycystic ovarian disease from hypogonadotrophic hypogonadism, as the former is characterized by amenorrhoea in the *presence* of oestrogen.

3. The following drugs can produce amenorrhoea:
   a. Phenothiazines   T
   Phenothiazines, metoclopramide, domperidone, and other drugs with dopamine antagonist properties can all increase serum prolactin and cause amenorrhoea. For the same reason, domperidone and metoclopramide are

inappropriate agents with which to treat bromocriptine-induced nausea (although they have been tried).

b. Ethinyloestradiol T

Eventually, breakthough bleeding may occur, but continual use of oestrogen keeps the endometrium in a chronically proliferated state.

c. Goserelin (a GnRH superagonist) T

After initial pituitary stimulation, these drugs down-regulate gonadotroph response to the superagonist as well as endogenous FSH and LH, and produce hypogonadotrophic hypogonadism, as long as they are taken.

d. Continuous use of the progesterone-only pill T

Often, intermenstrual 'spotting' occurs, but the patient may become amenorrhoeic.

e. Combined, cyclical oestrogen and progestogen contraceptive pill F

Post-pill amenorrhoea has not been substantiated as a genuine phenomenon on careful statistical analysis.

4. The following conditions are associated with oligomenorrhoea:

a. Polycystic ovarian disease T

Polycystic ovarian disease occurs in about 10 per cent of pre-menopausal women. Although the primary underlying mechanism is still unknown, it may well be a dominantly inherited trait associated with insulin resistance, with premature baldness as part of the male phenotype.

b. Thyrotoxicosis T

c. Hyperprolactinaemia T

d. Androgen-secreting ovarian neoplasms T

e. Anorexia nervosa T

5. Polycystic ovarian disease:

a. Is typically associated with fewer than six menstrual periods per year T

It is also one of the most common causes of subfertility and hirsutism. Ovarian ultrasound is not often required to make the diagnosis of polycystic ovarian disease. When used, the characteristic appearance of enlarged ovaries with prominent, echogenic stroma and more than 15 follicles, 2–10 mm in diameter, ranged around the edge of the organ is best seen transvaginally rather than transabdominally.

b. Is characterized by hypoandrogenization F

Androgen levels are typically raised and/or sex hormone binding globulin levels depressed. Insulin resistance is also often associated with polycystic ovarian disease, and by reducing IGFBP-1 (insulin-like growth factor binding protein-1) and increasing the bioavailability of IGF-I, hyperinsulinaemia may be implicated in the pathogenesis of this condition. It is thought that raised

IGF-I acts at the ovary and pituitary to exacerbate hyperandrogenism.

    c. Is an oestrogen-deficient state   F
        It is characterized by anovulation in the presence of oestrogens, hence the withdrawal bleed if a short course of progesterone is given (as medroxy-progesterone acetate (Provera®) 5 mg daily for 5 days).

    d. May be partly or completely reversed by weight gain   F
        Adipose tissue is thought to be instrumental in the perpetuation of PCOD. Adrenal and ovarian androgens are aromatized by peripheral adipose tissue to oestrone. High oestrone levels feed back at the pituitary, reduce FSH and result in arrest of follicle development. At the same time LH levels are enhanced, increasing androgen production by ovarian stroma and theca cells. Hence weight loss can ameliorate the condition and, for the majority of women, a 10–15 per cent reduction in body weight will result in return of menstrual periods. Unfortunately, perhaps because of hyperinsulinaemia, weight loss seems to be extremely difficult for the patients to accomplish.

    e. Tends to be associated with a high LH/FSH ratio   T
        It is (see the answer above), but LH levels are very variable, and many endocrinologists make a clinical diagnosis and check the FSH only (to exclude ovarian failure by ensuring that it is not high).

6. The pre-menstrual syndrome (pre-menstrual tension):

    a. Produces characteristic changes in hormone levels and fluid balance   F
        There are no consistent differences in hormone milieu from normal.

    b. Is recognized in all societies   F
        There are societies where the condition is not described, and symptoms related to menstruation cannot be elicited. This does not mean that the condition is not real.

    c. Can be ameliorated by blocking ovulation with the contraceptive pill   T
        Unfortunately a useful response to this is far from universal, and this treatment has often been tried before the patients are referred for a further opinion.

    d. May be bad enough to warrant oophorectomy   T
        The distress that premenstrual syndrome causes to some women can be gauged by the fact that the side-effects and risks of oestrogen withdrawal are less problematical to them.

    e. Can cause aggressive outbursts, headaches, and pyrexia   F
        Pyrexia is not associated with the condition. Uncontrolled aggression certainly is, and can be very troublesome for the patients and for their partners.

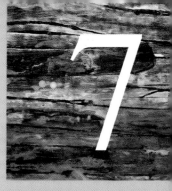

7

Fertility

- Summary

- Introduction

- Semen analysis

- Oligomenorrhoea and amenorrhoea

- Ovulation induction

- Key points

- Case history

- Multiple-choice questions

Summary

Normal function

- Sexual reproduction, the advantage of which is to allow a woman to produce offspring with fewer mutations than either parent.
- Fertility is assumed as a birthright, and its absence, affecting as many as 1 couple in 7, can be devastating.

Typical pathology

- Female
  - → Polycystic ovarian disease.
  - → 'Poor hypothalamic cycling mechanism' (usually caused by being underweight for height, or by severe mental or physical stress).
  - → Hyperprolactinaemia (usually microprolactinoma).
- Male
  - → Oligospermia.
  - → Hyperprolactinaemia (usually macroprolactinoma) causes erectile dysfunction rather than infertility, although oligospermia can occur.

'Typical clinical scenario'

- An anxious and disconsolate woman in her mid-30s who has failed to conceive after months or sometimes years of unprotected intercourse. Less often, the male partner also attends.
- A 26-year-old woman with mild polycystic ovarian disease who is concerned about hirsutes in the short term, but is also worried that her future fertility may be impaired.

Introduction

For the 10–15 per cent of couples affected, infertility can produce enormous emotional turmoil. Bereavement reactions, depression, feelings of hopelessness and victimization are compounded by the daily trauma of seeing parents leading flotillas of children around the streets and supermarkets.

Remarkable advances in the therapeutics of infertility, including ovulation induction with gonadotrophin injections, *in vitro* fertilization, ovum donation, and the availability of donor sperm banks for artificial insemination, have transformed the prospects for infertile couples and offered hope when none previously existed. Consultations, at least for the affluent, can now be upbeat.

The remit of the endocrinologist is to ensure, first, that suitable numbers of phenotypically normal spermatozoa are being deposited in the right place at an appropriate frequency and, secondly, to confirm that ovulation is occurring (i.e. by identifying raised progesterone levels in the middle of the luteal part of the cycle: see p. 110). Discrete enquiries about the frequency of intercourse are appropriate at the outset. The patient may not make it clear, for example, that the reason for the partner's failure to attend clinic is that he is working abroad.

The average pregnancy rate in couples not using any form of contraception is about 85 per cent per annum. Although there are no universally applicable figures, about 1 couple in 10 has problems conceiving successfully.

Semen analysis

As 'male factors' are responsible for 40 per cent of cases of infertility and semen analysis is such a simple, painless, and inexpensive investigation, this should be one of the first investigations to be carried out. This is particularly true if the female is having regular, spontaneous menstrual cycles, as these are likely to be ovulatory. Semen samples produced by masturbation (rather than coitus interruptus) should be collected into a clean container and examined microscopically once the clot has liquefied—between 30 and 60 min after ejaculation. The volume of ejaculate and the morphology, motility, and number of spermatozoa are readily quantified. However, the *quality* of the sperm, i.e. its ability to fertilize an

Table 7.1
Sperm transport, and ovum fertilization and implantation

Transport of sperm to the ovum is mediated by sperm flagellar movements, uterine contractions, and beating of the cilia in the uterus and fallopian tubes. Spermatozoa and the ovum have functional lives after ejaculation/ovulation of less than 48 and less than 24 hours respectively. The spermatozoa that fertilize the ovum usually take between 8 and 12 hours to arrive in its vicinity.

Within the female genital tract, spermatozoa rapidly undergo 'capitation' which allows an acrosome reaction and sperm/ovum membrane fusion to occur. The sperm head first adheres to the zona pellucida surrounding the ovum, penetrates it after 15–25 mins then almost immediately traverses the perivitelline space and membrane to form the male pronucleus. Access of other sperm to the perivitelline membrane is blocked by release of granules containing hydrolytic enzymes into the perivitelline space

At this stage the ovum undergoes the final stage of meiosis and extrudes a haploid set of chromosomes. The male and female pronuclei each containing a haploid set of chromosomes replicate, a mitotic spindle forms and the first division of the fertilized ovum occurs about 28 h after fertilization. The fertilized egg enters the uterine cavity as a 16-cell morula and implants at the blastocyst stage, 7 days after ovulation

ovum, cannot be assessed indirectly with accuracy. Semen analysis on more than one occasion produces more accurate results.

Oligomenorrhoea and amenorrhoea

The cause of amenorrhoea or oligomenorrhoea should be established in the normal way. If the patient has a microprolactinoma, the introduction of bromocriptine will often restore menstruation, ovulation, and fertility. If polycystic ovarian disease is present, it may be possible to induce ovulation with clomiphene citrate, 100 mg daily (or more in obese patients) for 5 days from the second day of progestogen-induced uterine bleeding. Clomiphene is best regarded as an anti-oestrogen that occupies oestrogen receptors in the hypothalamus and reduces feedback inhibition. It induces ovulation in 75 per cent of women, and pregnancy occurs in 30–50 per cent. Chorionic gonadotrophin (hCG, 1000–3000 U intramuscularly—the equivalent of LH) at mid cycle, can be used to stimulate ovulation if clomiphene alone is unsuccessful. If an LH level within the first week of the cycle exceeds 10 U/l, the incidence of early fetal loss after clomiphene-induced ovulation tends to be high and patients are best referred to specialist units for ovulation induction at the outset. If ovulation is occurring (i.e. the progesterone is elevated on days 19–21 of the cycle) but no pregnancy ensues after several months, structural problems should be excluded.

Ovulation induction

This is a specialist procedure that should only be carried out in dedicated endocrine or gynaecology clinics. Various protocols are used. Typically, intramuscular injections of gonadotrophins are given in daily doses governed by changes in the number and size of developing follicles and the thickness of the endometrium, determined by weekly pelvic ultrasound examinations. An injection of 5000–10 000 U hCG is then given (12–24 h after the last injection of FSH/LH) to bring about ovulation. Further hCG and/or progestogens (as pessaries, 200 mg daily) may be given to support the early pregnancy if luteinization is thought to be inadequate. In women with high LH/FSH ratios, it is becoming more common to use GnRH superagonists to turn off endogenous gonadotrophin production completely at the outset, before inducing follicular maturation. With this treatment, ovulation occurs in 90 per cent of hypogonadotrophic women and pregnancy rates exceed 50 per cent. There is a 20 per cent chance of multiple pregnancy. Ovulation induction using a GnRH pump to deliver 5–25 μg GnRH every 90–120 min subcutaneously for 10–20 days each cycle is now used less often.

Ovarian hyperstimulation syndrome is an unusual but potentially fatal complication of gonadotrophin-induced ovulation induction. It can result in the development of ascites, pleural and pericardial effusions, and lead to intractable vascular collapse.

Key points

- Male factors are responsible for 40 per cent of infertility.
- Clomiphene induces ovulation in up to 75 per cent of women with PCOD.
- Ovarian hyperstimulation syndrome is an unusual but potentially fatal complication of ovulation induction.

'My patient has been trying for a baby for 18 months without success. Please advise'

History

A 29-year-old woman in a stable relationship since the age of 22, had pursued a successful career in publishing. Two years previously the couple had decided to start a family, and after 7 years of continuous use, she duly stopped taking the contraceptive pill (containing 20 μg oestradiol and desogestrel 150 μg). Menstrual cycles did not return for 5 months, and then occurred every 5 to 6 weeks only.

Her menarche was at the age of 11 and as far as the patient could recall, menstrual cycles had been fairly regular before she started taking 'the pill'. She denied any excessive hair growth or dyspareunia.

Examination

Unremarkable.

Investigations

Her FSH and LH were 3.2 and 7 U/l (normal range 1–9 and 3–8 U/l, respectively). Sex hormone binding globulin was 30 nmol/l (normal range 40–135 nmol/l in females), prolactin was 750 mU/l (normal range < 800 mU/l), and testosterone 2.2 nmol/l (normal range 0.3–2.5 nmol/l in females).

Management

Two weeks after the first appointment she returned to clinic (alone) and was reassured to learn that no untreatable cause of subfertility had been unearthed. Her partner was unable to attend clinic owing to various business engagements. She was asked to have a further blood sample 19 days after the first day of the next menstrual cycle for progesterone estimation. The result, 5 nmol/l (normal range > 30 nmol/l during the luteal part of the cycle), confirming that a corpus luteum—and hence an ovulatory cycle—were absent. Although the diagnosis of mild polycystic ovarian disease was suspected, the importance of assessing her partner was stressed. When a sample of his semen was eventually obtained, analysis showed oligospermia and an increased proportion of abnormal forms. She was given a course of clomiphene citrate (100 mg daily for 5 days from day 2 of each cycle) and he was asked to moderate his (fairly heavy) alcohol intake. On the third cycle of clomiphene treatment, she conceived.

Explanation

As all of us as individuals are infertile, the importance of seeing an infertile couple together is obvious, not least because problems may exist with both parties. The period of amenorrhoea after the contraceptive pill was stopped, the history of reduced frequency of menstrual periods, and the slightly elevated LH/FSH ratio all suggest polycystic ovarian disease. The business life of the patient's partner led him to drink alcohol excessively and to take cannabis and other recreational drugs on occasion, all of which can adversely affect spermatogenesis. He also spent considerable periods away from home, further reducing chances of conception. 'Post-pill amenorrhoea', although widely adduced as a distinct diagnosis rather than a historical observation, probably has no statistical or physiological basis.

Multiple-choice questions

1. Causes of infertility include the following:
   a. Hyperprolactinaemia;
   b. Testosterone treatment in men;
   c. Oestrogen treatment in women;
   d. Long-acting GnRH agonists;
   e. Bilateral adrenalectomy.

2. Treatments to enhance fertility include:
   a. Cyproterone acetate;
   b. Bromocriptine;
   c. Clomiphene citrate;
   d. Continuous infusions of GnRH;
   e. Weight loss in women with polycystic ovarian disease.

3. Techniques to induce or enhance fertility include:
   a. Artificial insemination with porcine semen;
   b. Cryopreservation of unfertilized ova produced by superovulation in women about to undergo chemotherapy or radiotherapy;

    c. Injection of a single spermatozoon into an ovum *in vitro*;

    d. *In vitro* fertilization;

    e. Sperm concentration before artificial insemination.

4. Fertility can be enhanced by:

    a. Stopping smoking;

    b. Stopping drinking alcohol;

    c. Using a padded jockstrap to protect the testes;

    d. Stopping treatment with cimetidine;

    e. Only having sexual intercourse mid cycle.

Answers

1. Causes of infertility include the following:

    a. Hyperprolactinaemia   T

    This depresses gonadotrophin secretion and ovarian oestrogen production, and reduces the chances of fertility during breast feeding.

    b. Testosterone treatment in men   T

    This reduces gonadotrophin secretion, and restores libido and potency in hypogonadal patients, but reduces fertility. However, treatment with testosterone has not proved to be a reliable enough contraceptive to be used specifically for this purpose.

    c. Oestrogen treatment in women   T

    This is, of course, a major component of the contraceptive pill.

    d. Long-acting GnRH agonists   T

    After initial stimulation of gonadotrophin production, FSH and LH are rapidly 'turned off', leading to hypogonadotrophic hypogonadism. This treatment is used for exactly this purpose in premature puberty—not to reduce fertility, but to arrest progression through puberty.

    e. Bilateral adrenalectomy   F

    This has no effect on fertility, provided glucocorticoid replacement is given as per usual.

2. Treatments to enhance fertility include:

    a. Cyproterone acetate   F

    An anti-androgen used in polycystic ovarian disease. The drug is teratogenic and is used with oestrogens, principally to treat hirsutism and androgenization.

    b. Bromocriptine   T

    In hyperprolactinaemic patients, this is very effective. Bromocriptine or another dopamine agonist is first-line treatment for prolactinomas.

    c. Clomiphene citrate   T

    This appears to act principally by reducing oestrogen feedback at the level of the pituitary, so that FSH (and LH) secretion is enhanced. Treatment usually consists of a course of 100–150 mg clomiphene daily for 5 days from day 2 of each cycle.

    d. Continuous infusions of GnRH   F

        A continuous infusion of GnRH acts very much like a long acting 'super-agonist' and turns off gonadotrophin production. In fertility treatment, a GnRH pump must be used to deliver pulses of the peptide every 90–120 min. This treatment has been largely superseded by gonado-trophin injections, particularly as high multiple conception—one of the principal side-effects—is now treatable.

    e. Weight loss in women with polycystic ovarian disease   T

        Peripheral fat converts androgens to oestrogens. High oestrogen levels (oestrone) inhibit pituitary FSH release and have the opposite effect to clomiphene citrate, i.e. follicular development is arrested.

3. Techniques to induce or enhance fertility include:

    a. Artificial insemination with porcine semen   F

        The definition of a species is that fertility is maintained only within it. Sperm can now be effectively cryopreserved, selected to produce a suitable phenotype, and tested to ensure that it is infection-free.

    b. Cryopreservation of unfertilized ova produced by superovulation in women about to undergo chemotherapy or radiotherapy   F

        At present, unfertilized ova cannot be cryopreserved.

    c. Injection of a single spermatozoon into an ovum *in vitro*   T

        This has been performed but is currently only a research procedure.

    d. *In vitro* fertilization   T

        This is the classical protocol that was reduced to the 'test tube baby technique' by the tabloid press.

    e. Sperm concentration before artificial insemination   T

4. Fertility can be enhanced by:

    a. Stopping smoking   T

        Smoking has anti-oestrogenic effects as well as other poorly defined adverse effects on fertility.

    b. Stopping drinking alcohol   T

        This mechanism is unknown.

    c. Using a padded jockstrap to protect the testes   F

        Anything that might increase the ambient temperature of the testes will, if anything, reduce fertility.

    d. Stopping treatment with cimetidine   T

        This has mild anti-androgenic actions.

    e. Only having sexual intercourse mid cycle   F

        The presence of viable spermatozoa in the female genital tract throughout the cycle enhances fertility.

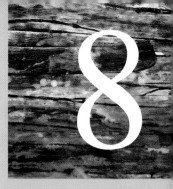

8

Pregnancy

- Summary

- Introduction

- Hormonal changes

- The thyroid in pregnancy

- Diabetes in pregnancy

- Adrenal problems in pregnancy

- Pituitary

- Key points

- Case history

- Multiple-choice questions

Summary

Normal function

- To nurture the fertilized ovum from implantation until delivery of the fetus at term.
- To prepare the breasts for lactation.
- To make appropriate modifications to the mother's psychological state and neuroendocrine responses to stress.

Typical pathology

- Gestational diabetes affects 5 per cent of pregnancies. Between 25 and 50 per cent of women with gestational diabetes develop full-blown diabetes within the subsequent 15 years.
- Postpartum thyroiditis, which affects up to 5 per cent of women during the year after delivery (see p. 65). Abnormal thyroid function is part of the differential diagnosis of postpartum depression.

'Typical clinical scenario'

- A 23-year-old and her partner with their 3-month-old baby. Until her GP checked her thyroid function tests, the couple thought that the mother's fatigue, insomnia, agitation, palpitations, and weight loss were related to the stress of looking after their new baby.

Introduction

Pregnancy is the most common cause of secondary amenorrhoea. Although now remarkably safe, labour and delivery remain one of most dangerous times in a woman's and her baby's life. The management of pregnancy and the problems associated with it are largely the province of the obstetrician. Nevertheless, a number of endocrine problems such as diabetes mellitus and thyroid disease can appear during pregnancy, or be adversely effected by pregnancy or by the rebound in immune competence that follows it.

It is also important to remember that the successful treatment of endocrine problems that have been maintaining *infertility*, such as hyperprolactinaemia in a patient with a prolactinoma, often abruptly restores fertility.

Hormonal changes

Placental progesterone and oestrogen output exceeds that of the maternal ovaries by more than tenfold, and 100-fold, respectively. Both of these hormones, and prolactin from the anterior pituitary, increase throughout pregnancy and peak at term.

Table 8.1
Placental development, hormone production, and permeability

Development

Seven days after fertilization the blastocyst consists of an inner cell which becomes the embryo and a surrounding layer of trophoblast cells that develop into the placenta. The outer layer of trophoblast becomes the syncytiotrophoblast, a continuous layer of multinucleate cytoplasm that progressively grows and thickens throughout pregnancy. The fetal capillaries are separated from the lakes of maternal blood by the endothelial cells of the fetal capillary wall, a layer of connective tissue that surrounds them, and by an outer layer of syncytiotrophoblast. To increase the surface area for gas and nutrient transfer, the fetal capillaries are arranged as (chorionic) villi. The placenta is a fetal organ: i.e. a male fetus has a genetically male placenta. Thus biopsy of the chorionic villi under ultrasound control, allows the integrity of the fetal genome to be examined at a very early stage of development

Hormone production

In addition to providing a barrier between fetal and maternal blood, the syncytiotrophoblast produces large amounts of steroid and polypeptide hormones

Using the preandrogens DHEA and androstenedione derived from fetal and maternal adrenals as substrate, the placenta produces oestrogens, most of which are secreted into the maternal circulation. For the first trimester, the corpus luteum is the major source of maternal progesterone production. After that time placental progesterone synthesis, using LDL cholesterol as a substrate, predominates. The high levels of progesterone maintain uterine quiescence until term

The placenta also produces a number of hormones that are similar in structure and function to those produced by the hypothalamus and pituitary. hCG (human chorionic gonadotrophin), for example, mimics the action of LH and is thought to maintain the corpus luteum in the early part of pregnancy

Permeability

The placenta is permeable to lipid soluble molecules, particularly small ones, but is impermeable to most peptide hormones such as insulin, GH, and parathyroid hormone. Some maternal immunoglobulins (such as those associated with Graves' disease) can cross the placenta, but glucocorticoids, thyroid hormones, and catecholamines are extensively metabolized as they pass through, with most cortisol and thyroxine being converted to inactive cortisone or reverse T_3, respectively

Chorionic gonadotrophin (hCG), the placental equivalent of LH, is maximal at around the tenth week after ovulation and declines thereafter. A raised level of hCG in the urine can be used to diagnose pregnancy as soon as 8 days after ovulation.

Human placental lactogen (human chorionic somatomammotrophin) has weak growth-promoting and lactogenic properties and is also anti-insulin. It is produced in prodigious amounts reaching up to 1 g/day—and may contribute to gestational diabetes.

The thyroid in pregnancy

Physiology

In pregnancy the thyroid gland enlarges and becomes more vascular, so that an overlying bruit is often heard. Total thyroxine may increase up to double normal, mainly as a result of the oestrogen-induced increase in binding proteins. However, in early pregnancy free thyroid hormones also increase despite a mild fall in TSH, possible due to the TSH-like action of hCG. Free thyroid hormones return to normal by about the twentieth week, matching the decline in hCG, and remain so until delivery.

Pathology

Hypothyroid patients taking thyroxine do not usually need to adjust their dose during pregnancy. Thyrotoxic patients should be carefully controlled, erring, if anything, towards undertreatment, as both carbimazole and propylthiouracil cross the placenta. Both drugs are also found at low levels in breast milk. Radioiodine is absolutely contraindicated during pregnancy but, if given at other times, has no effect on subsequent fertility.

During the year following delivery, up to 5 per cent of women experience 'postpartum thyroiditis'. The condition may present as thyrotoxicosis, hypothyroidism, or with a biphasic pattern, usually hyperthyroidism followed by hypothyroidism. Most women spontaneously return to euthyroidism.

Diabetes in pregnancy

The incidence of gestational diabetes is 5 per cent, and the infant mortality if the condition remains untreated is 7 per cent. All women are screened for glycosuria at their first visit to the antenatal visit, and more formally for gestational diabetes at 24–26 weeks' gestation using the same criteria applied to non-pregnant patients (see p. 257). During early pregnancy, insulin sensitivity is often slightly enhanced by circulating oestrogen and progesterone. Insulin resistance in later pregnancy may be related to the high levels of human placental lactogen.

The neonatal mortality of babies born to diabetic mothers is higher than normal, as is the incidence of congenital malformations. Optimal treatment means maintaining blood glucose between 4 and 7 mmol/l at all times with a glycosylated haemoglobin level (HbA 1c) of less than 6.5 per cent. Good blood glucose control early on in pregnancy halves the incidence of major malformations such as congenital heart disease. There is therefore an unequivocal place for pre-conception counselling and treatment in established diabetics. After delivery, 50 per cent or more of mothers revert to normal, but gestational diabetes may recur during subsequent pregnancies.

Adrenal problems in pregnancy

Pre-existing Addison's disease

The production of binding proteins for cortisol and hence circulating cortisol levels are increased in pregnancy. In patients with treated Addison's disease, however, glucocorticoid requirements are usually unchanged. Occasionally, the requirement for glucocorticoids increases slightly in the third trimester, and uncomplicated labour itself should be covered with 25 mg of intravenous hydrocortisone every 6 h. If labour is prolonged or difficult, the dose should be increased to 100 mg every 6 h, returning to normal levels within 3 days of delivery.

Pre-existing treatment with anti-androgens (for hirsutism)

Women of childbearing age should not be treated with an anti-androgen such as cyproterone acetate without concurrent use of a contraceptive dose of oestrogen. In the unlikely event of pregnancy in a woman being treated with an anti-androgen, virilization of a female fetus may occur and the pregnancy should be terminated.

Congenital adrenal hyperplasia in a previous child

As many forms of congenital adrenal hyperplasia are familial, if congenital adrenal hyperplasia has been diagnosed in a previous child, the mother should be given 20 μg/kg pre-pregnancy weight of dexamethasone daily in divided doses from the beginning of pregnancy. Dexamethasone will cross the placenta and prevent excessive ACTH-induced fetal adrenal androgen production from virilizing an affected female fetus. Once chorionic villus sampling or amniocentesis is carried out and the sex of the baby is known, treatment of male fetuses and unaffected females can be stopped.

Pituitary problems in pregnancy

Pituitary adenomas

As normal pituitary function is required for fertility, the presentation of new pituitary problems during pregnancy is very unusual. Bromocriptine treatment of pre-existing macroprolactinomas is usually stopped when pregnancy is diagnosed, exposing the patient to a small but real risk that the tumour will increase in size symptomatically during pregnancy. Close follow-up is instituted and, in the unlikely event that headaches or visual field changes occur, dopamine agonist treatment can be re-instituted to good effect. Bromocriptine is not teratogenic.

Pituitary failure

Sheehan's syndrome

The pituitary doubles in size during normal pregnancy, largely owing to oestrogen-induced hyperplasia and hypertrophy of lactotrophs. Under these circumstances a sudden drop in blood pressure (classically caused by a postpartum haemorrhage) can result in pituitary infarction. The resulting panhypopituitarism leads to failure of lactation, failure of return of menstruation, and to the development of hypothyroidism and hypoadrenalcorticalism, which may take some time to become clinically apparent.

Lymphocytic hypophysitis

This is a rare condition, confined to women, in which infiltration of the pituitary with lymphocytes can present with a pituitary mass, or pituitary failure. It mostly occurs during pregnancy or in the postpartum period. There is no specific treatment except for hormone replacement and, if visual fields are affected, transphenoidal surgery.

Key points

- Treatment of gestational diabetes halves the incidence of major congenital malformations.
- Postpartum thyroiditis is a common and often self-limiting cause of abnormal thyroid function in the year after delivery.
- Pregnancy does not usually affect the doses of thyroxine and hydrocortisone used for replacement therapy.

'My patient has felt increasingly run down since delivery of her baby. Please advise'

History

A 24-year-old female had felt increasingly tired and listless since the birth of her daughter 6 months previously. She breast fed initially, but the baby was clearly failing to thrive after the first week and formula feeds were substituted on the advice of the midwife. As far as the patient was aware, the pregnancy and delivery had been entirely unremarkable. She had put her tiredness down to the rigors of looking after a new baby. Her periods had not returned postpartum.

Examination

The patient was clinically moderately hypothyroid, but was also noted to be unusually pale. Her blood pressure was 102/70 mmHg sitting and 94/70 mmHg standing, with a regular pulse of 62 bpm.

Investigations

Tests of baseline pituitary function showed a TSH of 1.2 mU/l (normal range 0.3–6 mU/l), with an FSH of 1 U/l (normal range 1–9 U/l) and LH of less than 1 U/l (normal range 3–8 U/l). Prolactin was less than 50 mU/l (normal range <800 mU/l), random cortisol was 160 nmol/l (normal range 150–700 nmol/l) and the free T_4 was 7.4 pmol/l (normal range 10–23 nmol/l). A Synacthen test showed an inadequate adrenal response with cortisol rising from 140 to 200 nmol/l (normal response ≥ 495 nmol/l).

The obstetric records were requested and reviewed. The pregnancy and first and second part of labour (i.e. dilatation of the cervix to 10 cm and delivery of the baby) had indeed been uneventful. The patient, distracted by her new baby, had been unaware that following the third part of labour (placental delivery) a fairly brisk postpartum haemorrhage had occurred, amounting to the loss of about 1.2 l of blood.

Management

The diagnosis is Sheehan's syndrome—postpartum pituitary infarction. The patient was started on hydrocortisone, increased to a full replacement dose (15–20 mg/day, usually as 10–15 mg a.m., and 5 mg in the early afternoon) over a period of 1 month. She was also given thyroxine (112.5 μg/day, i.e. 100 μg and 125 μg on alternate days) and sex hormone replacement therapy.

Explanation

The pituitary almost doubles in size during pregnancy owing to the increased numbers of cells—particularly those that produce prolactin. The blood supply to these cells is often relatively tenuous so that if sudden hypotension occurs, for example, during a postpartum haemorrhage, pituitary infarction can result. The pallor is in part the result of low levels of ACTH. The clinical picture is typified by this case, although the diagnosis may not be made for many years after the event. The patient has secondary hypothyroidism, hypoadrenocorticalism, and hypogonadism. It is particularly important to recognize the condition as isolated thyroid hormone replacement could precipitate an Addisonian crisis in a patient who is also hypoadrenocortical. It is also important, particularly if the condition has been present for months or years, to introduce glucocorticoid replacement therapy with hydrocortisone slowly, as glucocorticoid-induced mental changes can be dramatic.

Multiple-choice questions

1. In postpartum thyroiditis:
   a. Pain in the neck is characteristic;
   b. A thyroid bruit is typical;
   c. The thyroid is typically unable to release stored thyroid hormones;
   d. Treatment with radioiodine is appropriate;
   e. Carbimazole is the treatment of choice.

2. In gestational diabetes:
   a. The screening tests used to diagnose normal glucose handling are more stringent than in non-pregnant individuals;
   b. If the woman is essentially asymptomatic, the baby is unlikely to come to any harm;
   c. Patient compliance with attempts to optimize diabetic control is usually good;
   d. Treatment with insulin is often recommended;
   e. Most women go on to full-blown diabetes after the pregnancy.

3. Oxytocin:
   a. Is produced by the posterior pituitary;
   b. Increases before suckling;

    c. Produced in response to suckling can cause uterine contractions;

    d. Given intravenously, is widely used to accelerate labour;

    e. Can cause water intoxication.

4. In pregnancy:

    a. Cyproterone acetate (an anti-androgen) is contraindicated;

    b. If the fetus is at risk of congenital adrenal hyperplasia, dexamethasone can be given to reduce adrenal inflammation;

    c. Bromocriptine has been found to be teratogenic;

    d. Prolactin levels do not increase until after the placenta has been delivered (third stage of labour);

    e. Hypothyroid patients usually need to increase their dose of thyroxine replacement.

Answers

1. In postpartum thyroiditis:

    a. Pain in the neck is characteristic   F

    It can certainly be true in some other kinds of thyroiditis, but any type of thyroiditis presenting with neck pain is rare, or at least rarely recognized in clinical practice.

    b. A thyroid bruit is typical   F

    This would be more typical of Graves' disease, as a bruit is associated with increased biosynthetic activity and blood flow through the gland. In postpartum thyroiditis, iodine uptake stops and synthetic activity is low. Thyrotoxicosis results from uncontrolled release of stored hormone.

    c. The thyroid is typically unable to release stored thyroid hormones   F

    There is usually uncontrolled discharge of thyroid hormones from the gland.

    d. Treatment with radioiodine is appropriate   F

    In postpartum thyroiditis iodine uptake (and therefore radioiodine uptake) is often greatly reduced, making this form of treatment ineffective. It would be an inappropriate treatment in any case, since it is irreversible and the condition may remit spontaneously. In addition, radioisotope treatment should be avoided in those who have very close contact with young children or babies, as the secondary dose may be high at close range. In postpartum thyroiditis, the uptake of technetium is reduced or completely blocked—a feature that is useful in distinguishing the condition from Graves' disease. Radioiodine does not adversely affect fertility.

    e. Carbimazole is the treatment of choice   F

    Carbimazole does not work well, because failure of iodine uptake is characteristic of the condition. As carbimazole and propylthiouracil both work by blocking iodine uptake, they tend to be ineffective. In many cases, treatment with beta-blockers such as propranolol is sufficient until the condition abates.

2. In gestational diabetes:
   a. The screening tests used to diagnose normal glucose handling are more stringent than in non-pregnant individuals   F
   The same criteria are used.
   b. If the woman is essentially asymptomatic, the baby is unlikely to come to any harm   F
   Stillbirths, perinatal mortality, pre-eclamptic toxaemia, and perinatal morbidity are all increased if the maximum blood sugar exceeds 7 mmol/l. The benefits of prenatal counselling and vigorous, effective treatment are dramatic and unequivocal.
   c. Patient compliance with attempts to optimize diabetic control is usually good   T
   Pregnant women are a highly motivated group.
   d. Treatment with insulin is often recommended   T
   e. Most women go on to full-blown diabetes after the pregnancy   F
   Up to 50 per cent eventually go on to diabetes over the subsequent 15 years. Gestational diabetes often recurs in subsequent pregnancies.

3. Oxytocin:
   a. Is produced by the posterior pituitary   F
   It is *released* from the posterior pituitary, but *synthesized* in the supraoptic and paraventricular nuclei of the hypothalamus.
   b. Increases before suckling   T
   Hearing a baby cry or even thinking about the infant can stimulate oxytocin release, producing myofibril contraction, the sensation of 'tingling' around the alveola and nipple, and milk 'letdown' or ejection. Oxytocin rises further following nipple stimulation.
   c. Produced in response to suckling can cause uterine contractions   T
   These can be extremely painful. Often not too pronounced with the first child, these so-called 'after pains', particularly within the first week or two of subsequent deliveries, can occasionally be as severe as labour pain itself and require opiate analgesia.
   d. Given intravenously, is widely used to accelerate labour   T
   Active management of labour depends on a 'partogram'—a graph of the expected pattern of cervical dilatation and fetal descent against time during the first stage of labour. If labour slows, intravenous infusions of oxytocin are used to accelerate it. Labours lasting for days are fortunately a thing of the past, as modern obstetric management of labour can essentially guarantee delivery (one way or another) within a set time.
   e. Can cause water intoxication   T
   Oxytocin has weak vasopressin-like activity. When given in pharmacological amounts to increase uterine contractility and accelerate labour, concurrent administration of large amounts of intravenous dextrose (i.e. free water) can result in profound hyponatraemia and water intoxication,

as the diuresis that would normally occur in response to falling osmolality and reduced vasopressin release from the posterior pituitary is inhibited.

4. In pregnancy:

a. Cyproterone acetate (an anti-androgen) is contraindicated   T
   It has the potential to feminize a male fetus.

b. If the fetus is at risk of congenital adrenal hyperplasia, dexamethasone can be given to reduce adrenal inflammation   F
   Dexamethasone is given to cross the placenta and reduce fetal pituitary ACTH production, and therefore the excessive drive to adrenal cortical pre-androgen and androgen synthesis

c. Bromocriptine has been found to be teratogenic   F
   There is no evidence that bromocriptine is teratogenic. Nevertheless, it is stopped when pregnancy is confirmed. Patients with macroprolactinomas have a 16 per cent chance of the tumour enlarging significantly (i.e. symptomatically) during pregnancy, and in these patients the drug can be re-introduced.

d. Prolactin levels do not increase until after the placenta has been delivered (third stage of labour)   F
   Prolactin levels gradually rise throughout pregnancy, but milk secretion is blocked by concurrent high levels of oestrogen and progesterone.

e. Hypothyroid patients usually need to increase their dose of thyroxine replacement   F
   Occasionally, a slight increase is required, but usually the dose required to keep TSH within the normal range remains unchanged.

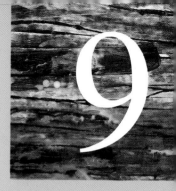

9

Contraception

- Summary
- Introduction
- Types of oral contraceptive
- Key points
- Multiple-choice questions

Summary

Normal function

- Protection from pregnancy
  - → Freedom from excessive fertility.
  - → During treatment with potential teratogens such as anti-androgens (i.e. for hirsutism).
  - → Before, and for 4–6 months after radioiodine treatment to allow thyrotoxicosis to be controlled.

Typical pathology

- Disabling side-effects with commonly used preparations.
- Contraindications to oestrogen-containing preparations such as a history of venous thrombosis or treated oestrogen-dependent tumours such as breast cancer.

'Typical clinical scenario'

- A 36-year-old smoker with migraine and a history of venous thrombosis in the left leg. Other problems related to contraception are usually seen by specialists in family planning clinics or GPs.

Introduction

Most contraceptive problems are dealt with in general practice and in family planning clinics. Few cases are referred to the endocrine clinic, not least because if different forms of oral contraceptive are found to be unsuitable, there are other forms of contraception that are almost as safe in preventing unwanted pregnancy. The overall risks of hormone contraceptive pills are much less than that of pregnancy. The combined pill provides excellent protection against pregnancy, reduces the incidence of menorrhagia, dysmenorrhoea, benign breast disease, pelvic inflammatory disease, functional ovarian cysts, and iron deficiency anaemia. The 'pill' reduces the incidence of ovarian and endometrial cancer and, of course, almost eliminates the risks and complications of pregnancy and abortion.

There is no upper age limit for use in healthy non-smokers, and the combined pill can be used even in patients with varicose veins or fibroids without interruption, from soon after the menarche until the end of reproductive life. Nevertheless, there is some (albeit inconsistent) evidence, that a slight increase in the risk of carcinoma of the breast exists in those taking it from a young age, and a possible increased risk of carcinoma of the cervix. The increased risks of myocardial infarction, venous thrombosis, and embolic events are virtually restricted to those with pre-existing cardiovascular disease and those who smoke. However, recent data suggest that certain types of progestogen may be associated with an enhanced risk of venous thrombosis.

Types of oral contraceptive

As the average dose of oestrogen has been reduced, the combined oral contraceptive pill has become increasingly free of side-effects. Almost all combinations use ethinyloestradiol as the oestrogen, along with one of six different progestogens. The newer derivates 'gestodene, desogestrel, and norgestimate' having a less marked adverse effect on blood pressure, lipids, and carbohydrate metabolism than their older counterparts, 'norethisterone, levonorgestrel, and ethynodiol'. Gestodene and desogestrel, however, may have an increased propensity to cause venous thrombosis, although these data await confirmation.

Monophasic pills

Most women are started on monophasic pills, providing a fixed dose of oestrogen (usually 20–35 μg of ethinyloestradiol daily) and progestogen throughout the active cycle. After each 21-day course, 7 placebo or pill-free days allow hormone concentrations to drop, inducing withdrawal bleeding. Exogenous oestrogens suppress ovarian activity and ovulation, and the progestogen, amongst other effects, makes cervical mucus almost impenetrable to sperm.

Biphasic and triphasic pills

If breakthough bleeding occurs with monophasic preparations, biphasic or triphasic pills, which attempt to mimic natural hormonal fluctuations by varying pill contents, may be useful. The side-effects of headache, breast tenderness, and irregular uterine bleeding usually resolve by the third cycle. If not, it is worth trying a pill which uses a different progestogen.

Progesterone-only pills

For smokers over the age of 35 years or patients with diabetes mellitus, hypertension, focal migraine, a history of thromboembolic disease, or who are breast feeding, the progesterone-only pill is suitable. There are six progesterone-only preparations, all of which are taken continuously. These provide less effective protection than oestrogen-containing pills and the tablets must be taken at the same time each day. The most commonly used types in the United Kingdom contain ethynodiol diacetate, levonorgestrel or norethisterone at very low doses. Concurrent treatment with antibiotics or enzyme-inducing drugs reduces protection in progestogen-only pills as well as combined pills. Contraindications to the progestogen-only pill are pre-existing pregnancy and serious cardiovascular disease. The pill is relatively contraindicated in patients with breast cancer.

Contraceptive implants

Subdermal implants, which gradually release their progestogens through the walls of one or more silastic tubes, provide protection for up to 5 years and are associated with a lower pregnancy rate than the progesterone-only pill. Many women experience one or more unwanted effects, such as irregular menstrual bleeding, and as many as 50 per cent consider having the silastic tubes containing the progestogen removed. The use of depot progestogen preparations may also result in a significant decrease in bone mineral density.

Postcoital contraception

Postcoital contraception is accomplished by taking two tablets of Ovran 50® within 72 h of unprotected intercourse, and repeating the dose exactly 12 h later. The pregnancy rate with this regimen is 2 per cent, but as the fetus is undamaged, an abortion need not be recommended. Most women experience some nausea during this treatment.

Key points

- Excess mortality in contraceptive pill users is largely confined to smokers over the age of 35 years.
- Monophasic 'pills' maintain the same oestrogen/progesterone ratio throughout the active, 21-day cycle.
- Biphasic or triphasic pills may be useful to prevent breakthrough bleeding with monophasic pills.
- The contraceptive pill, and the oestrogen/progesterone combinations used for sex hormone replacement therapy, are different in composition, dose, and function.

Multiple-choice questions

1. The combined oestrogen/progesterone contraceptive pill (containing the progestogen, norethisterone):
   a. Increases the risk of ovarian and endometrial neoplasia;
   b. Can be used in patients with varicose veins;
   c. Significantly increases the risk of venous thrombosis in non-smokers;
   d. Could equally well be used in older women for 'HRT' (hormone replacement therapy);
   e. Is suitable for use in some women aged 40.

2. In hormonal contraception:
   a. The combined pill is one of the most reliable methods of birth control;
   b. The annual death rate directly related to combined oral contraceptive use in smokers and non-smokers up to the age of 35 is similar;
   c. The relative risk of death from pregnancy and childbirth (i.e. no contraceptive used) is greater than that directly related to combined oral contraceptive use up to the age of 35;

    d. The progesterone-only pill is suitable for patients over the age of 35 who smoke;

    e. Care must be taken to take the combined oral contraceptive pill at the same time each day.

3. The combined oestrogen/progesterone contraceptive pill:

    a. Increases the risk of thromboembolic disease;

    b. Increases the risk of stroke;

    c. Usually causes a significant increase in blood pressure;

    d. Can cause post-pill amenorrhoea;

    e. Triples the incidence of breast cancer.

4. Absolute contraindications for oral contraceptive use include:

    a. Acute liver disease;

    b. Undiagnosed vaginal bleeding;

    c. History of cervical dysplasia;

    d. History of coronary artery disease;

    e. Diabetes mellitus.

5. Long-term contraception with progestogen implants (Norplant®):

    a. Progestogens work in part by decreasing cervical mucus viscosity;

    b. Is achieved by inserting a single levonorgestrel and cholesterol pellet subcutaneously;

    c. Rarely causes significant side-effects warranting removal of the implant;

    d. Return of fertility after removal of the implants is often incomplete and delayed;

    e. Are unsuitable for older women who smoke.

Answers

1. The combined oestrogen/progesterone contraceptive pill (containing the progestogen norethisterone):

    a. Increases the risk of ovarian and endometrial neoplasia   F
       The risk of each is reduced.

    b. Can be used in patients with varicose veins   T

    c. Significantly increases the risk of venous thrombosis in non-smokers   F
       The increased risk is confined to smokers over the age of 35 years.

    d. Could equally well be used in older women for 'HRT' (hormone replacement therapy)   F
       The combination, and particularly the doses used, are very different.

    e. Is suitable for use in some women aged 40   T
       If there is no history of coronary artery disease and the subjects do not smoke, there is no contraindication.

2. In hormonal contraception:
   a. The combined pill is one of the most reliable methods of birth control   T
   The risk of unwanted pregnancy is less than 10 per cent of that experienced by people using barrier methods. The only other method of comparable efficacy is male sterilization.
   b. The annual death rate directly related to combined oral contraceptive use in smokers and non-smokers up to the age of 35 is similar   F
   The risk in smokers is increased about four-fold at all ages.
   c. The relative risk of death from pregnancy and childbirth (i.e. no contraceptive used) is greater than that directly related to combined oral contraceptive use up to the age of 35   T
   This is the reason why the combined oral contraceptive pill is not contraindicated in smokers up to that age, even though the risk is higher than in non-smokers.
   d. The progesterone-only pill is suitable for patients over the age of 35 who smoke   T
   e. Care must be taken to take the combined oral contraceptive pill at the same time each day   F
   It is the progesterone-only pill where this is a particular concern, as the effect barely exceeds 24 h.

3. The combined oestrogen/progesterone contraceptive pill:
   a. Increases the risk of thromboembolic disease   T
   The risk does not seem to change with the duration of treatment, and disappears soon after the treatment is stopped.
   b. Increases the risk of stroke   T
   The risk of subarachnoid haemorrhage is increased, but the incidence is so low in young, non-smoking women, that it is not usually a consideration.
   c. Usually causes a significant increase in blood pressure   F
   The mean increase is 5/2 mmHg only. A significant increase in blood pressure (to >140/80 mmHg) is unusual. If the patient has been stabilized effectively on oral hypotensives, the addition of the oestrogen/progesterone contraceptive pill does not significantly disturb treatment
   d. Can cause post-pill amenorrhoea   F
   The incidence of amenorrhoea after discontinuation of the contraceptive pill is now believed to be the same as in women who have not been exposed to treatment. By 3 months, 80 per cent of women are menstruating normally.
   e. Triples the incidence of breast cancer   F
   There are conflicting data in the literature about the association between the combined pill and an increased risk of breast cancer. Most are agreed, however, that there is a small increased risk.

4. Absolute contraindications for oral contraceptive use include:
   a. Acute liver disease   T
   b. Undiagnosed vaginal bleeding   T
   c. History of cervical dysplasia   F
   d. History of coronary artery disease   T
   e. Diabetes mellitus   F

5. Long-term contraception with progestogen implants (Norplant®):
   a. Progestogens work in part by decreasing cervical mucus viscosity   F
      The mode of action of the contraceptive effect of progestogens is uncertain. However, *increased* cervical mucus viscosity, reduction in the mid-cycle LH surge, suppression of endometrial proliferation, and interference with implantation are all implicated.
   b. Is achieved by inserting a single levonorgestrel and cholesterol pellet subcutaneously   F
      The active ingredient, levonorgestrel, is packed into six silastic tubes, each 34 mm long by 2.44 mm in diameter, which are inserted in a fan shape subdermally in the upper, inner part of the woman's non-dominant arm. Newer designs use two rods of similar size, filled with levonorgestrel, or a single rod made of EVA-copolymer, filled with 3-keto-desogestrel crystals. A pellet is an uncoated plug of active ingredient such as that used to deliver the long-acting GnRH agonist, goserelin.
   c. Rarely causes significant side-effects warranting removal of the implant   F
      Between 25 and 50 per cent of women do not continue with the treatment for the full 5 years because of side-effects, such as weight gain, mood changes, acne, nausea, dizziness, changes in menstrual cycles, and local discomfort.
   d. Return of fertility after removal of the implants is often incomplete and delayed   F
      Fertility returns within days, and is complete.
   e. Are unsuitable for older women who smoke   F
      They are suitable for older women, smokers, and for those with hypertension or migraine.

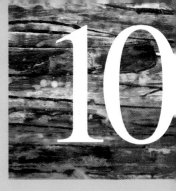

10

Hirsutism

- Summary
- Introduction
- Sources of androgens
- Response of hair follicles to androgens
- Key points
- Case history
- Multiple-choice questions

Summary

Normal function

- Appropriate distribution and arrangement of hair has no functional significance (except perhaps for the eyebrows and lashes), but enormous social and psychological importance.

Typical pathology

- Idiopathic hirsutism.
- Mild polycystic ovarian disease.

'Typical clinical scenario'

Two patients:
- The first is distraught. She is completely normal apart from a few hairs out of place on her lower abdomen between the pubis and umbilicus (the position of the male escutcheon).
- The second, also with idiopathic hirsutism, is coping very well, but has an almost full beard and marked body hair growth.

The extent of hirsutism, level of circulating androgens, and the patients' anxiety are poorly related.

Introduction

Hirsutism, the development of a characteristically male pattern of body and facial hair growth in women, is a common presenting complaint in the endocrine outpatient clinic. Although hirsutism is usually a cosmetic problem rather than a manifestation of major underlying pathology, the psychological trauma of perceived excessive hair growth should not be underestimated, even if scarcely a blade seems to be out of place.

The idealized female, a concept perpetuated by women's glossy magazines and pandered to by salons and supermarkets, has perfectly styled scalp hair and well-defined eyebrows and eyelashes. Except for pubic hair—retained as a badge of female sexuality but trimmed to be completely concealed by even the most revealing clothing—she may expect, or be expected to have, an essentially hair-free body.

Compared to these images, it is all too easy for a woman to believe that the icons of beauty she sees are natural, rather than the result of shaving, waxing, plucking, electrolysis, depilatory creams, cosmetics, and camouflage. This is particularly true for Asian women, who tend to be more hirsute than their American and North European counterparts.

Sources of androgens

There are two principal biologically active androgens: testosterone and its more active metabolite dihydrotestosterone. In women, the adrenals are responsible for most of the plasma pre-androgens, dehydroepiandrosterone (DHEA) and DHEA sulphate (DHEAS), and the ovaries produce most of the circulating testosterone (Fig. 10.1). Each contributes equally to the circulating androstenedione (AD) pool. Knowledge of the relative proportion of androgens from each different source is usually unhelpful in the management of hirsutism.

Response of hair follicles to androgens

The response of pilosebaceous units to androgens depends on the location of the follicle, the age of the individual, genetics, and other unknown factors. In the absence of androgens, scalp hair is not lost and sex hair does not appear. The effects of circulating androgens are modified by their interaction with sex hormone binding globulin (SHBG). Hair follicles have the curious potential to be either completely independent of circulating androgens (e.g. eyebrows, scalp hair at the back and sides), or to be increased or totally inhibited by them.

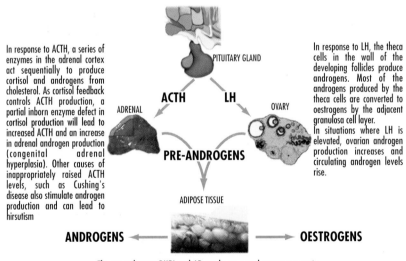

In response to ACTH, a series of enzymes in the adrenal cortex act sequentially to produce cortisol and androgens from cholesterol. As cortisol feedback controls ACTH production, a partial inborn enzyme defect in cortisol production will lead to increased ACTH and an increase in adrenal androgen production (congenital adrenal hyperplasia). Other causes of inappropriately raised ACTH levels, such as Cushing's disease also stimulate androgen production and can lead to hirsutism

PITUITARY GLAND

ACTH **LH**

ADRENAL OVARY

PRE-ANDROGENS

In response to LH, the theca cells in the wall of the developing follicles produce androgens. Most of the androgens produced by the theca cells are converted to oestrogens by the adjacent granulosa cell layer. In situations where LH is elevated, ovarian androgen production increases and circulating androgen levels rise.

ADIPOSE TISSUE

ANDROGENS ← → **OESTROGENS**

The pre-androgens DHEA and AD can be converted to testosterone in adipose tissue. The same tissue can also convert circulating androgens to oestrogens, primarily oestrone. Oestrone feedback at the pituitary gland increases LH release, in turn stimulating further androgen production by the ovaries. Overall, peripheral conversion tends to increase effective androgen levels, and the more adipose tissue there is, the greater the rate of peripheral androgen production.

Fig. 10.1 Androgen sources.

Table 10.1
Causes of hirsutism

Causes of true hirsutism	Causes of downy hair growth
Common	Common
Idiopathic	Glucocorticoids (often seen in
Racial or familial (i.e. East Indian)	iatrogenic Cushing's syndrome)
Polycystic ovarian disease	Minoxidil
Rare	Less common
Congenital adrenal hyperplasia	Cyclosporin
Ovarian tumours	
Adrenal tumours	

Table 10.2
Signs of hirsutism

Worry	Don't worry
Rapid onset, short history	Regular menstrual cycles
Signs of virilization	Mild, gradually progressive problem
Testosterone of over 6 nmol/l	Onset around the time of puberty or
(nr 0.3–2.5 nmol/l)	after stopping the contraceptive pill
DHEAS over 18.5 μmol/l	
(nr 5.4–9.2 μmol/l)	

nr, Normal range

Key points

- Hirsutism is common, distressing, but almost always benign.
- Most cases are idiopathic or related to polycystic ovarian disease.
- Medical treatment does not work well and the effects are reversed when it is stopped.
- Testosterone is primarily a gonadal marker—high levels imply ovarian disease.
- A serum testosterone of less than 6 nmol/l virtually rules out androgen-secreting tumours.
- Only a small proportion of hirsute women improve on the contraceptive pill alone.

Table 10.3
Investigations for hirsutism

Common	Investigations
Mild, longstanding hirsutes with regular periods	None
Progressive hirsutes with irregular or absent periods	Source of androgens is probably not important unless fertility is required Check LH, FSH, SHBG, and testosterone
Rare Marked hirsutes of rapid onset, with amenorrhoea ± virilism	Check LH, FSH, SHBG, testosterone, 17-hydroxyprogesterone (17OH-P), 17OH-P response to Synacthen®, and DHEAS. Consider ultrasound and CT of abdomen. If Cushing's syndrome is suspected, a short dexamethasone suppression test and 24 h urinary free cortisol excretion can be measured. Virilizing adrenal tumours (i.e. an ACTH-independent mechanism) can be excluded if excess adrenal steroids (DHEAS and urinary cortisol) are suppressed to normal by 3 mg of dexamethasone daily for 5 days

Table 10.4
Treatment options for hirsutism

General measures	
Reassurance	Reassurance is critical, not least because endocrine therapy acts very slowly, tends to produce a fairly modest improvement, and is completely reversed once treatment stops. In many women the severity of symptoms from PCOD tends to wane as they reach their 30s
Physical treatment	
Electrolysis	Electrolysis produces an immediate and relatively long-lasting effect. As only a few hairs can be removed at one time, however, a significant area may take many months to treat. It is very expensive, and tends to be uncomfortable. Scarring can occur if it is used injudiciously
Cosmetic disguise	Cosmetics work immediately, and can be very useful. Unfortunately, specialist help is very expensive, difficult to find, and not often available for this indication
Plucking, waxing, shaving	Plucking and waxing are immediately effective, but are painful and tend to cause a rash. Patients are often concerned that shaving will exacerbate hirsutes. It is more probable that women start to shave when hirsutes worsens, and that the association is spurious. The use of shaving soap or creams should be encouraged to minimize skin trauma
Laser	The use of a ruby laser, which produces light at a wavelength highly absorbed by hair but not by skin, is an experimental treatment that is currently undergoing clinical trials

continued next page

Endocrine treatment

Weight loss

Adipose tissue is able to convert pre-androgens to androgens and oestrone. Weight loss reduces androgen and oestrone formation and increases the chances of endocrine therapy working, or of the problem resolving of its own accord. Unfortunately, this is difficult and disheartening for patients to achieve. They may feel that they are being blamed.

Anti-androgens such as cyproterone acetate, (up to 100 mg/day on days 5–15 of the cycle) with oestrogens such as ethinyloestradiol, 50 μg on days 5–26)

Anti-androgens such as cyproterone acetate are effective but can potentially feminize a male fetus. Concurrent use of oestrogen protects against pregnancy and also increases hepatic sex hormone binding globulin production (which preferentially binds testosterone), further reducing free androgen levels. Doses are gradually reduced over several months, and can then be conveniently given as the combined contraceptive pill, Dianette®. Unfortunately any improvement may take 6 or 9 months and is lost once treatment stops. Side effects are bloating, nausea, breast tenderness, headaches, weight change, and depression

Glucocorticoids

Glucocorticoids reduce circulating ACTH by increasing negative feedback at the pituitary. Although a potentially useful treatment in hirsutes secondary to congenital adrenal hyperplasia, anti-androgens are just as effective and may have fewer side-effects

'My patient complains of facial hair growth. Does she have an endocrinopathy?'

History

A 30-year-old female was referred with excessive facial hair growth. She claimed that she had always been hairy but that for the past few years, she had found herself shaving her face more and more frequently. Menstrual cycles occur every 2–4 months, and had been irregular since her menarche at the age of 13. She denied any discomfort on sexual intercourse (dyspareunia) and, although worried about fertility, was not yet planning a family.

Examination

She was slightly overweight (BMI 28 kg/m^2) with stubble on her neck, chin, and sideboards. She had a few hairs around the areolae and on the lower abdomen, but no acanthosis nigricans, stigmata of Cushing's disease, or evidence of virilization (i.e. no deepening of her voice, male body habitus, temporal hair recession, etc.)

Investigations

LH, 9 U/l (normal range 3–8 U/l); FSH, 2.3 U/l (normal range 1–9 U/l); SHBG, 20 nmol/l (normal range 40–135 nmol/l in females); PRL, 350 mu/l (normal range < 800 mU/l); testosterone, 2.8 nmol/l (normal range 0.3–2.5 nmol/l).

Management

This is a typical history of mild polycystic ovarian disease and hyperandrogenism. The condition was explained to the patient and she chose to continue treating the hair growth with depilatory creams and shaving (having been reassured that the latter is in itself unlikely to increase the rate of hair growth). The patient was reassured that although she might need some hormonal encouragement to ovulate, her chances of fertility remained good.

Explanation

The presence of menstrual bleeding and lack of dyspareunia indicates that oestrogen levels are not suppressed. The high LH/FSH ratio and moderately raised testosterone with low sex hormone binding globulin (SHBG) is typical of polycystic ovarian disease. An ultrasound examination of the ovaries and further blood tests are not usually necessary. Had the patient requested hormonal treatment for hirsutism, she would have been warned that the response is usually delayed for many months and even then is often minimal. Some physicians believe that there is no advantage in high-dose treatment and that the combined pill, Dianette®, is adequate on its own.

Multiple-choice questions

1. The following have potentially useful anti-androgen effects:
   a. Spironolactone;
   b. ACTH;
   c. Cyproterone acetate;
   d. Ethinyloestradiol;
   e. Flutamide.

2. Endogenous androgens are derived from the following sources:
   a. The adrenal medulla;
   b. The granulosa cells of developing follicles;
   c. Peripheral fat;
   d. Sertoli cells;
   e. Kupffer cells of the liver.

3. Polycystic ovarian disease is typically associated with:
   a. Obesity;
   b. High LH and FSH levels;
   c. Multiple ovarian cysts in various stages of development;
   d. Reduced fertility;
   e. Increased risk of miscarriage.

4. Virilization is characterized by:
   a. Breast enlargement;
   b. Pectoral muscle wasting;
   c. Clitoromegaly;
   d. Deepening of the voice;
   e. Scalp hair recession.

Answers

1. The following have potentially useful anti-androgen effects:
   a. Spironolactone   T
      This is widely used for its anti-androgenic properties in the United States, where cyproterone is unlicensed.

The usual regimen is 25–100 mg twice daily, on which dose up to 75 per cent of women notice an improvement after 6 months.

b. ACTH   F

ACTH stimulates androgen (as well as cortisol) synthesis in the adrenal cortex. This is the reason why patients with Cushing's disease are hirsute.

c. Cyproterone acetate   T

This is a widely used anti-androgen. As it is not contraceptive on its own, it is always used with oestrogens to prevent potential feminization of a male fetus

d. Ethinyloestradiol   T

Although not directly anti-androgen, it has 'anti-androgenic effects' by inducing hepatic production of sex hormone binding globulin. If more androgens are 'bound' in the bloodstream, less is available to act on androgen receptors.

e. Flutamide   T

Flutamide is an anti-androgen used in prostatic cancer. At 125–250 mg twice daily (concurrent with an oral contraceptive, see (c) above), it has similar efficacy to spironolactone. Finasteride, a 5α-reductase inhibitor (i.e. blocks conversion of testosterone to dihydrotestosterone) at a dose of 5 mg daily (although 1 mg may be as good), is as effective as 100 mg spironolactone in reducing hair shaft thickness.

2. Endogenous androgens are derived from the following sources:

a. The adrenal medulla   F

The adrenal cortex is the source. The medulla makes catecholamines and gives rise to phaeochromocytomas rather than virilizing neoplasms.

b. The granulosa cells of developing follicles   F

The theca cells in the ovary are the source of androgens. They are 'aromatized'—converted to oestrogens—by the granulosa cells surrounding the developing follicles. Thus in the absence of developing follicles (i.e. in the pre-pubertal or postmenopausal ovary), there are no granulosa cells to convert androgens to oestrogens, and no oestrogen output by the ovary.

c. Peripheral fat   T

The pre-androgens DHEA and DHEAS are converted to testosterone by peripheral fat. Confusingly, peripheral fat also converts androgens to the oestrogen 'oestrone', which is thought to be involved in the self-perpetuation of polycystic ovarian disease.

d. Sertoli cells   F

The Leydig cells are the source of testosterone in the testes. The Sertoli cells produce inhibin, and stimulate the formation of spermatozoa from spermatogonia.

e. Kupffer cells of the liver   F

The principal sources of androgens in females are peripheral adipose tissue, the ovaries, and the adrenal glands, rather than the liver.

3. Polycystic ovarian disease is typically associated with:

   a. Obesity   T

The association with obesity is well known, but by no means invariable. If the patient manages to lose weight the condition often improves, as peripheral production of oestrone decreases.

   b. High LH and FSH levels   F

The LH tends to be high and the FSH normal. However, the LH/FSH ratio is not a sensitive or specific finding in PCOD.

   c. Multiple ovarian cysts in various stages of development   T

The characteristic appearance on transvaginal ultrasound is said to resemble a string of pearls—a series of immature follicles ranged around the periphery of the ovary.

   d. Reduced fertility   T

Anovulation is common.

   e. Increased risk of miscarriage   T

This is also true, though the reason is unclear. Particularly if the LH is persistently greater than 10U/l, the early miscarriage rate is high.

4. Virilization is characterized by:

   a. Breast enlargement   F

If anything, the opposite would be expected.

   b. Pectoral muscle wasting   F

The muscles tend to hypertrophy. A male body habitus is assumed.

   c. Clitoromegaly   T

Although true, it is very rarely helpful to examine for clitoromegaly in the adult clinic, as other obvious and less embarrassing signs of virilization are likely to be present.

   d. Deepening of the voice   T

This tends to be irreversible, like clitoromegaly.

   e. Scalp hair recession   T

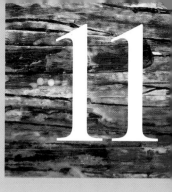

11

The breast

- Summary

- Introduction

- Lactation

- Galactorrhoea

- Breast pain (mastalgia)

- Key points

- Case history

- Multiple-choice questions

Summary

Normal function

- Lactation
- Oestrogen-primed (enlarged) breasts are a socially important sign identified with the female body form.

Typical pathology

- Female
  - → Galactorrhoea.
  - → Cyclical breast pain.
- Male
  - → Gynaecomastia. The development of tender, sub-areolar plaques during puberty is common. It usually resolves over a period of a few years but can cause considerable anxiety. Gynaecomastia secondary to oestrogen-secreting tumours is very rare.

'Typical clinical scenario'

- A 27-year-old with persistent galactorrhoea after cessation of nursing (breast feeding). A microprolactinoma was not found on pituitary MR scanning, but the problem resolved after treatment with bromocriptine.

Introduction

The form of male and female breasts can first be differentiated at puberty, when each successive cycle of ovarian follicular development and the associated prolonged pulse of oestrogen from the granulosa cells that surround them, stimulates breast ductal development and the laying down of fat and connective tissue. Formation of small pads of tissue beneath the nipple and areolae (breast buds) is the first sign of puberty in girls (Fig. 11.1). The delayed appearance of this sign can be psychologically traumatic. Appropriate breast enlargement, mediated by large doses of exogenous oestrogens and surgical augmentation, is a sought-after sign of femininity in male to female trans-sexuals.

Lactation

Exposure of the breasts to high levels of oestrogen in the presence of prolactin, promotes breast ductal growth. Progesterone acts synergistically with prolactin in the oestrogen-primed breast to induce lobuloalveolar development. Lactation itself is inhibited until the levels of oestrogen and progesterone drop precipitously following expulsion of the placenta.

High levels of prolactin are needed to induce lactation, and continued lactation depends on suckling-induced prolactin release. Stimulation of the breast or

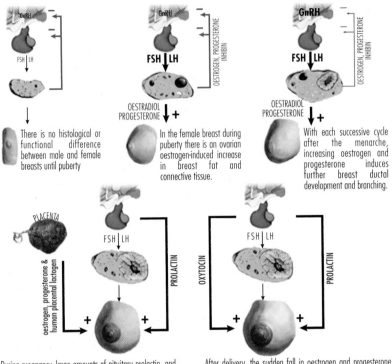

There is no histological or functional difference between male and female breasts until puberty

In the female breast during puberty there is an ovarian oestrogen-induced increase in breast fat and connective tissue.

With each successive cycle after the menarche, increasing oestrogen and progesterone induces further breast ductal development and branching.

During pregnancy, large amounts of pituitary prolactin, and high levels of oestrogen and progesterone from the placenta contribute to further breast growth, ductal development and alveolar differentiation

After delivery, the sudden fall in oestrogen and progesterone following expulsion of the placenta, allows prolactin to induce lactation in the primed breast tissue. Nipple stimulation enhances prolactin secretion. Expulsion of milk from the breast is mediated by oxytocin, which rises in anticipation of nursing, and further as a neuroendocrine response to nipple stimulation

Fig. 11.1 Breast development.

nipples of a nursing mother acutely increase prolactin levels up to tenfold. However, a month or two after delivery prolactin levels often fall to within the normal non-pregnant range between feeding episodes. Nevertheless, in most women, if prolactin levels are suppressed *below* normal by dopamine agonists, lactation ceases.

Oxytocin, unlike prolactin, rises in anticipation of nursing and, particularly near parturition, can produce painful uterine cramps, so called 'after pains'. Impairment of oxytocin release by stress or fright impairs lactation. In one-third of normal, menstruating women (who are not postpartum), stimulation of the breast or nipples can double prolactin levels.

Lactation-associated infertility is mediated by the antigonadotrophin effect of raised prolactin. Most women resume menstruation by 6 months postpartum even if they continue nursing, and fertility may return before menstruation. Contraception should recommence soon after delivery and certainly within

Table 11.1
Oxytocin

Is produced in the hypothalamus and released from the posterior pituitary

Stimulates uterine contractions at parturition

Stimulates smooth muscle contraction in the breast during suckling

Has the same effects on water homeostatis as vasopressin, but it is only 1/100 as strong. This weak antidiuretic effect of oxytocin, however, can be a problem when high levels (as Syntocinon®) are used to accelerate labour. Unless free water intake is controlled, water intoxication can occur, with subsequent convulsions

In almost all women who have been pregnant, the act of expressing milk will stimulate oxytocin production and perpetuate milk flow. This may become a problem if women repeatedly 'check to see whether galactorrhoea has stopped yet'

Suckling-induced oxytocin release can cause painful uterine contractions

5 weeks of delivery in mothers who breast feed, using a low-dose oestrogen preparation or a progesterone-only pill.

Galactorrhoea

Galactorrhoea may not necessarily need treatment other than explanation and reassurance. If, however, it is associated with amenorrhoea and other signs of low oestrogen levels, it should be treated directly with dopaminergic drugs such as bromocriptine or cabergoline. It is also appropriate to ask the patient to try to reduce nipple stimulation by avoiding excessive contact with her breasts (i.e. vig-

Table 11.2
Galactorrhoea

Common causes	Microprolactinomas that may be too small to identify on MR scanning
	Idiopathic— prolactin levels normal
	Prolonged postpartum lactation
Less common causes	Macroprolactinomas
	Treatment with phenothiazines or antiemetics such as domperidone
Rare causes	Mammosomatotroph adenomas, i.e. acromegaly with raised prolactin
	Hypothyroidism
	Surgery, trauma, or infections of chest wall
	Hypothalamic diseases such as sarcoidosis, Langerhans cell histiocytosis
	Self-manipulation of breasts

orous washing or wearing tight clothes), as this in itself can perpetuate the problem.

Breast pain (mastalgia)

Breast pain is often a diffuse ache that is initiated or exacerbated premenstrually. There is a high placebo response and treatment is often difficult. Oil of evening primrose and bromocriptine are both more effective than placebo, and danazol, an antigonadotrophic drug, is more effective than either but has major side-effects including menstrual irregularity, weight gain, and androgenic effects. Tamoxifen may be useful in mastalgia, but has not been subjected to clinical trials.

Key points

- Prolactin-induced milk accumulation requires breast tissue to be oestrogen-primed. For this reason, galactorrhoea in men with macroprolactinomas is very unusual.
- Between suckling episodes, maternal prolactin levels often fall to normal.
- Although prolactin inhibits gonadotrophin release, contraceptive precautions are necessary from 5 weeks postpartum. A progestogen-only product is suitable.
- The cause of mastalgia (breast pain) in adult women is rarely apparent and treatment is usually unsatisfactory.
- Galactorrhoea is typically caused by prolactinomas, some of which may be too small to see on MR imaging. In some cases, galactorrhoea is a continuation of postpartum lactation—the wet nurse phenomenon.

'My patient has stopped breast feeding, but still has galactorrhoea and amenorrhoea'

History

A healthy 24-year-old female complained of persistent 'leaking breasts' and amenorrhoea. She had a 10-month-old son who was breast fed until he was 5 months old. For the first 2 months after weaning, whenever he cried, there was spontaneous milk ejection. Although that had since stopped, she found herself still able to express milk manually and her clothes were often stained with milk.

Examination

Examination was not carried out. She was clearly healthy and there was nothing to gain by confirming her observation of galactorrhoea.

Investigations

A prolactin level was 150 mU/l (well within the normal range).

Management

The association between nipple stimulation and milk ejection was explained to the patient. She was advised to avoid inadvertant breast stimulating where possible and was prescribed bromocriptine (1–2.5 mg daily) for a few weeks to see whether galactorrhoea could be 'turned off'. As the patient was nauseated by the treatment, it was suggested that she use the oral tablets vaginally—a manoeuvre that slows absorption and reduces side-effects.

Explanation

The most likely problem is the 'wet nurse' phenomenon. Lactation is inhibited until after delivery and is then perpetuated by suckling-induced prolactin release. Nipple or breast stimulation acutely increases circulating prolactin by up to tenfold, even though levels between feeds are often normal. By 'checking to see whether the problem was still there', the patient simulated on-going demand for breast milk. The episodic elevation of prolactin continued to suppress her oestrogen levels, resulting in amenorrhoea.

Multiple-choice questions

1. In breast development:
   a. Differences in the male and female breast are evident in babies and young children;
   b. Breast ductal development is mostly prolactin mediated;
   c. Breast alveolar development is mediated almost entirely by progesterone;
   d. High levels of hormones during pregnancy result in enhanced ductal and alveolar growth;
   e. The onset of lactation at the end of pregnancy is mediated by a sudden increase in prolactin.

2. Galactorrhoea:
   a. Can be caused by daily manipulation of the nipples in women who have never been pregnant;

b. Can occur with normal prolactin levels;
c. Can occur in men with high prolactin levels;
d. Can occur in acromegaly;
e. Can be associated with hypothyroidism.

3. In galactorrhoea:
   a. Lactation that persists for some time after an infant has been weaned is one of the most common causes of galactorrhoea;
   b. Herpes zoster of the chest wall may be responsible;
   c. Checking to see whether the problem persists may perpetuate the condition;
   d. The absence of a pituitary abnormality on MR scanning means that a prolactinoma is not responsible;
   e. Bromocriptine may be useful even if prolactin levels are normal.

Answers

1. In breast development:
   a. Differences in the male and female breast are evident in babies and young children   F
      There are no discernable differences until puberty.
   b. Breast ductal development is mostly prolactin mediated   F
      It is oestrogen mediated.
   c. Breast alveolar development is mediated almost entirely by progesterone   F
      Progesterone and prolactin are equally involved.
   d. High levels of hormones during pregnancy result in enhanced ductal and alveolar growth   T
   e. The onset of lactation at the end of pregnancy is mediated by a sudden increase in prolactin   F
      The sudden fall in oestrogen and progesterone levels allows the pre-existing high levels of prolactin to induce lactation.

2. Galactorrhoea
   a. Can be caused by daily manipulation of the nipples in women who have never been pregnant   F
      This would be unusual. The breasts need to have been primed by the high levels of oestrogen, progesterone, and prolactin during a previous pregnancy.
   b. Can occur with normal prolactin levels   T
      This situation occurs in the majority of nursing mothers a few months postpartum.
   c. Can occur in men with high prolactin levels   T
      It can, but it is extremely rare, unless the male breast has been oestrogen-primed.

d. Can occur in acromegaly   T

Mostly, galactorrhoea is associated with prolactinomas. It can occur in pituitary stalk compression, although prolactin levels are usually not high enough to initiate the process. Some somatotroph adenomas 'mammo-somatotroph' to be precise, can produce high levels of prolactin as well as growth hormone, and galactorrhoea is associated with these, particularly in women.

e. Can be associated with hypothyroidism   T

Hyperprolactinaemia is certainly associated with hypothyroidism as TRH stimulates prolactin secretion (see Fig. 1.1), but galactorrhoea in these circumstances is very unusual.

3. In galactorrhoea:

a. Lactation that persists for some time after an infant has been weaned is one of the most common causes of galactorrhoea   T

In some women who do not breast feed their babies, persistent amenorrhoea and galactorrhoea can last for more than 6 months postpartum. Many cases are probably the result of small prolactinomas, and untreated, amenorrhoea persists in as many as 50 per cent.

b. Herpes zoster of the chest wall may be responsible   T

This is true, but extremely rare. Stress can also increase prolactin levels, and both painful infections and trauma are major stressors.

c. Checking to see whether the problem persists may perpetuate the condition   T

Breast stimulation is the way that babies manage it.

d. The absence of a pituitary abnormality on MR scanning means that a prolactinoma is not responsible   F

The tumour may well be too small to see.

e. Bromocriptine may be useful even if prolactin levels are normal   T

A short course of bromocriptine is often sufficient to stop worrisome galactorrhoea that has no serious underlying cause.

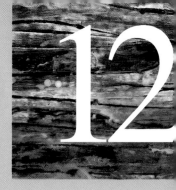

12

The testis

- Summary

- Introduction

- Testicular function

- Key points

- Case history

- Multiple-choice questions

Summary

Normal function

- Production of androgens, particularly testosterone and dihydrotestosterone.
- Spermatogenesis.
- The fetal testes produce Müllerian-inhibiting hormone.

Typical pathology

- Mumps and surgical problems such as torsion of the testis are the most common identifiable causes of testicular failure.
- Idiopathic oligospermia or azoospermia.
- Secondary hypogonadism due to the development of a pituitary adenoma or following transphenoidal surgery for the same.
- Hypogonadotrophic hypogonadism caused by a developmental defect in hypothalamic GnRH neurone development (Kallmann's syndrome). This usually presents as pubertal failure and is often associated with anosmia.

'Typical clinical scenario'

- A 46-year-old man with hypogonadism secondary to an endocrinologically inactive pituitary adenoma. His complaint is of lack of energy and loss of libido. He is also having difficulty sustaining an erection.

Table 12.1
Testicular descent

Determination of gonadal sex (i.e. progression from the undifferentiated gonad of early gestation to the testis or ovary) and the embryological development of the internal and external genitalia are discussed in chapter 5. At the level of the developing testis and above, the mesonephros (the ridge of tissue at the back of the body cavity that becomes the kidney and gonads) degenerates almost entirely, while below that level it forms the gubernaculum. By the beginning of the third month of pregnancy the rapid growth of the body, not matched by the gubernaculum, brings the inguinal region to the level of the testes (thus far 'ascent of the body', rather than 'descent of the testes'. The testes remain there until the seventh month of pregnancy then continue their descent through the inguinal ring, over the pubic bone, and into the scrotum by a mechanism that is currently unknown. As some testes remain in the inguinal canal or high in the scrotum until 3 months of age, failure of descent cannot be diagnosed with certainty until after that time

Introduction

The main functions of the testes in adult life are to produce spermatozoa and androgens. The testes also produce a unique peptide *in utero*—Müllerian-inhibiting hormone—which is responsible for the involution of Müllerian structures in early fetal life. The testes develop on the posterior abdominal wall and migrate through the deep inguinal ring to the scrotum during development (Table 12.1) Their increase in size from 2 ml in volume (approximately 2 cm in length) is the first sign of puberty. By the age of 16 to 19 years the testes reach adult proportions of 4.6 ± 1 cm in length, 12 to 25 ml in volume.

Testicular tumours secreting oestrogens and giving rise to the rapid development of painful gynaecomastia are very rare.

In most cases both the diagnosis of gonadal failure and the likely causes are clear from the history, and can usually be confirmed by measuring testosterone and gonadotrophin (FSH and LH) levels. If the gonadotrophins are elevated and testosterone is low, primary gonadal failure is present.

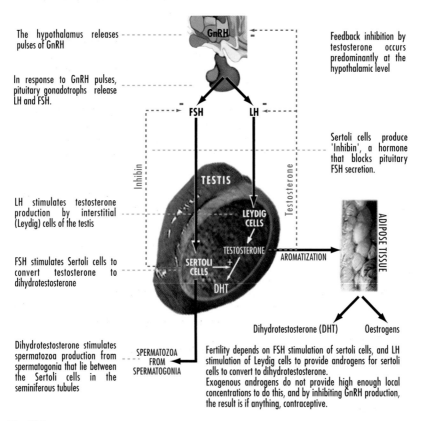

The hypothalamus releases pulses of GnRH

GnRH

Feedback inhibition by testosterone occurs predominantly at the hypothalamic level

In response to GnRH pulses, pituitary gonadotrophs release LH and FSH.

FSH **LH**

Sertoli cells produce 'Inhibin', a hormone that blocks pituitary FSH secretion.

Inhibin

Testosterone

TESTIS

LH stimulates testosterone production by interstitial (Leydig) cells of the testis

LEYDIG CELLS

ADIPOSE TISSUE

FSH stimulates Sertoli cells to convert testosterone to dihydrotestosterone

TESTOSTERONE

SERTOLI CELLS +

AROMATIZATION

DHT

Dihydrotestosterone (DHT)   Oestrogens

Dihydrotestosterone stimulates spermatozoa production from spermatogonia that lie between the Sertoli cells in the seminiferous tubules

SPERMATOZOA FROM SPERMATOGONIA

Fertility depends on FSH stimulation of sertoli cells, and LH stimulation of Leydig cells to provide androgens for sertoli cells to convert to dihydrotestosterone.
Exogenous androgens do not provide high enough local concentrations to do this, and by inhibiting GnRH production, the result is if anything, contraceptive.

Fig. 12.1

Table 12.2
Major effects of androgens

Linear growth and epiphyseal fusion	Excessive levels before puberty result in rapid growth but an even more rapid advance in bone age. Premature epiphyseal fusion results in marked loss of final adult height
Spinal growth	Spinal growth is sex hormone rather than growth hormone dependent. Lack of androgens results in a short trunk but long limbs (eunuchoid habitus) as epiphyseal fusion is delayed
Male pattern of hair growth	Scalp hair loss cannot be reversed. Beard growth, once established, takes years to slow down even if androgen levels are minimal
Increased muscle Strength	Supraphysiological doses further enhance this. An observation exploited (at some peril) by body builders and athletes
Penile enlargement and scrotal rugosity	As the testes are the predominant source of androgen and penile growth is androgen dependent, the testes enlarge *before* the phallus at the onset of puberty.
Libido and potency	Potency is rapidly restored by androgen replacement. After chronic insufficiency, abrupt provision of normal androgen levels can produce distressing aggression and excessively heightened libido
Indirect effect on bone mineral density	Bone mineral density may be oestrogen dependent in men as well as women. If testosterone is very low (≤ 3 nmol/l), insufficient oestrogen will be generated by aromatization to protect the skeleton. Testosterone may also have a direct effect on the skeleton
Laryngeal enlargement	An irreversible phenomenon that most male trans-sexuals have to bear, although there are surgical procedures to raise the voice pitch

Table 12.3
Common causes of male hypogonadism

Pituitary tumours or treatment of the same causing hypopituitarism
Hyperprolactinaemia
Klinefelter's syndrome (1 : 600) (typically small, hard testes)
Kallmann's syndrome (see p. 129)
Delayed puberty
Viral orchitis
Alcoholism

Hypogonadism (Table 12.3) from before puberty results in eunuchoidism. In eunuchs, failure of sex hormone-induced epiphyseal closure allows growth to continue into the middle of the third decade. The result is patients of average height or above, in whom span exceeds height and heel–pubis length exceeds pubis–crown length by 5 cm or more.

Testicular function

Testicular examination

Unless the testes have suddenly changed in size, their examination is limited to an assessment of overall size and consistency. Klinfelter's testes tend to be small and hard; those of an alcoholic, or a man with secondary gonadal failure (hypogonadotrophic hypogonadism—as in pituitary failure or hyperprolactinaemia), small and soft. Orchidometers, a series of avoid standards (Fig. 12.2), may be used to provide a more objective estimation of testicular size.

Table 12.4
Spermatogenesis

Approximately 95 per cent of the 12–25 ml volume of normal adult testes is made up of seminiferous tubules. LH-induced Leydig cell androgen production and FSH stimulation of the Sertoli cells within the tubules (which convert testosterone to dihydrotestosterone) are both vital for the initiation of spermatogenesis. Maintenance of spermatogenesis is then possible with LH alone

Spermatogenesis involves multiplication of germ cells (spermatogonia), meiosis to reduce the number of chromosomes to the haploid state (to form spermatids), and formation of the structural elements of the mature spermatozoa to protect and transport the male chromosomes to the ovum. Spermatogenesis takes approximately 10 weeks, and from puberty to old age the process produces 200 million sperm daily

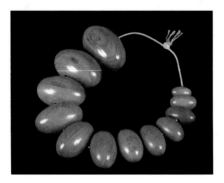

Fig. 12.2 An orchidometer, used to estimate testicular size by direct comparison.

Table 12.5
Androgens status in men

Questions to ask	Reason for asking
Has there been any change in libido?	No androgens, no libido: a maxim the holds true for both sexes. Sex drive progressively falls following castration
Are you still able to achieve a climax?	Potency, as distinct from libido, is the ability to have an erection and achieve (biologically) successful intercourse. Only 1 in 5 cases of impotence (at most) are related to hormonal abnormalities
Any change in shaving frequency?	Patients rarely volunteer that beard growth has slowed, or that they have never had to shave more than once or twice a week
Have you noticed any breast pain or enlargement?	Increased endogenous oestrogen/androgen ratio or an acute increase in absolute oestrogen level. This occurs with oestrogen- or hCG-secreting (usually testicular) tumours or aromatization of large amounts of exogenous androgen (a side-effect noted by body builders and other athletes taking supraphysiological doses of anabolic androgens)
Do you have a past history of pituitary disease?	Prolactin suppresses sex hormone production. Macroadenomas may also cause hypopituitarism by compressing the pituitary. Pituitary surgery ± radiotherapy is the most common cause of hypogonadism

continued next page

Were you normal at birth?	3 per cent of normal full-term male infants have at least one cryptorchid testis at birth, and 0.5 per cent remain undescended (usually unilaterally) at puberty
Is your sense of smell normal?	Kallmann's syndrome is isolated hypogonadotrophic hypogonadism. It is usually associated with anosmia. The male to female ratio is 5:1
Have you had viral orchitis or trauma?	Recovery is usually complete after mumps orchitis, but testicular atrophy may ensue
Have you ever had radio-therapy or chemotherapy?	Chemotherapy before, but not after, puberty usually has no effect on testicular function. Attempts to return patients to a pre-pubescent state before chemotherapy to protect the testes have been unsuccessful
Do you take drugs or use marijuana?	Spironolactone, cimetidine, cardiac glycosides, anti-androgens, alcohol, anabolic steroids, or other 'body building drug combinations', etc.
Have your testes decreased in size?	Damage to seminiferous tubules before puberty results in small, firm testes. Postpubertal damage leads to small, soft testes
Has there been any testicular pain or enlargement?	Testicular tumours are the most common solid tumours in men aged 20–35 years. Cryptorchidism increases the risk five-tenfold. They are often bilateral, one following the other some time later. 95 per cent are seminomas

Semen analysis

There is only one test and one result, pregnancy, that establishes whether a semen sample has the potential to fertilize a human ovum *in vivo*. Semen analysis is an imperfect art that currently depends on microscopic examination of a sample 30–60 min after ejaculation. The total number of spermatozoa and morphological features (immature and abnormal forms) are commonly used. Functional tests, such as penetration through bovine cervical mucus and penetration of zona pellucida-stripped hamster eggs, are not generally available.

Androgen replacement

Oral androgens are extensively destroyed by first-pass metabolism in the liver. A variety of parenteral preparations are used (see p. 52).

Key points

- Although, ideally, three blood samples taken at 15–20 min intervals should be pooled to give mean circulating testosterone, a single sample is fairly representative.
- In hypopituitary patients, exogenous androgens do not restore fertility.
- Oral androgens are poorly absorbed.

'My male patient complains of tender gynaecomastia'

History

A 23-year-old man, anxious to meet the physical criteria required to be considered for membership of one of the more elite sections of the armed forces, had been training hard since his teenage years and had a torso that was considered 'cut' (i.e. muscular outlines well defined). Nevertheless, in his ever-increasing attempts to reach the prerequisite weight and size, he had purchased a course of androgens and anabolic steroids from contacts in the gym. These included weekly injections of Deca-Durabolin® and Sustanon®, with daily oral tamoxifen.

Examination

On examination he was very fit-looking, with enviable muscular development. However tender masses approximately 2 cm in diameter were present deep to the breast areolae bilaterally, and although his phallus was normal, his testes were small and soft.

Investigations

No investigations were carried out.

Management

He hardly needed to be told that the cause of the problem was the treatment he had self-administered, and that the correct course of action was to stop.

Explanation

At physiological doses, exogenous testosterone feeds back at the level of the hypothalamus and to a lesser extent at the pituitary, to reduce pulsatile release of GnRH and secretion of FSH and LH. Without gonadotrophin stimulation, testicular interstitial cells atrophy and as local levels of testosterone and dihydrotestosterone fall, spermatogenesis decreases and the testes become smaller and softer. This patient was taking enormously high doses of the anabolic steroid nandrolone (Deca-Durabolin®) and a mixture of testosterone esters (Sustanon®), the latter alone at a level at least three times that routinely used for male sex hormone replacement. Concurrent treatment with tamoxifen (an oestrogen receptor antagonist) was insufficient to prevent oestrogens formed by peripheral aromatization of androgens from causing gynaecomastia and breast tenderness.

The reduction in testicular size and the appearance of gynaecomastia, which often takes a considerable time to resolve, was enough to make the patient stop taking the treatments. The association of these drugs with hepatic tumours was also explained.

Multiple-choice questions

1. Testicular function:
   a. Exogenous testosterone (Sustanon®) stimulates spermatogenesis;
   b. Sertoli cells convert endogenous testosterone produced by Leydig cells to dihydrotestosterone;

c. Development from spermatogonia to mature spermatozoa takes about 6 weeks;

d. In hypogonadotrophic hypogonadism, daily intramuscular injections of gonadotrophins (FSH and LH) are required to induce spermatogenesis;

e. Until puberty, the testes have no significant endocrine function.

2. The following drugs interfere with spermatogenesis:
   a. Cyclophosphamide;
   b. Nonoxinol;
   c. Atenolol;
   d. Anabolic steroids;
   e. Suphasalazine.

3. Testicular function can be impaired by the following:
   a. Spironolactone;
   b. Maldescent (cryptorchidism);
   c. Wearing tight clothes;
   d. Testicular radiotherapy for acute lymphoblastic leukaemia;
   e. Hyperprolactinaemia.

4. Semen:
   a. For analysis should ideally be collected in a condom at intercourse;
   b. The specimen should be examined after an hour, when it has fully liquified;
   c. Is routinely examined for motility and density (number/ml) only;
   d. After abstaining from intercourse for 6 days, the first ejaculate contains four times as many sperm as usual if sex occurs daily;
   e. A postcoital test is analysis of ejaculate obtained by masturbation within 12 h of intercourse.

Answers

1. Testicular function:
   a. Exogenous testosterone (Sustanon®) stimulates spermatogenesis   F
      The opposite effect is achieved. Exogenous testosterone cannot achieve the high local levels of testosterone needed for Sertoli cells to stimulate spermatogenesis. The effect of exogenous testosterone, if anything, is to suppress pituitary gonadotrophin production and to act as a contraceptive.
   b. Sertoli cells convert endogenous testosterone produced by Leydig cells to dihydrotestosterone   T
   c. Development from spermatogonia to mature spermatozoa takes about 6 weeks   F
      It takes 6 months or more, hence the long course of intramuscular gonadotrophin (FSH and LH) treatment required to restore fertility to patients with hypogonadotrophic hypogonadism.

d. In hypogonadotrophic hypogonadism, daily intramuscular injections of gonadotrophins (FSH and LH) are required to induce spermatogenesis   T
    FSH and LH stimulate Sertoli and Leydig cells as illustrated above.

e. Until puberty, the testes have no significant endocrine function   F
    Although high levels of androgen production do not occur until puberty, the testes produce Müllerian-inhibiting hormone during early fetal life, without which the uterus and Fallopian tubes would not involute. There is a curious, but not unduly rare, condition called 'vanishing testis' syndrome, in which the phenotype is entirely male, but no testes—either descended or otherwise—seem to be present. In these patients, the absence of Müllerian structures indicates that during fetal life, a source of Müllerian-inhibiting hormone (presumably testicular) must have been present.

2. The following drugs interfere with spermatogenesis:
   a. Cyclophosphamide   T
       Antineoplastic and chemotherapeutic drugs have a dramatic effect, rendering postpubertal males azoospermic or severely oligospermic within a few weeks. About half of the patients treated regain spermatogenesis, but even then, it may take several years to return. Spermatogenesis in males treated pre-pubertally is usually not effected.

   b. Nonoxinol   F
       This is the spermicide used in gels and creams for added protection during intercourse. It is not an effective contraceptive when used alone, and is certainly not taken internally.

   c. Atenolol   F
       β-Adrenergic drugs interfere with erectile competence but not with spermatogenesis.

   d. Anabolic steroids   T
       Contrary to expectations, body builders who abuse their bodies by taking large amounts of androgens and anabolic steroids rapidly achieve small, soft testes with feeble sperm counts. These drugs turn off pituitary gonadotrophin synthesis. Rather than ask directly about drug habits, it is useful to approach the subject obliquely by asking 'What sports or pastimes do you enjoy?'

   e. Suphasalazine   T
       It effects spermatogenesis and sperm motility.

3. Testicular function can be impaired by the following:
   a. Spironolactone   T
       It is a reasonably powerful anti-androgen.

   b. Maldescent (cryptorchidism)   T
       The assumption that undescended testes do not function well purely because their ambient temperature is too high, may be an over-

simplification. Testicular morphology and descent may be connected. The rate of testicular tumours in undescended tests is five-tenfold higher than normal. Androgen secretion from undescended testes is preserved.

c. Wearing tight clothes   T

If the testes are held tight to the body, they may not be able to operate at their preferred temperature. Why there should be an evolutionary advantage in having optimal spermatogenesis at a temperature below core temperature is not known.

d. Testicular radiotherapy for acute lymphoblastic leukaemia   T

This can severely affect spermatogenesis and androgen function, irrespective of the age at which treatment is undertaken.

e. Hyperprolactinaemia   T

The mechanism is similar to that causing amenorrhoea in women.

4. Semen:

a. For analysis should ideally be collected in a condom at intercourse   F

Coitus interruptus can produce a contaminated or incomplete sample. The use of condoms is also counterproductive as they contain chemicals that inhibit spermotozoa activity. The sample should be collected by masturbation into a clean glass or plastic container.

b. The specimen should be examined after an hour, when it has fully liquified   F

Liquefaction occurs within 15–30 min, and the sample should be analysed *within* 1 h.

c. Is routinely examined for motility and density (number/ml) only   F

Motility, density, and morphology is routinely graded. The sperm count should be greater than 20×10^6/ml, with a total ejaculate count of greater than 60×10^6. At least 60 per cent of sperm should have normal morphology.

d. After abstaining from intercourse for 6 days, the first ejaculate contains four times as many sperm as usual if sex occurs daily   T

e. A postcoital test is analysis of ejaculate obtained by masturbation within 12 h of intercourse   F

A postcoital test is the analysis of sperm penetration through the partner's cervical mucus. The sample is obtained by taking a cervical smear after intercourse.

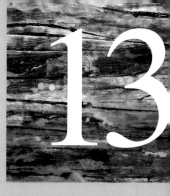

13

Erectile dysfunction

- Summary

- Introduction

- Mechanism of penile engorgement (tumescence)

- Priapism

- Key points

- Case history

- Multiple-choice questions

Intracorporeal injections	Vasodilators, usually prostaglandin E_1 (alprostadil, 2.5–90 mg ± phentolamine, 1 mg), self-injected through a fine-bore (≤25 g) needle into one of the corpora cavernosa at the base of the penis (Fig. 13.1), will produce a satisfactory erection after 10–20 min. Patients must be warned about local pain and trauma, priapism, and the potential for fibrosis and reduced efficacy following prolonged use. Their written consent should be obtained before treatment is initiated, and clear instructions given in case priapism ensues
Surgery for 'venous leaks'	Complete erectile failure and/or hypotension following intracorporeal injection, suggests that arteriovenous shunts or 'venous leaks' are present. These are sometimes amenable to surgical treatment. Although often adduced as a cause of impotence, venous leaks are rare
Implants	The insertion of implants into the corpora is more commonly performed than surgery for venous leaks. Both semi-rigid and inflatable implants cause problems, and neither type is able to protect the glans penis from trauma as neither cause the glans to become turgid
Testosterone and other androgens	There is no evidence that the moderately depressed testosterone levels found in many middle-aged to elderly men (6–10 nmol/l) is responsible for impotence. Neither, unfortunately, is there any evidence that giving exogenous androgens to these men increases potency. In contrast, impotence associated with true hypogonadism and very low testosterone levels can be very effectively treated with exogenous androgens

Key points

- The brain is the most important sex organ.
- The treatment of erectile dysfunction is not possible unless the patient or doctor raises the subject.
- The presence of 'morning erections' excludes an organic cause of erectile dysfunction.
- Erectile dysfunction is eminently amenable to treatment.

'My patient is impotent. His testosterone is low. Does he have an endocrine problem?'

History

A 55-year-old man complained of a 3-year history of erectile failure. Otherwise he claimed to be fit and well with no known history of diabetes, heart disease, or other vascular problems. When asked directly, it was clear that he occasionally had erections, but that they were not of sufficient quality to allow successful intercourse. Masturbation was more often successful, and he did have morning erections. He denied excessive alcohol intake and was taking no medication.

Examination

Unremarkable.

Investigations

Prolactin 740 mu/l (normal range < 800 mu/l), repeat testosterone was 9 nmol/l (normal range 10–35 nmol/l).

Management

The following explanation was offered. Psychogenic impotence—the diagnosis here—is something of a misnomer, as all erections are psychogenic. However, the implication is that other causes of erectile dysfunction, such as structural anomolies, neuropathies, endocrine, or vascular problems are not present, as they would preclude erections at any time.

The use of erotic stimuli and torniquets was suggested but did not prove particularly effective. A small dose of intracorporeal alprostadil (increased in 2 mg increments, leaving 10 min between each addition) was tried, and a total of 6 mg was successful in clinic. The patient used the same dose at home on two occasions, and, his confidence restored, found that he could manage well without it.

Explanation

Erections are associated with rapid eye movement (REM) sleep, and if the patient wakes during this phase of sleep, an erection will often be present. In this patient there was therefore little point in undertaking extensive investigations. The slightly low testosterone is typical, and inconsequential. The incidence of impotence in acromegaly and prolactinoma is no less than 70 per cent, compared to an incidence in alcoholism and renal failure of about 45 per cent.

Multiple-choice questions

1. The following drugs may produce or exacerbate erectile failure:
   a. Doxazosin (an alpha-adrenergic blocker);
   b. Atenolol;
   c. Spironolactone;
   d. Goserelin (a GnRH analogue);
   e. Alcohol.

2. Treatments for erectile dysfunction include:
   a. Intravenous injections with papaverine;
   b. Testosterone implants to increase androgen levels from low normal to high normal levels;
   c. Intracorporeal injections with prostaglandins;
   d. The use of proprietary creams;
   e. Marijuana.

3. Treatments for drug-induced priapism include:
   a. Running up and down stairs;
   b. Intravenous injection of alpha-adrenergic stimulants;
   c. Inserting a 19 g butterfly needle through the glans into one of the corpora cavernosa;
   d. Surgical decompression;
   e. Withdrawing blood under gravity flow.

4. In the treatment of erectile dysfunction:
   a. Implants protect the glans from trauma;
   b. Injections of papaverine or alprostadil (prostaglandin E_1) are made near the glans for best effect;
   c. The dose of intracorporeal papaverine is reduced in diabetes;
   d. Surgery for venous leaks is commonly carried out;
   e. An episode of priapism may render the patient permanently impotent.

Answers

1. The following drugs may produce or exacerbate erectile failure:
   a. Doxazosin (an alpha-adrenergic blocker)   F
   The drug usually has no effect on erectile function but, if anything, it might be expected to improve the quality of tumescence.
   b. Atenolol   T
   c. Spironolactone   T
   Many antihypertensives (perhaps with the exception of alpha-blockers) can produce impotence. Spironolactone, in particular, as well as being an aldosterone antagonist, has anti-androgenic properties and is widely used in the treatment of hirsutism in the United States, where cyproterone is unlicensed.
   d. Goserelin (a GnRH analogue)   T
   This is used in prostatic cancer to turn off pituitary gonadotrophin production and reduce circulating testosterone.
   e. Alcohol   T
   'It provokes the desire, but it takes away the performance' (*Macbeth*, II. iii. 34).

2. Treatments for erectile dysfunction include:
   a. Intravenous injections with papaverine   F
   The papaverine is injected intracorporeally, where its properties as a powerful vasodilator produce an erection over a period of about 20 mins. About 17 per cent of patients experience some discomfort in the penis during erection, and there are other problems such as fibrosis and priapism that make written consent before the procedure, and a low starting dose, worthwhile.
   b. Testosterone implants to increase androgen levels from low-normal to high-normal levels   F
   Unless the patient is profoundly hypogonadal, testosterone has no effect on erectile ability or frequency
   c. Intracorporeal injections with prostaglandins   T
   Alprostadil, prostaglandin E_1 (Caverject®), is now licensed for use in impotence and is likely to become more widely used than papaverine. However, it is expensive (£10/injection), and primary-care physicians may be unwilling to prescribe it.

   d. The use of proprietary creams   F

It probably depends on who rubs it in, but there are no known agents that will effectively produce an erection pharmacologically by this route. Enhanced erectile competence is occasionally experienced as a side-effect of alpha-adrenoreceptor blockers such as doxazosin. Early results of trials in diabetics with erectile dysfunction suggest that Sildenafil®, a cyclic phosphodiesterase inhibitor designed for angina prophylaxis, may be useful taken orally.

   e. Marijuana   F

Impotence is one of the side-effects of this so-called 'harmless' drug.

3. Treatments for drug-induced priapism include:

   a. Running up and down stairs   T

This increases blood flow to the penis and is believed to wash out the vasodilator.

   b. Intravenous injection of alpha-adrenergic stimulants   F

Metaraminol, an alpha-agonist is used, but injected intracorporeally (into the shaft of the penis).

   c. Inserting a 19 g butterfly needle through the glans into one of the corpora cavernosa   T

This is standard treatment, being careful to avoid the urethra, and is carried out without anaesthetic. The resulting shunt from the cavernosa into the spongiosum adds further to the venous drainage.

   d. Surgical decompression   T

This has to be carried out with some haste to prevent the formation.of fibrous tissue that may render the patient impotent subsequently.

   e. Withdrawing blood under gravity flow   T

This may work better than using the syringe piston to generate high negative pressures.

4. In the treatment of erectile dysfunction:

   a. Implants protect the glans from trauma   F

The glans is the distended distal end of the corpus spongiosum. It cannot be made 'rigid' by an implant, and therefore may be subject to trauma during intercourse.

   b. Injections of papaverine or alprostadil (prostaglandin E_1) are made near the glans for best effect   F

They are injected near the base of the penis.

   c. The dose of intracorporeal papaverine is reduced in diabetes   F

The dose tends to be higher. Nevertheless, a low starting dose is advised.

   d. Surgery for venous leaks is commonly carried out   F

Implant surgery is carried out more commonly.

   e. An episode of priapism may render the patient permanently impotent   T

Unless priapism is avoided or dealt with correctly and with due haste, this may indeed occur.

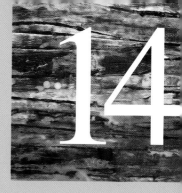

14

Puberty

- Summary

- Introduction

- Mechanisms of puberty

- Key points

- Case history

- Multiple-choice questions

Summary

Normal function

- Attainment of final adult height following the adolescent growth spurt.
- Development of secondary sexual characteristics.
- Achievement of fertility.
- Psychological changes associated with the development of independence.

Typical pathology

- Constitutional delay. Late entry into puberty in a child with no identifiable problems, who subsequently enters and progresses normally through puberty. Constitutional delay may produce adverse psychological effects that persist in the long term. The late rise in sex hormones may also predispose to osteoporosis in later life.
- Being underweight for height tends to delay the onset of pulsatile secretion of GnRH from the hypothalamus.
- Turner's syndrome.

'Typical clinical scenario'

- A short, but otherwise normal-looking 15- or 16-year-old girl with Turner's syndrome, accompanied by her anxious mother or parents. The incidence of Turner's is more than 100-fold higher than that of acromegaly.

Introduction

Entry into puberty and progression through puberty is, for the majority of individuals, a fairly seemless process during which secondary sexual characteristics develop, the adolescent growth spurt occurs, and fertility and independence are achieved.

Pubertal problems are not often encountered by the endocrinologist dealing with adult patients. If the patient with delayed puberty survives the trauma of peer pressure at school and parental anxiety without seeking medical help, he (and they are almost invariably male) is unlikely to present with pubertal failure until his late teens or early twenties. The usual impetus then comes from a rejection by a potential employer, such as the armed forces, on the grounds of lack of pubertal development.

The main diagnostic dilemmas are distinguishing patients with delayed puberty due to occult chronic disease or hypogonadotrophic hypogonadism from those with 'constitutional delay'. Most children with late onset of puberty have constitutional delay, compounded in at least 25 per cent of girls by being underweight for height. Chronic disease and Turner's syndrome account for most of the remainder, along with an increasing number of patients who have been treated for childhood malignancies with radiotherapy or chemotherapy. With the exception of inflammatory bowel disease, gluten-induced enteropathy (coeliac disease), and renal disease, chronic conditions severe enough to cause poor growth or delayed puberty are usually apparent clinically. The prevalence of behavioural problems, family conflict, anxiety, depression, and other neuroses in 'normal' puberty is between 10 and 20 per cent.

Mechanism of puberty

Puberty is a centrally mediated mechanism controlled by changes in feedback sensitivity to testosterone or oestrogen. Immediately prior to the onset of puberty, the sensitivity of gonadotrophin (FSH and LH) production to feedback inhibition by gonadal steroids (testosterone or oestrogen) falls dramatically. As central mechanisms become less sensitive to feedback inhibition, sex hormone levels rise and puberty is entered. The various phenotypic changes of puberty—breast development in girls (thelarche), the development of sexual hair (adrenarche), and the stages of male genital development—are graded '1' (pre-adolescent), to '5' (full adult development). The critical stage is progression from stage 1 to stage 2, i.e. entry into puberty. As puberty approaches, adrenal androgen production begins largely under the control of ACTH. As this is independent of the GnRH mechanisms, premature adrenarche—development of axillary and pubic hair before the age of 8—can be independent of premature puberty.

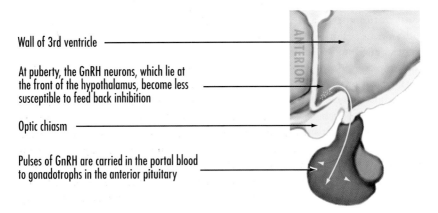

Wall of 3rd ventricle

At puberty, the GnRH neurons, which lie at the front of the hypothalamus, become less susceptible to feed back inhibition

Optic chiasm

Pulses of GnRH are carried in the portal blood to gonadotrophs in the anterior pituitary

ANTERIOR

Fig. 14.1 The pattern of release of hypothalamic gonadotrophin-releasing hormone (GnRH or LHRH—which stimulates FSH and LH release from gonadotrophs) is highly relevant physiologically and therapeutically. It is involved in the control of sexual development and maturation through puberty, and the subsequent attainment of fertility. Pharmacological blockade of the effects of GnRH on gonadotrophs is used in cancer chemotherapy and in the treatment of precocious puberty.

Normal puberty

Table 14.1
The pineal gland

The pineal gland is a small, neurosecretory gland that lies in the midline against the superior colliculi at the back of the midbrain. In lower vertebrates the pineal is light sensitive, but in man this function has been lost. The pineal has sympathetic innervation which is responsible, via an elaborate route, for light-dark entrainment. Its function is not well established in man, but in rodents and other vertebrates the pineal gland is responsible for down-regulation of the gonadal axis and gonadal atrophy that occurs in response to being kept in the dark. The pineal gland produces a number of biologically active peptides in addition to melatonin, a hormone that may set the hypothalamic clock mechanism. During the night, melatonin production and secretion is high. Oral melatonin is said to reduce the effect of jet lag, perhaps by resetting the hypothalamic time clock

Delayed puberty

The age at which investigations are undertaken for delayed puberty depends on the sex of the patient and often on the extent of anxiety engendered in the patient and his or her parents by the perceived delay. In general, the absence of signs of puberty by the age of 13 years in girls or by the age of 15 or 16 years in boys is worthy of further investigation. In most cases, no specific cause will be identified (constitutional delay) and puberty will occur spontaneously.

If no abnormality is identified after taking the history and examining the patient, it is often appropriate to reassure the patient and his or her parents, and observe for 6 months.

Constitutional delay of puberty occurs more commonly in boys rather than girls, who tend to be shorter in stature than their peers at school but otherwise normal in appearance. As growth tends to slow before puberty, they often 'drop off the centiles'. If the delay in physical and mental maturation is clearly causing emotional problems with disruptive behaviour or bullying, boys can be offered one or two courses of intramuscular testosterone enanthate, 125 mg monthly for 4–6 months, or oral oxandrolone 1.5–2.5 mg/day. This treatment 'borrows' height from later on, and has no adverse effects on adult stature. Girls with constitutional delay can be offered a 6–12 month course of ethinyloestradiol, 2–5 μg orally/day.

If signs of puberty regress in either sex after these treatments are stopped, it suggests that the patient has hypogonadotrophic hypogonadism.

If atypical features are evident at the outset, or if growth velocity remains low after 6 months, further investigations may be appropriate (Fig. 14.2).

Table 14.2
Puberty

	Females	Males
Mean age of entry	95 per cent of girls enter puberty between the ages of 8 and 13 years (mean 10.8 years)	95 per cent of boys enter puberty between the age of 9 and 14 years (mean 11.5 years)
First sign	The appearance of breast buds A 'breast bud' is an elevation of the papilla and breast as a small mound. It may be asymmetrical at first	Growth of the testes and scrotum When the testes exceed 4 ml in volume (2.4 cm length), pubertal enlargement has begun
Stages	Breast buds (stage 2) 8.9–12.9 years (may be asymmetrical at first), and menarche 12.7 ± 1.9 years, typically when weight reaches 48 kg (7.5 stone). The appearance of sexual pubic hair at a mean of 11.9 ± 2.2 years, is not an event of much importance	Testes 4 ml (stage 2) 11.5 ± 2 years, sexual pubic hair 13.1 ± 2 years, testes ≥ 12 ml, 14 ± 2.5 years
Age of peak growth velocity	Girls grow fastest at the beginning of puberty, with peak velocity occurring at, or soon after the breast bud stage, usually at around 12 years of age	Boys grow fastest at the end of puberty. Velocity peaks at age 14. A rapid increase in shoe size often heralds the onset of the growth spurt
Duration	Between 2 and 5 years (mean 4.2 years)	Between 2 and 6 years (mean 3.5 years)
Prevalence of constitutional delay	Uncommon If there is no sign of breast buds by 13 years, they should be investigated	Common Even to the age of 17, investigation is not required unless there are other clinical indications

Table 14.3
Delayed puberty

Girls ≥13 years History Boys ≥16 years	Examination
Is there a family history of late puberty?	Is the patient's general appearance normal?
Is there evidence of chronic diseases such as asthma?	Is the standing height and weight normal?
Is the patient slimming or weight watching?	In oncology patients, is the sitting height normal?
Is there any evidence of emotional deprivation?	Are the testes and phallus size normal?
Is the patient keeping up intellectually at school?	Is breast shape and the amount of glandular tissue normal?
Does the patient enjoy much strenuous physical activity?	Is the sense of smell normal?

THYROID FUNCTION	FSH & PROLACTIN		SCREEN FOR OCCULT DISEASE	KARYOTYPE
HYPOTHYROIDISM Low FT4 (with high TSH unless there is a pituitary or hypothalamic problem)	**HYPERGONADOTROPHIC HYPOGONADISM** FSH & LH high. A pelvic ultrasound is useful in females	**HYPOGONADOTROPHIC HYPOGONADISM** FSH, LH & gonadal hormones low	**OCCULT CHRONIC DISEASE** CRP, Creatinine, Antigliadin antibodies Bicarbonate & Potassium	**ANEUPLOIDY** particularly important in females with pubertal delay

HYPOTHYROIDISM	FUNCTIONAL	TO EXCLUDE....	TURNER'S SUNDROME
• These children often appear rather porcine, facially, and 'square built', as reduction in height velocity usually exceeds reduction in weight gain. • The replacement dose of T4 in children is similar to that of adults ie. high on wt/wt basis	• Puberty does not usually commence until body weight reaches a critical mass - 48kg. • Reversible hypogonadotrophic hypogonadism can be caused by a ≥ 5-10% weight-for-height deficit • Strenuous physical activity	• Crohn's disease • Coeliac disease • Impaired renal glomerular or tubular function • Renal tubular acidosis & • Bartter's syndrome.	• 1 in 2,500 live births • Usually < 5' tall. • Sparse pubic hair • Little breast development • In 10%, puberty & menarche can occur, and in ≤ 1%, pregnancy, depending on the extent of X chromosome deletion.

GONADAL FAILURE	OTHER		KLINEFELTER'S SYNDROME
• Chemotherapy or radiotherapy • Turner's syndrome • Klinefelter's syndrome • Primary testicular failure • Gonadal dysgenesis measuring gonadal hormones is often unhelpful	• Idiopathic hypogonadotrophic hypogonadism (Kallman's:1 in 7500 males, 1:50,000 females) • Hypothalamic tumours ie. Craniopharyngiomas Astrocytomas & Gliomas • Prolactinomas in this age group are very rare		• 1:500 live births • Small, firm testes ≤ 3.5cm long • Small phallus • Gynaecomastia in 50% • Eunuchoid proportions • Often disproportionately tall.

Fig. 14.2 Investigation of pubertal delay.

Table 14.4
Precocious sexual maturation (girls ≤8 years; boys ≤9 years)

Characteristics

Precocious puberty, early activation of the hypothalamic pituitary gonadal axis, is 10 times more common in girls than boys

In girls it is usually idiopathic (66 per cent), but in girls under 3 years old, between 30 and 50 per cent have hamartomas of the posterior hypothalamus

It is more common in children who have had cerebral insults, or who have malformation of the brain of any kind

In boys it is more sinister: 80 per cent result from hypothalamic tumours and a further 5 per cent from congenital adrenal hyperplasia. It is rarely idiopathic

Premature thelarche (breast development) is oestrogen dependent and occurs in isolation in 1:5000 children

Premature pubarche or adrenarch (appearance of pubic or axillary hair) is an adrenal androgen-dependent phenomenon that can occur in isolation, i.e. without any other evidence of puberty

Investigations

MRI scan of the brain in boys and in those girls with new CNS signs or symptoms

Pelvic ultrasound in girls to confirm an increase in size of both ovaries (≥1–2 ml volume)

Before using a long-acting GnRH analogue to inhibit puberty, it is appropriate to:

1. check baseline bone age so that the effectiveness of treatment can be monitored;

2. carry out a GnRH test (100 μg of GnRH iv) to confirm that there is the expected increase in gonadotrophin release (LH usually rising to ≥7.6 iu/l within 20–30 min)

Treatment

Treatment depends on the primary problem

To inhibit puberty, a long-acting GnRH analogue is given.

Consequences

Excessive height early on is followed by short stature, as bone age can advance exceedingly rapidly—by as much as a year every month or two

The onset of behavioural problems associated with puberty also occur prematurely and can severely disrupts family life.

Precocious puberty

This term implies activation of the normal hypothalamic pituitary axis at an abnormally young age. In boys, this is spermatogenesis before the age of 9 years, and in girls, cyclical ovarian activity and menstruation before the age of 8 years. It is caused by premature activation of cyclical GnRH secretion by the hypothalamus, the cause of which may or may not be identifiable. When no cause is identified, the condition is called 'idiopathic sexual precocity', and premature sexual development resulting from the primary secretion of androgens or oestrogens by tumours (with low gonadotrophins) is termed 'pseudoprecocious puberty'.

Key points

- Delayed puberty is usually constitutional.
- If there is no sign of breast bud development (elevation of breast and papilla as a small mound) by the age of 13 in girls, they should be investigated.
- The first sign of puberty in boys is an increase in testicular size to 4 ml.
- Formal investigation of delayed puberty in boys, if there is no obvious illness or abnormality, can often be delayed until they are 16 years old or even later.
- Unless there is an obvious cause of sexual precocity, such as central nervous system trauma, precocious sexual maturation needs investigation.

'My patient is 16 years old. She has no signs of puberty. Please advise'

History

The 16-year-old patient appeared to be fairly indifferent, but clear evidence of puberty in her younger sister (age 11) had finally driven her mother to seek medical advice for short stature and delayed puberty on her behalf. There was no history of ill health or school problems, and no family history of delayed puberty or social problems. She was now one of the shortest in the class.

Examination

The patient was $4'11\frac{1}{2}''$ tall (1.51 m) and appeared normal but pre-pubertal, with no evidence of breast development and rather sparse pubic hair. Her mother and father were 1.63 m $(5'4'')$ and 1.78 m $(5'10'')$, respectively.

Investigations

FSH was 12 U/l (normal range 1–9 U/l) with an LH of 16 U/l (normal range 3–8 U/l) and oestradiol < 50 pmol/l (normal range 110–180 pmol/l follicular and 550–850 pmol/l luteal). Karyotype analysis identified a partial deletion of the long arm of her X chromosome rather than the classical 'XO' genotype. Further investigations consisted of an radiograph of her wrist, which showed almost complete epiphyseal fusion, and an abdominal ultrasound which identified small, but otherwise normal-looking, ovaries, one of which contained a single, small follicle.

Management

The nature of Turner's syndrome was sympathetically explained to the patient and her mother. Sex hormone replacement therapy in the form of low-dose oestradiol (increasing gradually from 2 μg daily) was initiated to take her through puberty, with a view to continuing treatment in the longer term. Her mother was particularly concerned about the prospects of fertility. Advice from a medical geneticist was sought and in this particular case, the degree of partial X chromosome deletion was estimated to give the patient a small chance of spontaneous fertility. The possibility of ovum donation for future fertility was raised. Her mother immediately volunteered but was told that thus far, successful cryopreservation of unfertilized ova has not been achieved. In view of the patient's relatively advanced bone age, growth hormone treatment was not considered a useful option in this case.

Explanation

The classical Turner's syndrome phenotype of short stature, increased carrying angle (cubitus valgus), webbed neck, absence of breast development (shield chest), short neck, low posterior hair line, and short fourth metacarpal become more pronounced as the length of X chromosome long-arm deletion increases. In many cases the diagnosis is made at birth or in early childhood as a result of lymphoedema. These children are successfully treated with growth hormone, and later, oestrogen and progesterone to achieve an acceptable adult height and transition through puberty at an appropriate age. Fertility is usually not achieved, unless the length of X chromosome deletion is very small.

Multiple-choice questions

1. Puberty:
   a. The mean age of onset of puberty is earlier in males than females;
   b. Puberty is characterized in girls by an early growth spurt;
   c. The average height added during the growth spurt (including the year either side) in boys is about 30 cm (1 foot);
   d. The first sign of normal puberty in girls is the appearance of fine pubic hair around the labia;
   e. The first sign of puberty in boys is elongation of the phallus.

2. In delayed puberty:
   a. The absence of signs of puberty in either sex by the age of 15 warrants investigation;
   b. Constitutional delay is the most common 'cause';
   c. Oral androgens can be useful in advancing the signs of puberty in boys who are being teased at school;
   d. The bone age is often delayed;
   e. It may be worth asking patients if they have a sense of smell.

3. Causes of delayed puberty include:
   a. McCune–Albright syndrome: polyostotic fibrous dysplasia, café au lait spots, etc.;
   b. Neonatal hydrocephalus;
   c. Hypogonadotrophic hypogonadism;
   d. Turner's syndrome;
   e. Crohn's disease.

4. Common investigations in the diagnosis of causes of delayed puberty include:
   a. MRI scan of pituitary and hypothalamus;
   b. Antigliadin antibodies;
   c. Karyotype;
   d. Gonadal ultrasound;
   e. Gonadotrophins.

Answers

1. Puberty:
   a. The mean age of onset of puberty is earlier in males than females   F
   The mean age in boys is 11.5 years and in girls 10.8 years.
   b. Puberty is characterized in girls by an early growth spurt   T
   In boys, the growth spurt occurs near the end of puberty.
   c. The average height added during the growth spurt (including the year either side) in boys is about 30 cm (1 foot)   F
   It is less than this in both sexes—about 23 cm (just over 9″) in boys and 20 cm (just under 8″) in girls.

    d. The first sign of normal puberty in girls is the appearance of fine pubic hair around the labia   F

        Breast 'buds' are usually the first sign of normal puberty in girls.

    e. The first sign of puberty in boys is elongation of the phallus   F

        Elongation of the phallus, increased scrotal rugosity, and other signs of puberty are androgen-dependent, and as androgens come from the testes, it is testicular enlargement that precedes other changes.

2. In delayed puberty:

    a. The absence of signs of puberty in either sex by the age of 15 warrants investigation   F

        Certainly in girls, investigation would be warranted, but in boys, this is not too unusual, and it might be worth waiting a little longer.

    b. Constitutional delay is the most common 'cause'   T

        In most cases, no cause is found for delayed puberty and the child enters puberty spontaneously without recourse to unpleasant and unhelpful investigations.

    c. Oral androgens can be useful in advancing the signs of puberty in boys who are being teased at school   T

        Worries about the effects of low-dose androgens on final height have not been substantiated, and the effect of oral oxandrolone is to 'borrow height' from later on.

    d. The bone age is often delayed: T

        Many textbooks suggest that in 'constitutional delay of puberty', bone age and chronological age coincide. However, the statistical link between bone age and puberty is poor. At the onset of puberty, bone age in girls is on average lower than that in boys. Bone age can be 3 or even 4 years retarded in constitutional delay of puberty, and is frequently 2 years behind chronological age in patients who present with short stature.

    e. It may be worth asking patients if they have a sense of smell   T

        Kallmann's syndrome is hypogonadotrophic hypogonadism. Eighty-five per cent of patients are anosmic. The male to female ratio is 5:1, and the incidence about one-third that of Turner's syndrome.

3. Causes of delayed puberty include:

    a. McCune–Albright syndrome: polyostotic fibrous dysplasia, café au lait spots, etc.   F

        The third of the triad of signs is isosexual (i.e. appropriate for phenotype) precocious puberty. Interestingly, the mutation responsible for this (the *gsp* oncogene) is the same as that found in 40 per cent of somatotroph adenomas. The difference is that in McCune–Albright syndrome, the mutation occurs early on in fetal life and is found in a number of different tissues rather than just pituitary adenoma cells.

    b. Neonatal hydrocephalus   F

This tends to cause precocious puberty. Trauma to the central nervous system at birth or during early childhood is one of the most common causes of precocious puberty. A careful history should be taken to disclose these problems.

    c. Hypogonadotrophic hypogonadism   T

Of course. No gonadotrophins (FSH and LH) = no gonadal function.

    d. Turner's syndrome   T

Ovarian development is impaired (streak ovaries) in the full-blown syndrome, and ovarian function may be compromised if only part of one X chromosome is missing.

    e. Crohn's disease   T

Any chronic, active condition that causes systemic disturbance, such as asthma or inflammatory bowel disease, can delay puberty.

4. Common investigations in the diagnosis of causes of delayed puberty include:

    a. MRI scan of pituitary and hypothalamus   F

This is not usually necessary.

    b. Antigliadin antibodies   T

Coeliac disease (gluten-induced enteropathy) can be occult.

    c. Karyotype   T

Turner's syndrome and Klinefelter's syndrome are relatively common. Deletions of part of an X chromosome in Turner's syndrome can affect puberty and fertility. Other, more typical phenotypic characteristics, such as neck webbing, may be absent.

    d. Gonadal ultrasound   F

This is rarely necessary. The functional state of the gonads can be determined by physical examination, karyotype, and gonadotrophin estimation.

    e. Gonadotrophins   T

FSH and LH levels can be very informative in this situation. If the gonadotrophins are high, but there is no sign of puberty, this would suggest primary gonadal failure.

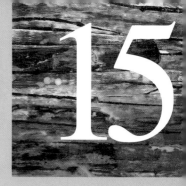

15

Short and tall stature

- Summary

- Introduction

- Assessment

- Growth hormone deficiency

- Excessive height

- Key points

- Case history

- Multiple-choice questions

Summary

Normal function of growth

- To allow a child to achieve his or her full genetic growth potential.
- To allow a child to attain an adult stature that does not impede the achievement of his or her chosen roll in life and in society.

Typical pathology

- Short stature
    → Idiopathic pubertal delay. Adolescent boys 'temporarily left behind' by their peers in terms of height, physical development and emotional maturity.
    → Turner's syndrome.

'Typical clinical scenario'

- A short teenager referred on from the paediatric clinic, who is currently receiving daily growth hormone injections. According to his latest bone age estimate, there is very little growth potential left.

Introduction

Short stature, a height more than two standard deviations below the mean for age, is a major social disadvantage. The usual causes are short parents, poor nutrition, social or emotional deprivation, or chronic conditions such as coeliac disease, renal impairment, asthma or colitis. Growth hormone deficiency as a cause of short stature is quite rare and, even when identified and treated appropriately, achievement of an acceptable adult height is far from certain.

Table 15.1
The insulin-like growth factors

Although there are growth hormone receptors in many tissues, most of the body's response to GH occurs through the intermediary of the insulin-like growth factors (IGFs, formerly somatomedins), which are produced in response to GH. Both IGF-I and IGF-II (which is not under the control of GH), are single-chain peptides, but otherwise similar in structure to insulin. These growth factors are bound to specific binding proteins in the plasma, but are cleaved to the active peptide at tissue level. IGF-I levels are increased in acromegaly and decreased in liver disease, cachexia, and hypopituitarism

Table 15.2
Short stature

History	Rationale
Parental height	Although a child can be expected to grow along the percentile tramlines defined in the '1990 Nine Centile UK Charts', and has a 95 per cent probability of achieving a final height within 8.5 cm of the height predicted from the mean parental height (predicted height = (maternal + paternal height) cm/2 + 9.5 cm for boys or -9.5 cm for girls), it should be borne in mind that some familial conditions can lead to treatable short stature. On average, the parents of GH-deficient children are slightly shorter than normal
Birth weight and mode; perinatal problems; school record	A history of perinatal asphyxia or breech delivery is more common in patients with growth hormone deficiency secondary to hypothalamic malfunction than in controls. For reasons that are unclear, both mental retardation and low birth weight are associated with short stature
Growth history and milestones	As human growth is at the best of times a little slow, any reliable data of earlier heights and weights, or comparisons with peer groups is useful
History of chronic disease	Asthma, cystic fibrosis, or severe eczema are usually obvious. Chronic renal failure and Crohn's disease can be more difficult to diagnose, and coeliac disease can be so subtle that only a jejunal biopsy reveals the diagnosis. A history of polyuria, nocturia, or polydypsia, suggesting renal failure, should be sought
Nutritional history	Anorexia nervosa and other causes of nutritional deficiency are potent causes of short stature. Adoption of a more Western' diet has dramatically increased the mean stature of the Japanese
Pubertal stage; age of entry into puberty	Precocious puberty, although causing an initial increase in growth rate, results in a very rapid advancement of bone age that limits final adult height
Social circumstances	Psychosocial problems and emotional deprivation limit height

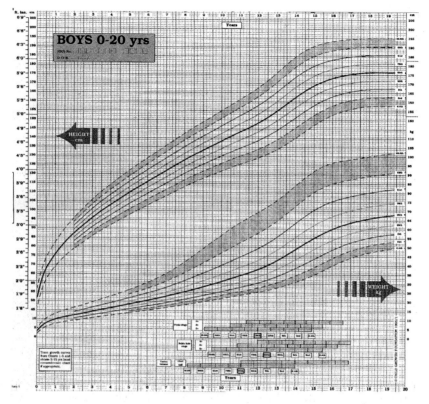

Fig. 15.1 An example of one of the new 'nine-centile' charts designed and published by the Child Growth Foundation (©), London, available from Harlow Printing Ltd, Tyne and Wear, UK.

Assessment

Up-to-date centile charts of stature and growth velocity derived from an appropriate population are vital for the assessment of growth, as growth through childhood from the age of 2 until puberty, although variable in absolute terms, is remarkably stable within a percentile channel. Boys enter puberty later than girls and achieve peak velocity at a mean of 14 years rather than 12 years. This allows for a more prolonged period of pre-pubertal growth (which mostly affects the limbs) followed by a more intense growth spurt, which adds, on average, 23 cm (peak velocity 10 cm/year) to male adult height compared to 20 cm (peak velocity 9 cm/year) in girls. Together these account for the greater mean adult height in men. Careful measurements of height and growth rate (i.e. auxological data) are indispensable in diagnosing GH deficiency, and are more useful than laboratory tests of induced GH secretion, which are uncomfortable, arbitrary, and not without risk. The diagnosis of GH deficiency is based on short stature and slow growth velocity in the absence of any other independent treatable abnormalities.

Measuring height

Carried out with care at approximately the same time of day using a stadiometer checked for accuracy on a daily basis, this critical measurement should be reproducible to within 3 mm or so. Without shoes, and with heels, bottom, and

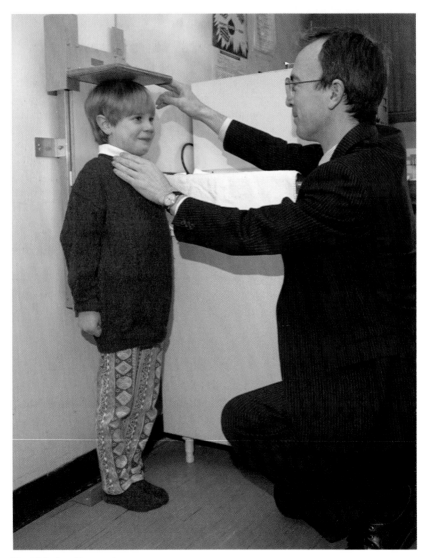

Fig. 15.2 A stadiometer in use.

shoulders touching the back plate, the head is positioned so that a line joining the lower border of the eye socket and the external auditory meatus is horizontal (90° to the stadiometer) (Fig. 15.2). The platen is then gently lowered once or twice to touch the vertex, and the height read off. Sitting height is estimated by having the patient sit against the stadiometer on a stool of known height. Body weight should be related to height rather than chronological age. The standard clinic weighing machine with a (loose) wooden bar, while adequate for estimating body mass index in a diabetic clinic, is a positive impediment to the assessment and treatment of disorders of growth.

Growth hormone deficiency

Idiopathic growth hormone deficiency is an unusual cause of short stature, affecting approximately 1 in 5000 children. The duration of GH treatment before puberty and the mean frequency of GH injections are good independent predictors of outcome in GH-deficient children. It is not surprising, therefore, that if therapy is delayed until the age of 8, achievement of normal adult height is unusual. However, with appropriate treatment the median final height in children entering puberty spontaneously is above −1.5 SD, and this is further increased to only 0.6 SD below normal in children requiring induction of puberty, as the treatment duration can be increased.

Treatment

Treat underlying problems. The replacement dose of thyroxine in children is surprisingly high—about 125 μg daily, and in very young children and neonates the dose on a weight-to-weight basis is even higher (up to 8 μg/kg daily). In true GH deficiency, weight-adjusted replacement doses are given as single daily injections (0.5–0.7 U/kg.week). The potential benefit of GH treatment must be

Table 15.3
Characteristics of GH deficiency

Incidence is 1 in 4–10 000 children

Often grow ≤3 cm/year

Progressively fall off the centiles

Overweight for height (abdominal obesity)

Often have a micro-phallus if onset early in life

Midline fusion defects and visual problems are common

Small or triangular face

Even with treatment, normal adult height may not be achieved

Table 15.4
Growth hormone stimulation tests

The diagnosis of GH deficiency is made on the basis of short stature and slow growth, with no other abnormality found

There is no 'gold standard' test

There are over 34 different GH stimulation tests in current use. In the UK, a combination of insulin and arginine tests are used more frequently, but none is well validated. In each, a GH of <10–15 mU/l is probably deficient; 17–20 mU/l, borderline and >20 mU/l normal	L-Arginine 0.5 g/kg over 30 min iv: measure GH after 1 h and 2 h
	Insulin-induced hypoglycaemia (glucose ≤2 mmol/l)
	Exercising to exhaustion increases GH in 70 per cent of normal children
	GH 1 h after the onset of sleep: >19 mU/l in 60 per cent of normals
	Clonidine, $4\mu g$/kg orally: measure GH after 1 h and 2 h

Table 15.5
Investigations for short stature

Height	Tests	Rationale
AT OR ABOVE THE 2nd PERCENTILE (WITHIN 2SD OF MEAN - OLD CHARTS) Looks normal, growing normally	No investigations	Although the chance of finding an organic problem is small, a careful history may reveal other problems at home. If signs of puberty are present in teenage boys with short stature, they can usually be reassured that their growth spurt will allow them to catch up.
BELOW THE 2nd PERCENTILE LINE (BETWEEN 2 & 3 SD OF MEAN - OLD CHARTS) Analyse growth from all available data	Urinalysis & U&E + bicarbonate	These would allow chronic renal problems, such as renal acidosis & Bartter's syndrome (see page 100) to be identified.
	Calcium, phosphate & alkaline phosphatase	These help identify pseudohypoparathyroidism, malnutrition or malabsorption leading to subclinical rickets. The absence of antigliadin antibodies make coeliac disease unlikely.
	TSH, FT3 & FT4	Hypothyroidism usually, but not invariably, leads to a short, plump child, as linear growth tends to be retarded more than weight gain.
	FBC, ESR, B12 & folate	Malabsorption, inflammatory bowel disease & haemoglobinopathies such as sickle cell anaemia should be disclosed by these tests.
	IGF-I	IGFI is of limited value. It is thought to be an index of GH secretion & nutrition, & tends to match bone age. A level of ≤ 1U/mL in early puberty or 1.5U/mL at mid-puberty is probably abnormal.
	Bone age (X-ray of left hand & wrist)	Bone age allows growth potential to be assessed, but is not very useful diagnostically as bone age & height are often retarded by the same disorder. If bone age & chronological age match, however, GH deficiency is unlikely.
	Karyotype if female	Depending on the amount of X chromosome missing, girls with Turner's syndrome may be phenotypically normal, apart from short stature. Other genetic anomalies can also cause short stature, but associated problems are usually of much greater consequence.
BELOW THE 0.4th PERCENTILE LINE (> 3 SD BELOW MEAN HEIGHT FOR AGE - OLD CHARTS, or VELOCITY LESS THAN 25th PERCENTILE FOR AGE)	Assess pituitary growth hormone reserves in addition to the above.	Many different tests are used to assess pituitary GH reserves (see page 232). In small children who are growing slowly, a rapid increase in growth velocity in response to GH treatment is a reassuring confirmatory sign of GH deficiency.

weighed up against the trauma of chronic daily injection and cost. In young children, GH treatment is economical because the response is often better and their body mass (and therefore the total dose of the peptide required) is smaller.

In Turner's syndrome, GH therapy (at a slightly higher dose than above— 1 U/kg.week) accelerates growth and adds, on average, about 6 cm to adult height. It also allows sex hormone replacement therapy to be introduced at a more appropriate time, without worrying about further compromising growth. Short children who are otherwise normal do not respond well to GH. Although growth may be more rapid initially, there is little evidence that final adult height is increased.

Excessive height

Although there are as many cases of constitutional tall stature as there are short, the same social stigma is not attached and patients are rarely referred to the endocrine clinic. Tall parents is the most common cause, but chromosomal problems such as XXY (Klinefelter's) or XYY, thyrotoxicosis, Marfan's syndrome, and homocystinuria should be considered. Tall stature from GH excess—pituitary gigantism—is very rare. Most pathological causes of tall stature are associated with reduced body mass index. Tall, fat children are almost always the result of overnutrition.

If the problem is identified in time, sex steroids can be given to advance the growth spurt and reduce adult height.

Key points

- Short stature resulting from growth hormone deficiency is rare.
- A child who is below the 0.4th percentile (more than 3 SD below mean height for age), has a 50 per cent chance of having organic disease.
- In establishing the diagnosis of GH deficiency, basal GH levels are one of the least helpful parameters.
- Bone age allows growth potential to be assessed.

'My 3-year-old son is short'

History

The patient was 3 years and 1 month old. His father explained that James was already the shortest in his infant school class and that as he, too, was short and bullied at school, he did not want the same to happen to his son. Both parents had heard about growth hormone and wondered if it would help. James's two elder siblings were normal height for age. Pregnancy had apparently been uneventful, and delivery of a healthy baby, weighing 6 lb 13 oz, straightforward. Like his siblings, James had had a few chest infections and the odd bout of diarrhoea, but no other significant problems.

Examination

The father was 5′ 3½″ (161 cm) (measured in clinic) and his wife, 5′ 5″ (165 cm) (according to the father). Unfortunately, no previous height information was available for the patient, but on the day he attended clinic, he was accurately measured at 2′ 10½″ (88 cm), i.e. just above the 3rd percentile. James appeared to be completely normal, with nothing to suggest a chronic disease. Overall he seemed happy and healthy.

Management

The following explanation was offered to his parents. First, growth hormone treatment does not work well in normal children, and James was very likely to be normal. It was also pointed out that growth hormone treatment may be counter-productive, as giving a child daily injections for a number of years is not a 'no lose situation'. No investigations were carried out. The plan was to see them again in 4 months so that growth velocity could be estimated. At the second appointment, James's height was 90 cm and he was clearly tracking along the 3rd percentile. His parents were less willing to accept the 'no treatment' option, however, and would not be reassured without 'investigations'. These included a full blood count, B_{12} and folate, urea, creatinine and electrolytes, bicarbonate, calcium, phosphate, viscosity, and thyroid function tests, all of which were normal.

Explanation

The mean parental height was 163 cm, and the expected adult height for the patient 5′ 8″ (172.5 cm, ~35th percentile (163 + 9.5 cm)). Although the patient was more than 2 SD below the mean for his age, he looked healthy. There is probably very little to gain from treating normal children with growth hormone. Had he been falling off the percentiles, however, a therapeutic trial with growth hormone might have been appropriate.

Multiple-choice questions

1. In GH deficiency:
   a. The parents of children with GH deficiency are often smaller than average;
   b. An injection of GH three times per week is now considered inadequate;
   c. A growth hormone series (GH levels every 30 min throughout the day) and IGF-I levels provide an accurate estimate of GH status;
   d. There is an association with hearing impairment;
   e. GH therapy results in normal or near normal height.

2. Causes of short stature include:
   a. Klinefelter's syndrome;
   b. Osteoporosis;
   c. Coeliac disease;
   d. Overnutrition;
   e. Intrauterine growth retardation.

3. Adult stature is reduced by:
   a. Having parents who smoke;
   b. Measles;
   c. Being fostered;
   d. Chronic, poorly controlled asthma in childhood;
   e. Premature puberty.

4. Growth in stature:
   a. Tends to track within the centile tramlines after the age of 2 years;
   b. Occurs in small microspurts interspersed with periods of absent growth;
   c. Measurements are made in stockinged rather than bare feet;
   d. Often occurs in adulthood;
   e. *In utero* is GH dependent.

Answers

1. In GH deficiency:
   a. The parents of children with GH deficiency are often smaller than average T
      The mid-parental height turns out to be about 0.5 SD below the mean. This needs to be kept in mind when the height outcome of GH-deficient children is considered.
   b. An injection of GH three times per week is now considered inadequate T
      Treatment is now carried out with daily injections.
   c. A growth hormone series (GH levels every 30 min throughout the day) and IGF-I levels provide an accurate estimate of GH status F
      The diagnosis of GH deficiency is auxological, i.e. dependent on measurements of height and calculations of growth velocity. Short stature and slow growth in the absence of any other causes are the signs to look for. There are at least 34 different provocative tests of GH secretion in use at the present time. In the future it might be that IGF-I and IGFBP-3, which are reduced in unequivocal GH deficiency, may reflect GH status more accurately than provocative tests. At present, however, it should be borne in mind that 18 per cent of those with 'unequivocally low GH levels' are 'normal' on retesting.
   d. There is an association with hearing impairment F
      There is an association of GH deficiency with visual impairment—the same midline fusion defects presumably being responsible for developmental problems involving both the visual pathway and pituitary.
   e. GH therapy results in normal or near normal height F
      It is unusual for GH therapy to be started early enough and aggressively enough to achieve genetic height potential. Until the recommended frequency of GH injections was increased, only 50 per cent of boys and 15 per cent of girls achieved an adult height above the 3rd percentile.

2. Causes of short stature include:
   a. Klinefelter's syndrome   F
      These patients tend to be on the tall side, as puberty is often delayed and they have more time to grow before their reduced androgen levels fuse their epiphyses.
   b. Osteoporosis   T
      Several inches can be lost in recurrent spinal fractures due to osteoporosis. Therefore, strictly speaking, a patient who was merely rather petite before, could be reduced to the 'short stature range'.
   c. Coeliac disease   T
      Any chronic disease can reduce growth. Total body irradiation for leukaemia in childhood, for example, can cause short stature through adverse effects on spinal growth and pituitary function, and by pre-disposing to premature puberty. Chemotherapy for leukaemias does not seem to produce much reduction in height, however, as the children are so ill that their bone age does not advance during treatment.
   d. Overnutrition   F
      This probably has little bearing on final adult height, but if anything tends to be associated with excessive height (and weight) early on.
   e. Intrauterine growth retardation   T
      Although there is some 'catch up' growth in these babies, they are, on average, smaller than their normal-sized peers. There is also a phenomenon of 'catch down' growth in particularly large babies.

3. Adult stature is reduced by:
   a. Having parents who smoke   T
      Passive smoking *in utero* and in childhood reduces final adult height.
   b. Measles   T
      Major childhood infections such as measles, are thought to reduce final adult height by as much as 25 mm, even in those who recover fairly rapidly from the condition.
   c. Being fostered   T
      Emotional and psychosocial deprivation are potent causes of short stature.
   d. Chronic, poorly controlled asthma in childhood   T
      Many chronic diseases can do this.
   e. Premature puberty   T
      Although these children may tower over their peers in childhood because their growth spurt is advanced, their bone age races ahead so that their metaphyses fuse early.

4. Growth in stature
   a. Tends to track within the centile tramlines after the age of 2 years   T
   b. Occurs in small microspurts interspersed with periods of absent growth   T
      When extremely careful measurements are taken, this pattern of growth in childhood seems to be normal.

c. Measurements are made in stockinged rather than bare feet   T

This is acceptable, but the measurement of growth should not be delegated to inadequately trained personnel, as inaccurate records can greatly complicate diagnosis and obscure the response to treatment.

d. Often occurs in adulthood   F

It is very rare for this to happen in man because sex hormones induce metaphyseal fusion. If, however, a patient has a somatotroph adenoma (secreting GH), that also compresses the normal pituitary and results in concurrent hypogonadotrophic hypogonadism, there will be a continual supply of GH and no male hormone to bring about bone fusion. The result is gigantism, an extremely rare condition characterized by very long limbs (GH dependent) but, as sex hormone-dependent spinal growth is reduced, a fairly normal sitting height.

e. *In utero* is GH dependent   F

We are not sure how this happens, but it appears to be independent of both sex hormones and GH.

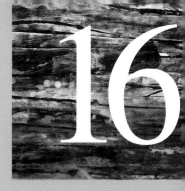

Food and energy

- Summary

- Introduction

- Metabolism of food

- Obesity

- Key points

- Case history

- Multiple-choice questions

Summary

Normal function

- The normal function of hunger and satiety is to induce an individual to consume an amount of food consistent with health.

Typical pathology

- Obesity
  - → Patients who believe that metabolic rather than dietary factors are responsible for their ectomorphic physique.
  - → Patients with hirsutism, oligomenorrhoea, and insulin resistance related to polycystic ovarian disease.
  - → Poorly controlled, non-insulin-dependent diabetics who continue to put on weight.
  - →Patients with hypothalamic damage following transcranial, subfrontal surgery.
- Underweight
  - → Patients who are 'fashionably slim' and develop hypothalamically mediated amenorrhoea.
  - → Thyrotoxic patients who lose weight despite an increase in appetite.

'Typical clinical scenario'

- An obese, middle-aged woman who categorically denies past or present excessive calorie intake, and who has been referred so that 'a glandular problem' as a cause of obesity can be excluded. With the possible exception of hypothyroidism, primary endocrine problems such as Cushing's syndrome leading to a presentation with weight gain are rare.

  In clinical terms, the way food is handled biochemically is of little practical significance. The long-term outcome of medical and/or dietary treatment for obesity is disappointing, as hunger and eating are closely allied to pain and pleasure, respectively.

Introduction

Food has important social, symbolic, and metabolic functions, and the sensation of hunger is highly successful in inducing people to seek food, or, in the case of neonates and young children, to have someone seek food on their behalf. Being able to consume the food you choose as often as you would like to, is for many people the epitome of affluence and social well-being. Partly as a consequence of this, the prevalence of young women trying to lose weight is always substantial, and the proportion of endocrine causes of obesity, minimal.

Table 16.1
Major peptide hormones produced by the gastrointestinal tract

The total mass of endocrine cells in the gastrointestinal tract exceeds that of all other endocrine tissue combined. Many of the gut peptide hormones are produced by a number of different tissues both within and outside the gastrointestinal tract. They are often present in more than one molecular form and tend to have multiple actions, including in some cases (such as somatostatin) those of peptidergic neurotransmitters

Secretin holds the distinction of being the first substance to be identified as a hormone. It is released from the duodenal and jejunal mucosa in response to food and the resulting increase in acid secretion. It is the most powerful stimulant of water and bicarbonate secretion by the pancreas

Gastrin is produced by small clusters of cells within the gastric antrum and released in response to food intake (particularly protein) and vagal stimulation. It stimulates gastric acid and intrinsic factor release from parietal cells of the stomach, and pepsin release from the gastric mucosa. It has other, less powerful, actions on smooth muscle which result in slowing of gastric emptying

Cholecystokinin–pancreozymin (CCK) duplicates many of the actions of gastrin. It is released from the duodenal and jejunal mucosa in response to gastric acid, long-chain fatty acids, and some of the essential amino acids. Its principal actions are stimulation of pancreatic enzyme secretion and gallbladder contraction. Release of CCK is inhibited by somatostatin—explaining the cholestasis and increase in gallstone formation in patients treated with somatostatin analogues

Vasoactive intestinal polypeptide (VIP), released from the pancreas in response to parasympathetic stimulation, enhances the effect of secretin

Somatostatin inhibits the secretion of multiple hormones and is produced by a number of tissues throughout the body, including the hypothalamus, pancreas, and the antral mucosal endocrine cells of the stomach. Paracrine effects of somatostatin produced by the latter are thought to inhibit gastrin secretion

As much of life revolves directly or indirectly around the acquisition, preparation, and consumption of food, it is not surprising that the long-term outcome of medical and/or dietary treatment for obesity is almost always disappointing. For the endocrinologist, dietary manipulation is often one of the most difficult and frustrating aspects of the management of hyperlipidaemia, diabetes mellitus, polycystic ovarian disease in obese patients, and delayed puberty or amenorrhoea in underweight girls or women.

In clinical terms, the way food is handled biochemically is of little practical significance. Water, a source of energy, nine essential amino acids, two fatty acids, 13 vitamins, and 15 inorganic compounds are all that are necessary for health. The minimal amount of each is the 'requirement', and as this is believed to vary somewhat between individuals, (Table 16.2) the 'recommended amount' exceeds the 'requirement' by a modest safety margin.

Table 16.2
Important nutrient requirements

Nutrient	Average requirement	Effects of insufficiency	Notes
Vitamin A	0.9 mg/day	Xerophthalmia, follicular hyperkeratosis	High levels found in liver, fish, and carrots, and added by law to margarines
Vitamin D	5–10 μg/day	Rickets and growth failure in children. Osteomalacea in adults	Excess causes hypercalcaemia and renal impairment. Found in fish and dairy products
Vitamin C	60 mg/day	Scurvy, characterized by extensive petechiae and bruising, and bleeding gums	Widely distributed but labile in storage and cooking
Vitamin B$_{12}$	3 μg/day	Pernicious anaemia, subacute combined degeneration	Found in liver, cheese, eggs, beef
Calcium	0.8–1.2 g/day	Rickets, growth failure, osteomalacea	High levels found in sardines, milk, cheese, and white (but not wholemeal) bread
Folic acid	0.4 mg/day	Pernicious anaemia	Widely distributed
Iron	10–18 mg/day	Anaemia	Liver, kidney, and wholemeal bread
Thiamin	1–1.5 mg/day	Beriberi—muscle aching and weakness. Cardiomyopathy	Found in most foods except oils, refined sugar, refined rice, and beer. Symptoms of deficiency can begin within a week
Riboflavin (vitamin B$_2$)	1.2–1.7 mg/day	Angular stomatitis, skin rash	Milk, meat, and eggs are the main sources

continued below

Nutrient	Average requirement	Effects of insufficiency	Notes
Nicotinic acid (niacin)	13–19 mg/day	Pellagra. This is a chronic wasting disease that cannot be diagnosed biochemically. It is characterized by dermatitis, diarrhoea, and dementia	In carcinoid syndrome the metabolism of tryptophan is greatly increased, predisposing to pellagra. The diagnosis of pellagra is based on the response to treatment
Pyridoxine (vitamin B_6)	1.8–2 mg/day	Glossitis, skin rashes, convulsions	
Zinc	15 ng/day	Psoriasiform rash, hypogonadism, and hypogonadism, and pubertal delay, slow wound healing	Widely distributed in association with protein in foods
Iodine	150 μg/day	Hypothyroidism and goitre	Excess causes hypothyroidism and goitre. Occasionally thyrotoxicosis occurs. Sea food and iodized salt are the main sources. The amount in meat and cereals depends on the food and soil that they were exposed to

Metabolism of food

After a meal, excess fuel is stored as glycogen and fat under the influence of insulin. Between meals, or in other catabolic states, glucagon and other counter-regulatory hormones such as catecholamines induce glycogen breakdown and mobilize fatty acids as substrates for gluconeogenesis and ketogenesis, respectively.

Table 16.3
Leptin

Leptin after λεπτοσ (leptos), Greek for thin, is a circulating protein derived from a gene expressed exclusively in white adipose tissue. By acting through specific, high-affinity receptors in the hypothalamus (and choroid plexus), leptin reduces food intake and increases energy expenditure. Under normal circumstances leptin is decreased by fasting and increased by eating, in parallel with (and possibly mediated by) changes in insulin levels

Plasma leptin levels are correlated with body mass index: obese subjects tend to have high leptin levels, suggesting that they are relatively insensitive to the hormone or more likely, that they are ignoring signals to stop eating. The exact relationship between insulin resistance, leptin resistance (if it exists in humans), hunger, weight gain, and fertility remains to be established.

Table 16.4
Causes of obesity

Common
   Previous or current excessive calorie intake

Relatively uncommon
   Hypothyroidism—either spontaneous or secondary to overuse of antithyroid drugs
   Iatrogenic Cushing's syndrome—pharmacological doses of glucocorticoids
   Polycystic ovarian disease
   Transcranial surgery for craniopharyngiomas or pituitary macroadenomas

Very rare
   Growth hormone deficiency and hypothyroidism in children retard linear growth more
      than weight gain
   Prader–Willi and Laurence–Moon–Biedl syndromes
   Cushing's disease
   Hypothalamic lesions
   Pseudohypoparathyroidism
   Hypogonadism
   Insulinoma

Obesity

The cultural association between obesity and wealth is no longer prevalent in developed society. While it is true that if somebody looks fat (or starts adducing 'a large frame size'), they invariably are fat, the most useful clinical definition of obesity is the body mass index (BMI = weight/height^2 (kg/m^2)) at or above which life insurance data show a significantly increased risk. Mortality rates increase gradually once the BMI has exceeded 25 kg/m^2 and become significantly elevated when the BMI equals or exceeds 30 kg/m^2. When BMI approximates 40 kg/m^2, the mortality from anaesthesia rises exponentially from about threefold.

All fat is not equal, however. A waist/hip ratio exceeding 1 in men and 0.9 in women (where the waist is the narrowest part between the iliac crests and ribs,

Table 16.5
Obesity and overweight

Prevalence	39 per cent of men and 32 per cent of women have a BMI >25 kg/m^2
	5–15 per cent of men and 8–25 per cent of women are obese
	Obesity is more common in lower socio-economic groups
Family history	72 per cent of obese adults had at least one fat parent
Racial effects	Obesity is more common in white men than black men
	Obesity is more common in black women than white women
Duration of obesity	Obesity from youth tends to lead to central and peripheral obesity
	Obesity developing in adulthood tends to be central
	Fat babies have an enhanced risk of becoming fat adults
	25 per cent of fat children become fat adults
Effects of exercise	It is unusual for reduced activity to lead to obesity unless caloric intake is high
	Once obesity is established, however, reduced exercise can maintain obesity in the face of normal caloric intake
	Exercise-induced thermogenesis is not impaired in obesity
	A brisk, 1 hour walk loses only about 300 kcal
Risks of disease	The increased risk associated with obesity is predominantly cardiovascular
	The risk of hypertension and of carcinoma of the colon, rectum, prostate, breast, uterus, and cervix is also increased
Prognosis of obesity	Fat people almost invariably remain fat for long periods, or for life
	If weight loss is achieved, its maintenance seems almost impossible
Metabolism and metabolic rate	A negative balance of 7500 kcal is required to lose 1 kg in weight. Therefore a daily deficit of 100 kcal will lead to a 5 kg weight loss over a 1 year period
	Obesity only occurs as a result of sustained and excessive intake of calories
	In absolute terms, obese subjects generate more heat that lean people at rest

Table 16.6
Eating disorders

	Anorexia nervosa	Bulimia
Prevalence	As high as 1 per cent	As high as 1 per cent
Sex dominance	95 per cent female	>95 per cent female
Behavioural and psychological characteristics	Fixed, distorted body image, and attitude towards eating and weight, involving hoarding of food and enjoyment of weight loss. Fear of fatness. Food restriction through reduced intake and ritualized exercise	Increased incidence of episodes of self-harm, antisocial behaviour such as stealing, the use of alcohol and drugs, and generally chaotic eating habits. Weight control through vomiting with binge eating. Ritualized exercise rare
Physical characteristics	Onset before 25 years old Weight loss ≥15 per cent body weight Presence of two or more of: amenorrhoea, lanugo hair, bradycardia, periods of overactivity, episodes of bulimia, and emesis	Often rapid fluctuations in weight. Many bulimic patients are thin, but emaciation is unusual Most are within 15 per cent of their ideal body weight
Endocrine characteristics	Sick euthyroid syndrome (see p. 79) Amenorrhoea Failure of dexamethasone suppression with normal 24 h urinary cortisol Osteoporosis: suppressed oestrogen, compounded by dietary deficiency of calcium ± vitamin D Prolactin normal and GH sometimes slightly raised	Amenorrhoea in about 50 per cent Literature on evaluation of the endocrine system in these patients has not systematically ruled out the possibility of an endocrine problem
Prognosis at 2 years	50 per cent normal weight, 20 per cent underweight 20 per cent unchanged, 5 per cent obese and 5 per cent mortality Heart disease is a potentially fatal complication	Suicides twice as common as in anorexia Aspiration pneumonia, gastric or oesophageal rupture, pancreatitis, and acute gastric erosions contribute to the mortality rate

and the hips are the widest point of the buttocks) almost trebles the relative risk of people with identical BMIs developing diabetes.

Obesity also causes morbidity indirectly. Women with Cushing's disease, for example, often find the response of others to their 'descent' into obesity one of the most distressing features of the condition.

Treatment

Unless an endocrine cause of obesity such as hypothyroidism or Cushing's disease is diagnosed, therapy for obesity is not often successful. If a very disordered pattern of eating is evident, referral to a psychiatrist with a special interest in eating disorders is warranted. In all cases realistic goals need to be set, as the patient may well be non-compliant from the outset if demands are perceived as unreasonable.

There are no safe drugs that increase energy expenditure. However, where BMI exceeds 35 kg/m², dexfenfluramine (a 5-hydroxytryptamine (5-HT) agonist that is not a controlled drug, does not produce dependence, and is not a centrally acting stimulant) can be used to reduce appetite for up to 3 months as an adjunct to the dietary treatment of severe obesity (15 mg daily increasing to 15 mg twice a day after 1 week). The long-term efficacy of dexfenfluramine is disappointing.

Key points

- Endocrine pathology is a very rare cause of obesity.
- Treatment of obesity is rarely effective.
- Central obesity carries a higher risk of diabetes than peripheral obesity.

'My patient is obese and eats almost nothing. Is there an endocrine cause?'

History

The 35-year-old patient had been obese for years and was absolutely convinced that she ate much less than other people. Despite this she continued to gain weight and although her own doctor had tried to convince her many times that there was no underlying cause, he had finally been persuaded to refer her along for a second opinion. She was an obese child but claims to have eaten the same as her parents and siblings, none of whom was obese. The reason for presenting now, was that she was too embarrassed to take her 5-year-old daughter swimming.

Examination

Her BMI was 33 kg/m². Pink-coloured striae were present on her lower abdomen and there was a pad of excess fat on the back of her neck. Her skin was not thinned, however, there was no bruising and she was able to stand from squatting five times in succession without assistance. Her tendon reflexes were brisk. Mentally she was quite normal, and she was clinically euthyroid.

Investigation

The history of obesity from childhood without mental changes, proximal myopathy, thinned skin, and bruising makes Cushing's disease very unlikely. Often the patient and doctor feel that *something* should be done, however, and in the event the patient was given a single 1 mg tablet of dexamethasone to take at home at 11 p.m., and a biochemistry request form for a cortisol estimation and TSH (for convenience) to be drawn at 9 a.m. the following morning.

Her cortisol was less than 50 nmol/l (normal suppression ranges to < 138 nmol/l (usually to < 50 nmol/l)) and her TSH was 2.5 mU/l (normal range 0.3–6 mU/l).

Management

The normal TSH, and normal cortisol suppression following dexamethasone, exclude both Cushing's syndrome and hypothyroidism. The diagnosis is obesity secondary to excessive calorie intake. These patients tend to eat very little at meal times when others are present, but presumably consume much larger amounts at other times. Weight reduction targets should always be modest, for example, to lose 1 kg in a month, at least initially.

Multiple-choice questions

1. Obesity:
   a. Is typically associated with thyrotoxicosis;
   b. Can be caused by hypothyroidism;
   c. Is associated with polycystic ovarian disease;
   d. Is often associated with acromegaly;
   e. Is associated with development of an insulinoma (an insulin-secreting pancreatic tumour).

2. Effective and safe treatments for obesity include:
   a. Thyroxine in euthyroid individuals;
   b. Chlorpropamide;
   c. Right hemicolectomy;
   d. Bromocriptine;
   e. Jaw wiring.

3. Obesity is a risk factor for:
   a. Osteoporosis;
   b. Surgery under general anaesthetic;
   c. Insulin resistance;
   d. Anaemia;
   e. Cardiovascular disease.

4. In obesity:
   a. Thin babies have a similar risk to fat babies of becoming fat adults;
   b. A family history of obesity is unusual;
   c. Exercise-induced thermogenesis is impaired;
   d. A large proportion of fat people eventually manage to lose weight successfully;
   e. Black men are affected more than white men.

Answers

1. Obesity:
   a. Is typically associated with thyrotoxicosis   **F**
      Rarely, appetite may be so enhanced in thyrotoxicosis that calorie intake outstrips increased energy expenditure. Usually, however, the opposite is true.
   b. Can be caused by hypothyroidism   **T**
   c. Is associated with polycystic ovarian disease   **T**
   d. Is often associated with acromegaly   **F**
      There are certain characteristic changes, but obesity is not associated.
   e. Is associated with development of an insulinoma (an insulin-secreting pancreatic tumour)   **T**

Excess production of an appetite-stimulating, anabolic hormone. A very rare tumour often associated with MEN 1.

2. Effective and safe treatments for obesity include:
   a. Thyroxine in euthyroid individuals   F
   This was used at one time but the risks outweight the benefits and thyroxine is no longer used in this context.
   b. Chlorpropamide   F
   Sulphonylureas tend to make patients put on weight rather than lose it. Metformin is the only oral hypoglycaemic that does not cause weight gain.
   c. Right hemicolectomy   F
   Jejunoileal bypass, gastric bypass, gastric plication, jaw wiring, and placement of gastric balloons are all used in morbid obesity, and all have complications.
   d. Bromocriptine   F
   It has been tried but found to be unsuccessful. hCG, opioid antagonists, and levodopa have also been tried.
   e. Jaw wiring   F
   Deaths have been reported from aspiration of vomit, and patients rarely maintain weight loss after the wires are removed.

3. Obesity is a risk factor for:
   a. Osteoporosis   F
   The increased fat mass converts adrenal androgens to oestrogens, and by maintaining higher ambient oestrogen levels, tends, if anything, to protect against osteoporosis.
   b. Surgery under general anaesthetic   T
   The risks increase enormously in morbid obesity.
   c. Insulin resistance   T
   The threshold for development of insulin resistance is as low as 120 per cent of ideal body weight and is maximal when 30 per cent of body weight is adipose tissue.
   d. Anaemia   F
   Marked obesity leads to a diminished response to both hypoxia and hypercapnia. This in turn can result in pulmonary hypertension and polycythaemia, rather than anaemia.
   e. Cardiovascular disease   T

4. In obesity
   a. Thin babies have a similar risk to fat babies of becoming fat adults   F
   Fat babies are significantly more likely to become fat adults.
   b. A family history of obesity is unusual   F
   More than 50 per cent have at least one fat parent.
   c. Exercise-induced thermogenesis is impaired   F
   It is the same as normal.

d. A large proportion of fat people eventually manage to lose weight successfully   F
   Alas no. Most of them remain fat throughout life. Very recently, there
   have been some interesting advances in understanding of appetite control
   derived from work on the obese (*ob/ob*) mouse. The gene thought to be
   responsible for this phenotype is expressed only in adipose tissue and the
   protein product, released from fat, is thought to act centrally at the level
   of the hypothalamus as an appetite regulator.

e. Black men are affected more than white men   F
   But black women are affected more than white women.

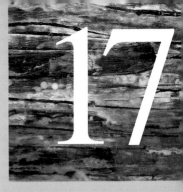

17

Diabetes mellitus

- Summary

- Introduction

- Diagnosis

- Objectives of diabetic care

- Targets

- Diet

- Drug treatment

- Special management situations

- Diabetic complications

- Special aspects of care

- Key points

- Case histories

- Multiple choice questions

Summary

Normal function

- Insulin is an anabolic hormone released from pancreatic islet beta cells in response to a rise in blood glucose level. By facilitating glucose uptake into cells, it keeps blood glucose within tightly controlled limits.
- The remarkably high prevalence of non-insulin-dependent diabetes in some societies suggests that the condition may have conferred an evolutionary advantage, although the nature of this remains obscure.

Typical pathology

- Inadequate insulin effect for whatever reason (i.e. insufficient quantity released or resistance to its actions), impairs glucose utilization as an energy source and allows blood glucose to rise. Untreated, this can result in the development of lethal complications such as ketoacidosis or hyperosmolar coma. Hypoglycaemia is a common complication of insulin treatment and, even when treatment is optimal, the patient is predisposed to heart disease and strokes, hypertension and peripheral vascular disease, blindness, renal failure, neuropathy, and premature death. New management strategies are making major inroads into the above problems.
  - → Non-insulin-dependent diabetes, typically in older, overweight patients.
  - → Insulin-dependent diabetes, typically in younger patients who lose weight prior to the diagnosis being made.
  - → Gestational diabetes. Diabetes in pregnancy occurs in 5 per cent of women and is associated with an increased risk of the subsequent development of non-insulin-dependent diabetes.

'Typical clinical scenario'

- An obese 64-year-old non-insulin-dependent diabetic with '+' of proteinuria on routine urine stick testing, an HbA1c of 10.2 per cent, total cholesterol of 7.2 mmol/l, and blood pressure of 178/94 mmHg. His blood glucose record book—had he remembered to bring it—would have shown readings in the range of 9–18 mmol/l, and his diet could be described as 'relaxed'.

  The strategy is to enable patients to achieve the best blood sugar control that they can within the life style they find acceptable, and for the diabetic clinic staff to ensure that risks are minimized and management of complications optimized, i.e. education and negotiation rather than remonstration.

Introduction

Diabetes mellitus is a chronic disease with a strong familial predisposition, frequently associated with time consuming, painful, and intrusive treatment, and a reduced life expectancy often punctuated by metabolic catastrophes and frightful complications. There is now unequivocal evidence that optimizing control of blood sugar reduces the risk of developing diabetic complications. The essence of management is to bring this about with minimal disruption to the diabetic's chosen life style.

Part of risk reduction is achieved by addressing the patient's blood glucose directly, and a larger part by educating the patient to adopt a life style that is compatible with the condition. In addition to controlling blood glucose, the risks of macrovascular disease are minimized by treating hypertension and hyper-lipidaemia aggressively, by ensuring that the patients are not passive or active cigarette smokers, and, in post-menopausal women, by replacing oestrogens. The strategy should be 'a negotiated settlement'.

Until insulin became available in the early 1920s, the diagnosis of diabetes in childhood predicted a decline into acidotic coma and death within at most a few months. Although we know that type 1 diabetes (Table 17.1) is caused by autoimmune destruction of pancreatic islet beta cells (triggered in genetically susceptible people by an unknown environmental agent), we cannot yet prevent or cure the disease.

The mortality rate for young diabetics is at least tenfold higher than normal. Heart disease accounts for 50 per cent, and strokes for a further 25 per cent of deaths in patients with diabetes or impaired glucose tolerance. Smoking doubles and hypertension quadruples the risk of heart disease and stroke in diabetes. Coronary artery bypass grafting is complicated by the early development of diffuse and extensive atherosclerosis.

Table 17.1
Diabetes mellitus

Insulin-dependent diabetes (type 1)	Non-insulin-dependent diabetes (type 2)
Need insulin to survive	Do not need insulin to survive
Common in youth	Common in later life
Annual incidence in youth is up to about 0.03 per cent	Annual incidence in the UK is about 1 per cent
Prevalence (under 30) is about 0.2 per cent	Prevalence is highly variable, up to 40 per cent in some societies
Familial risk low (<4 per cent of first-degree relatives affected)	Familial risk high (25 per cent have an affected first-degree relative)
Antibodies to islet cell cytoplasm present in 70–80 per cent	Antibodies to islet cell cytoplasm present in 0.1–1 per cent
Inflammatory cells around islets followed by a decline in insulin production to zero over about 3 years	Islets are normal and continue to secrete normal insulin, but for whatever reason, insulin output is insufficient for needs

After 30 years' duration of the disease, at least 50 per cent of diabetics are hypertensive and, in addition to remaining the most common cause of blindness in the working population, at whatever age diabetes is diagnosed it continues to reduce life expectancy by about 30 per cent.

Diagnosis

In many cases, the clinical diagnosis of diabetes is obvious, and can be confirmed readily by a single random test of urine and/or blood glucose. A random venous blood glucose of greater than 12 mmol/l, or two fasting levels of greater than 7.8 mmol/l indicate diabetes, and a fasting glucose of less than 6.7 mmol/l indicates normality (Fig. 17.1). The criteria for gestational diabetes are identical, although the condition needs to be reclassified after delivery. If in doubt, a 2 h glucose tolerance test is diagnostic (see below).

Glycosuria

Glycosuria is not diagnostic of diabetes mellitus, and the absence of glycosuria does not exclude diabetes mellitus. The renal threshold for glucose reabsorption (the level above which filtered glucose begins to escape renal reabsorption) varies between individuals, and in some it is low enough for glucose to appear in the urine without concomitant hyperglycaemia. Conversely, in many non-insulin-dependent diabetics, the renal threshold may be high enough to exclude glycosuria even when blood glucose levels are consistently around 18 mmol/l. For this reason, urinary glucose stick tests are infrequently used.

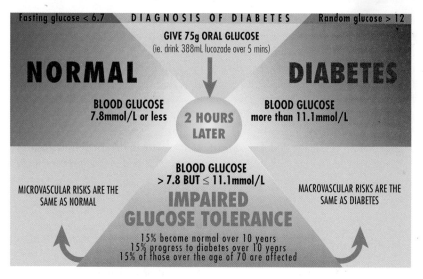

Fig. 17.1 The diagnosis of diabetes mellitus.

Objectives of diabetic care

To optimize metabolic control and minimize complications without forcing the patients to sacrifice what they consider to be an acceptable life style. This goal depends on education, which should be graded, tailored to suit the individual, repeated, reinforced, and ideally carried out by an enthusiast who has been taught how to do it. Risk factors such as hypertension, obesity, and hyperlipidaemia need to be treated, and complications such as visual impairment, renal failure, and foot ulceration should be prevented, or identified as early as possible so that treatment minimizes their extent. The dangers of smoking should be explained and the patient encouraged to stop.

Targets

Except perhaps for pregnant women, who are usually highly motivated and 'in for a 9-month sentence rather than "life"', setting targets that the patients cannot attain or feel that they cannot attain is entirely counterproductive. A diabetic who is found to have fasting and postprandial glucoses of less than 7 mmol/l and less than 11 mmol/l, respectively, on treatment; an HbA1c of less than 6.5 per cent; low density lipoprotein (LDL) and high density lipoprotein (HDL) cholesterols of less than 5.2 mmol/l and greater than 0.9 mmol/l; a triglyceride of less than 2.3 mmol/l; body mass index of less than 25 kg/m^2 (weight/height^2); no evidence of microalbuminuria; and a blood pressure of less than 140/90 has little need for intervention on metabolic grounds.

Diet

Much of life is taken up by working to earn money to buy food, choosing food, buying food, bringing it home, storing it, cooking it, eating it, clearing up after it, and wondering what to cook next. It is no wonder that insistence on dietary changes and restrictions that the patient finds uncomfortable are unproductive. Often, the whole family needs to change its eating habits. The emphasis should be on a balanced diet of good, whole food, with complex carbohydrates such as jacket potatoes, wholemeal bread, pasta, and whole-grain rice making up at least 50 per cent of calorie intake. Quick fixes of readily absorbed sugars should be avoided. However, if the odd, 'surreptitious' chocolate bar is enough to make the patient stop smoking and take his or her antihypertensive medication as prescribed, the payoff may be worthwhile.

Drug treatment

Insulin

Although insulin itself has changed little from that originally isolated, the use of a standardized concentration and the ready availability of stable mixtures and prefilled cartridges has done much to improve the efficacy and safety of insulin treatment. Asking patients to prepare their own insulin mixture is a thing of the past. In what other circumstances would a doctor suggest that a patient mix their own dangerous drugs?

Superfine needles are now less than 0.36 mm in outside diameter and extremely sharp. The injection pen devices are robust and can be easily used by all, including children and the blind. Although the needles generally supplied are very slightly thicker than the standard superfine needles on disposable insulin syringes, they stay sharper for longer because they are only used to penetrate the patient's skin, not the rubber bungs on insulin vials.

Older regimens of two injections of a 30 : 70 or 50 : 50 mixture of short- and long-acting insulin twice daily (with approximately two-thirds of the daily dose in the morning) are being superceded in new diabetics and younger patients by the more physiological and adaptable single injection of long-acting insulin once daily (to provide 24 h baseline cover), with boluses of soluble insulin 20 min before each meal. New, very rapidly acting analogues (insulin lispro (Humalog®)) are also now available.

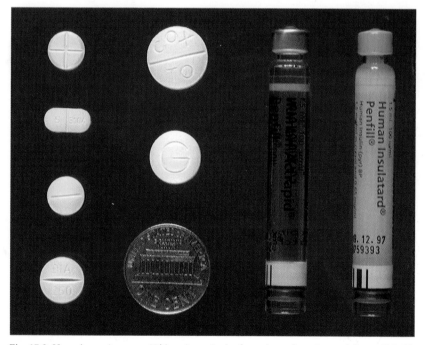

Fig. 17.2 Hypoglycaemic agents. Tablets shown in the first column from the top left are gliclazide (80 mg), glibenclamide (5 mg), glipizide (5 mg), and chlorpropamide (250 mg). In the second column, tolbutamide (500 mg) and metformin (500 mg) are above the coin. The cartridges are Mixtard® and Actrapid® penfills.

Insulin treatment for non-insulin-dependent diabetics is required if diet and tablets alone are insufficient. After months or years of poor control, these patients (insulin *treated*, rather than insulin *dependent*) not infrequently experience a marked sense of well-being on insulin, and sometimes regret their reluctance to agree to 'injections' earlier. Unfortunately, insulin is remarkably potent at making people gain weight.

Tablets

Sulphonylureas and biguanides

For non-obese patients, a sulphonylurea such as gliclazide (40–80 mg), glipizide (2.5–10 mg), or glibenclamide (2.5–10 mg) can be used. The original sulphonylurea, chlorpropamide (250 mg/day) is also enjoying a renaissance. It is often more useful to add metformin (500 mg three times a day or 850 mg twice a day) than increase the sulphonylureas to the maximum permissible doses. In obese patients, metformin is used as first-line treatment (500 mg three times a day or 850 mg twice a day), and the addition of sulphonylureas—though often necessary—is usually counterproductive, as they make the patient pile on even more weight.

Table 17.2
Glycosylated haemoglobin and blood glucose stix measurement

Glycosylated haemoglobin (HbA1c)

When protein and glucose are incubated together in solution, some of the protein becomes glycosylated, or irreversibly bound to the glucose. The rate at which this occurs is proportional to the concentration of glucose. Haemoglobin is the protein chosen to assess for glycosylation because it is cleared from the blood at a constant rate (in proportion to the average life of a red cell) and is easily sampled. While a single blood glucose estimation tells you relatively little about diabetic control, the percentage of glycosylated haemoglobin provides a fairly reliable representation of the mean blood glucose over the previous 6–12 weeks. The 'A1c' component of haemoglobin is chosen for technical reasons. If red cell half-life is unusually short or long, for example in patients with haemolytic anaemia or hereditary persistence of fetal haemoglobin, the percentage of HbA1c will be misleadingly low or high, respectively

Blood glucose stix measurement

The accuracy of blood glucose stix measurements can be affected, amongst other things, by poor technique such as the use of an inadequate blood sample and by the presence of glucose on the finger (e.g. handling commercial confectionary, which often contains glucose syrup). Samples for blood glucose obtained simultaneously should be sent to the biochemistry laboratory to confirm glucose stix findings in the emergency situation

Other drugs

α-Glucosidase inhibitors

Acarbose (Glucobay® 50 mg daily–50 mg three times a day) is a competitive, reversible inhibitor of small bowel α-glucosidase activity. It delays conversion of non-absorbable dietary starch and sucrose into monosaccharides when chewed with the first mouthful of a meal containing these carbohydrates. Unfortunately, undigested carbohydrates then ferment in the large bowel causing flatulence, bloating, and diarrhoea in 60 per cent of patients.

Guar gum

A non-digested complex carbohydrate that, in sufficient quantities, retards glucose absorption and results in much the same side-effects as the preparation above.

Both are used almost exclusively in non-insulin-dependent diabetics who are already taking oral hypoglycaemics, particularly if control remains poor or the use of sulphonylureas is causing excessive weight gain.

Special management situations

Diabetes in children

The differences between insulin-dependent diabetes in childhood and adulthood do not arise merely from the particular mind set of adolescence. There are also physical changes such as rapid growth, increase in lean body mass, and rapid changes in metabolic demands. These are compounded by feelings of victimization, rebelliousness, bereavement at loss of immortality, and fatalism, which combine to produce a turbulent mix that requires particular skills to handle well.

It is particularly important to view episodes of poor control as a weakness in the treatment regimen rather than the result of failure to comply with treatment or lack of understanding. As lack of parental support during adolescence is associated with poor control, it is important that both parents are included in diabetic education.

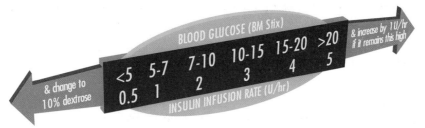

Fig. 17.3 Control of blood sugar—sliding scale.

Diabetes in pregnancy

Pre-natal counselling for diabetics or for those with previous experience of gestation diabetes is useful.

Table 17.3
Gestational diabetes

All pregnant women should be screened at 24–26 weeks	
Incidence	5 per cent of pregnancies
Diagnosis	At the end of the second trimester, a blood glucose of ≥7.2 mmol/l 1 h after 50 g oral glucose calls for a formal 75 g glucose tolerance test. This is normal if the 1 h and 2 h levels are <11.1 mmol/l and <7.8 mmol/l respectively
Maternal risks if untreated	Predisposition to pre-eclamptic toxaemia and polyhydramnios. There is also an increase in the Caesarean section rate
Fetal risks if untreated	Predisposition to miscarriage, fetal growth disturbance, and stillbirth, and an increase in perinatal morbidity and mortality
Long-term prognosis	Incidence of diabetes developing within the next 15 years is between 25 and 50 per cent. Risks of macrovascular disease are also enhanced
Management during pregnancy	Control blood sugar between 4 and 7 mmol/l at all times
Management during labour	Use a 5 per cent dextrose infusion (+20 mmol KCl) 1 l 8 hourly, plus insulin by syringe pump (1 unit/ml saline) according to hourly BM stix

Table 17.4
Diabetes and surgery

Diet controlled	If blood glucose measurements are all <10 mmol/l, treat as normal, but monitor blood glucose 4 hourly. Consider a glucose and insulin infusion if glucose levels inexorably rise (i.e. >1 mmol/l.h). Aim for a blood glucose of between 4 and 10 mmol/l
Diet and tablets	Discontinue oral hypoglycaemics on the day of surgery. Start infusions of insulin and glucose ≥2 h before theatre. Continue until the patient is able to eat and drink
Insulin-treated	Reduce evening long-acting insulin the day before surgery by 20 per cent, then treat as above. Change to four injections of insulin/day postoperatively before returning to usual regimen

Diabetic complications

Emergencies

Ketoacidosis

Pathogenesis

Lack of insulin leads to a rapid rise in hepatic glucose output and a fall in peripheral glucose uptake. When glucose reaches about 16 mmol/l, concentration-driven glucose uptake into cells and glycosuria match hepatic glucose production. Glucose levels rise above this in response to increased glucagon (driven by low insulin), cortisol, and catecholamines. Subsequently hyperglycaemia itself decreases peripheral glucose utilization.

Free fatty acids from adipose stores are the primary substrate for ketone body formation. Under normal circumstances the liver converts free fatty acids to triglycerides or to very low density lipoproteins (VLDL) which are released back into the circulation. In the presence of insulin deficiency and high levels of counter-regulatory hormones (particularly glucagon), enhanced peripheral lipolysis and hepatic fatty acid oxidation lead to the formation and release of high

Table 17.5
Diabetic ketoacidosis

Symptoms		Signs	Diagnostic tests
Osmotic	Other	Tachycardia	Blood glucose usually
Polyuria	Nausea	Hypotension	>15 mmol/l
Thirst	Vomiting	Deep and rapid breathing	Arterial blood pH <7.25
Nocturia	Abdominal pain	Warm skin	Bicarbonate <15 mmol/l
Polydipsia		Decreased core temperature	Urine ketones
Dehydration		Odour of ketones on the breath	
U&E		**FBC**	**Urine**
Hyperglycaemia masks hypernatraemia. For every 3 mmol/l that the glucose exceeds 5 mmol/l, serum sodium is underestimated by 1 mmol/l		Leucocytosis correlates with degree of ketoacidosis, rather than infection. Nevertheless, blood and throat swabs should be cultured	Should be sent for culture. Note that the presence of ketones does *not* make the diagnosis of ketoacidosis. Fasting ± vomiting make normal people ketotic

levels of acetoacetic and β-hydroxybutyric acids. This happens in both ketotic and 'non-ketotic' hyperglycaemia, but is only pronounced enough to cause acidosis in the former.

Demography

Between 20 and 30 per cent of new insulin-dependent diabetics present with ketoacidosis, but mostly the condition occurs in known diabetics (0.2–2 per cent/yr) who fail to take their insulin properly. In many cases, therefore, the condition is symptomatic of a failure of eduction. Patients need to be told that they need insulin all the time, even when they are not eating and, if anything, more so when they are under stress. Persistent vomiting, which can cause or be caused by ketosis, requires admission to hospital. Only 10 per cent of patients now present with coma, but the mortality remains 5–10 per cent.

Diagnosis

Management

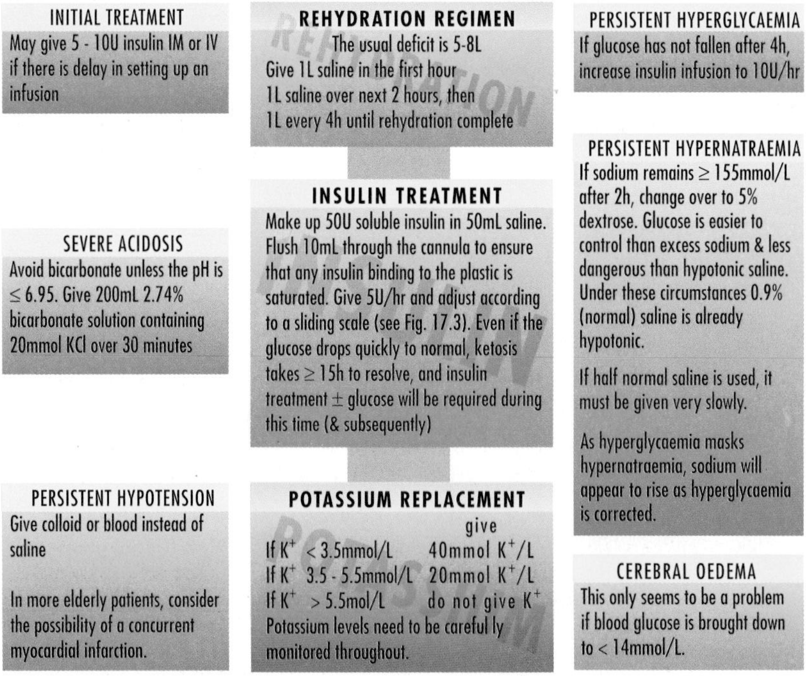

INITIAL TREATMENT
May give 5 - 10U insulin IM or IV if there is delay in setting up an infusion

REHYDRATION REGIMEN
The usual deficit is 5-8L
Give 1L saline in the first hour
1L saline over next 2 hours, then
1L every 4h until rehydration complete

PERSISTENT HYPERGLYCAEMIA
If glucose has not fallen after 4h, increase insulin infusion to 10U/hr

INSULIN TREATMENT
Make up 50U soluble insulin in 50mL saline. Flush 10mL through the cannula to ensure that any insulin binding to the plastic is saturated. Give 5U/hr and adjust according to a sliding scale (see Fig. 17.3). Even if the glucose drops quickly to normal, ketosis takes $\geq$ 15h to resolve, and insulin treatment $\pm$ glucose will be required during this time (& subsequently)

SEVERE ACIDOSIS
Avoid bicarbonate unless the pH is $\leq$ 6.95. Give 200mL 2.74% bicarbonate solution containing 20mmol KCl over 30 minutes

PERSISTENT HYPERNATRAEMIA
If sodium remains $\geq$ 155mmol/L after 2h, change over to 5% dextrose. Glucose is easier to control than excess sodium & less dangerous than hypotonic saline. Under these circumstances 0.9% (normal) saline is already hypotonic.

If half normal saline is used, it must be given very slowly.

As hyperglycaemia masks hypernatraemia, sodium will appear to rise as hyperglycaemia is corrected.

PERSISTENT HYPOTENSION
Give colloid or blood instead of saline

In more elderly patients, consider the possibility of a concurrent myocardial infarction.

POTASSIUM REPLACEMENT
give
If K$^+$ < 3.5mmol/L   40mmol K$^+$/L
If K$^+$ 3.5 - 5.5mmol/L   20mmol K$^+$/L
If K$^+$ > 5.5mol/L   do not give K$^+$
Potassium levels need to be carefully monitored throughout.

CEREBRAL OEDEMA
This only seems to be a problem if blood glucose is brought down to < 14mmol/L.

Fig. 17.4 Management of ketoacidosis.

Hyperosmolar non-ketotic coma

Hyperosmolar non-ketotic coma is a complication of non-insulin-dependent diabetes, and occurs when sustained osmotic diuresis cannot be matched by increased fluid intake. The treatment of hyperosmolar non-ketotic coma is similar to that of ketoacidosis, although as the condition is likely to have developed slowly, many clinicians would rehydrate the patient and treat the hyperglycaemia more gently. A high suspicion of infection requires blood and CSF cultures, and as hyperosmolar coma is thought by many to be a hypercoagulable state, patients are generally given intravenous heparin in addition to insulin and fluids. The mortality exceeds 50 per cent.

Osmolality is calculated as follows: $(Na^+ + K^+) \times 2 +$ urea + glucose (all biochemical values in mmol/l). In hyperosmolar non-ketotic coma the value is generally greater than or equal to 320 mOsm/l.

Lactic acidosis

Lactic acidosis is caused by failure of oxygen delivery or utilization by tissues. It rapidly resolves when liver perfusion is restored towards normal and oxygenation of tissues is improved. The association of lactic acidosis with ketoacidosis (in which glucagon and adrenaline stimulate glycolysis) and the biguanide phenformin, has led to the condition being associated with diabetes. More often, lactic acidosis is induced by cardiogenic shock, strenuous muscle exercise (fits, shivering, etc.), or ethanol ingestion.

Overt lactic acidosis is very rare, and there are no specific treatments other than vigorous management of the acidosis and of associated conditions such as cardiogenic shock and hyperglycaemia.

Hypoglycaemia

Many patients claim that they feel 'hypo' when their blood sugar is suddenly reduced from the hyperglycaemic range to normal (e.g. from 15 to 4 mmol/l). Unequivocal counter-regulatory changes do not appear until blood glucose descends to 2–3 mmol/l or less. The longer the duration of diabetes, the more likely symptoms of hypoglycaemia are to be muted or completely absent. Even though the diagnosis is often obvious to the patient, the loss of physical control can be very frightening, and good diabetic control is often time consuming to re-establish.

Patients with diabetes need to notify the Driver and Vehicle Licensing Agency (DVLA) and their insurance companies. Insulin treatment is not compatible with driving heavy goods vehicles. A hypoglycaemia-induced road traffic accident is a catastrophe classified as 'driving under the influence of drugs'.

Table 17.6
Hypoglycaemia

Demography	Signs	Treatment
Recurrent problem in ≥3 per cent	None—after many years of diabetes	Glucose or sucrose to drink or absorb through buccal mucosa if conscious
10 per cent experience coma annually	Sweating and/or tremor	Intramuscular glucagon, 1 mg—followed by oral glucose on awakening. This is a very useful (but underused) treatment
30 per cent experience at least one coma	Confusion or aggression	
Mortality is 0.2 per cent	Headaches on waking or night sweats	
May occur with glibenclamide	Focal neurological signs mimicking 'stroke'	250 ml of 10 per cent dextrose iv. 50 per cent dextrose is grossly hypertonic causes severe phlebitis and may obliterate a vein needed for future use. For these reasons it is now less commonly used
Consider that it may be a suicide attempt	Coma	

Notes

Always save sample for blood glucose (±C peptide) before treatment is started

Hypoglycaemia does not occur with metformin, and is very unusual with weaker sulphonylureas. Overdoses of chlorpropamide or glibenclamide are often lethal

Exclude alcoholism, hypoadrenalcorticalism, insulinomas, and insulin overdose

Microvascular complications

Retinopathy

The longer the duration of diabetes and the worse the control, the higher the prevalence and severity of retinopathy. Tightening diabetic control improves the long-term prognosis in retinopathy: the more rapid advancement of retinopathy in the short term is now known to be transient and more than compensated for in the longer term.

In the average diabetic out-patient clinic there is often scarcely enough time to dilate the pupils, let alone accurately diagnose early macular oedema or other conditions that might only be fully disclosed in a suitably lit, quiet environment by a specialist. Visual acuity should be carefully checked at each clinic attendance and any unexplained decline, irrespective of the fundoscopic findings (or lack of them), should prompt referral for an ophthalmological opinion.

The use of routine retinal photography is becoming more widespread. The difference between the field of view provided by the direct ophthalmoscope and

Table 17.7
Retinopathy

Prevalence	Signs	Treatment
At diagnosis: age 20–40 1.5%	Vascular	Optimize blood glucose control
age 60 10%	Capillary dilatation and closure	
After 5 years' diabetes ≥20%		Progression of retinopathy may accelerate for a year or two, but after that time, the benefits are unequivocal and well worth striving for
After 20 years' diabetes ≥80%	Venous dilatation and beading	
Endstage renal failure:	New vessel formation	
Proliferative retinopathy 75%	Extravascular	
Background only 100%	Soft exudates (arteriolar occlusion)	Laser treatment. Field loss occurs but acuity is preserved. It can be an uncomfortable procedure and result in altered colour perception and glare owing to internal reflections from white scar tissue
All of these figures should come down as overall control improves	Hard exudates (dilated leaking capillaries) Haemorrhages Microaneurysms Macular oedema New vessel formation Cataracts	

retinal camera is shown in Fig. 17.5a–d. Fluorescein angiography highlights areas of ischaemia, oedema, and other abnormalities that are otherwise difficult to identify (Fig. 17.5e).

Nephropathy

Diabetic nephropathy, like neuropathy and retinopathy, is related to duration of diabetes and degree of control. Detectable histological changes take at least 3 years to develop, and clinically significant proteinuria (i.e. > 0.5 g/day: three to four times normal loss) seldom occurs before the patient has had diabetes for 15 years. Proteinuria at around 0.5 g/day predicts endstage renal failure or death within 5 years. When protein loss exceeds 5 g/day, patient mortality at 2 years increases to 50 per cent, much of the increase being due to coronary heart disease. Nephropathy is the cause of death in 25–30 per cent of diabetics diagnosed before they are 30 years old. The presence of microalbuminuria, a level of albumin excretion above normal, but below that at which standard dipsticks become positive, is a very powerful predictor of diabetic nephropathy, endstage renal disease, cardiovascular disease, and premature death. Screening for micro-albuminuria and treatment with ACE inhibitors, particularly in young patients (irrespective of blood pressure), slows progression of nephropathy and improves outcome.

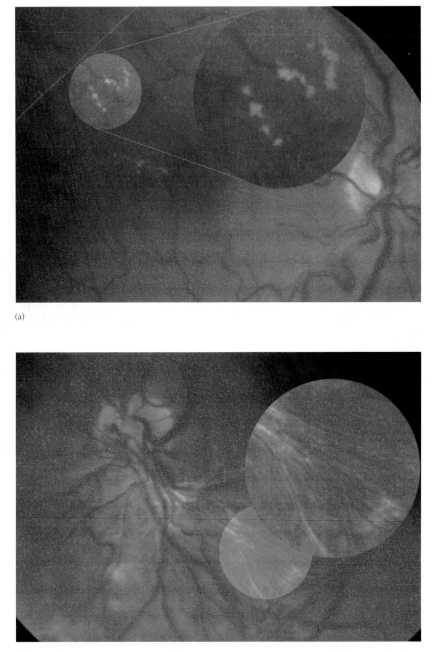

(a)

(b)

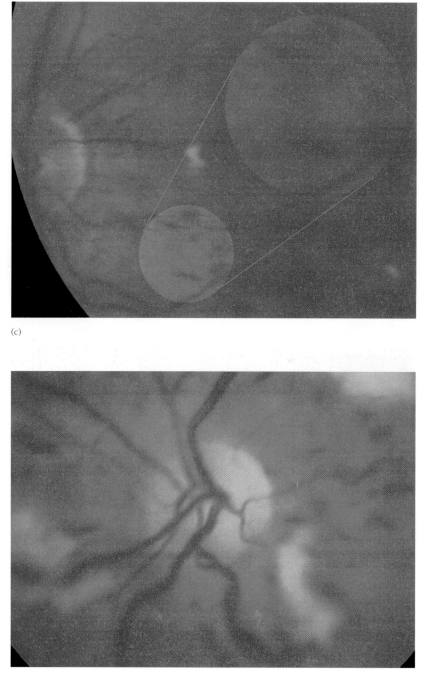

(c)

(d)

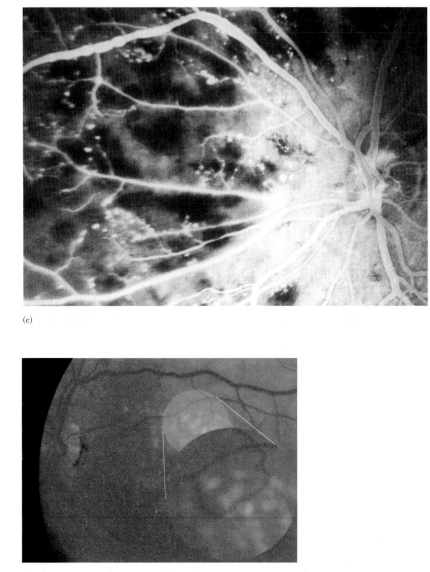

(e)

(f)

Fig. 17.5 Retinal photographs showing the field of view normally afforded by direct ophthalmoscopy in the clinic. (a) Hard exudates; (b) new vessels; (c) haemorrhages; (d) soft exudates; (e) fluorescein angiogram showing microaneurysms (appearing as white beads) and areas of ischaemia (black patches) that would be difficult to detect by ophthalmoscopy alone; and (f) photocoagulation scars (laser burns).

Table 17.8
Diabetic neuropathy

Peripheral neuropathy (very common)

So-called 'glove and stocking' neuropathy after its distribution. Affects particularly older patients with longer duration of disease

Signs

Symmetrical, usually sensory and confined to lower limbs, although absence of ankle jerks and wasting of small hand muscles is common

Symptoms

Numbness, tingling, burning, lacinating pain—sometimes severe and unremitting. Pain eventually vanishes as the nerves are destroyed

Complications

Absence of pain, vibration, and proprioception leads to unperceived injuries to skin and joints, calluses, ulceration, and Charcot's (neuropathic) joints

Erectile dysfunction (impotence)

Eventually affects 75 per cent of male diabetics. Combination of vascular disease with destruction of the nervi erigentes—the parasympathetic nerves that dilate the penile arteries. The problem is usually irreversible but far from untreatable (see page 204)

Autonomic neuropathy (common)

Absence of beat-to-beat variation on deep breathing or during a Valsalva manoeuvre

Orthostatic hypotension can occur

Erectile dysfunction and motility disturbances of the bladder and gut, are also common

Improved diabetic control has moderate beneficial effects on all types of neuropathy. Treatment with amitriptyline or other tricyclics is sometimes effective

Gastroenteropathy

Vagal neuropathy delays gastric emptying, the usual peristaltic 'sweeping' action of the gut is impaired. Constipation, sometimes alternating with diarrhoea, occurs in 66 per cent of diabetics, and in 90 per cent of those with extensive neuropathy

Mononeuropathy (rare)

Thought to be due to ischaemic injury of a nerve (i.e. arteriolar occlusion)

Peripheral or cranial nerves affected. Sudden wrist- or foot-drop, third, fourth or sixth nerve palsy, sometimes multiple

Radiculopathy is a rare cause of chest or abdominal wall pain, usually in patients who have had diabetes for 20 years or more

Apart from ensuring that blood glucose control is optimized, hypertension should be controlled vigorously. Target blood pressure in patients without nephropathy is less than 160/90 mmHg, and with proteinuria, 140/90 mmHg or probably less. ACE inhibitors appear to improve the prognosis even if the patient is not hypertensive.

Special aspects of care

Diabetic feet

Claudication is five times more common and gangrene 60 times more common in diabetics than in the rest of the population. Half of all amputations are carried out in diabetics. Neuropathy and microvascular changes contribute, but advanced atheroma is a major cause, and hypertension is a major cause of that. The primary objective is to retain a healthy diabetic foot at the end of every diabetic leg. Optimizing blood glucose control and minimizing macrovascular disease by education, preventing smoking, and controlling hypertension and hyperlipidaemia, will maximize the chance of this goal being achieved. Basic elements

Table 17.9
Features of diabetic feet

Neuropathic ulceration	Ischaemic ulceration
Warm, pink foot	Cold foot that blanches on elevation and is red when dependent
Bounding pulses	Absent pulses as atherosclerosis obliterates distal vessels
Diminished sensation, therefore little pain from the lesions	Pain, particularly local pain. Claudication ± diffuse pain at rest
Callus formation around the ulcer	No callus formation around painful ulcers
Other features	Other features
Evidence of mechanical or thermal injuries	Greatly increased chance of foot loss within 3 months
Charcot's joint—warm, swollen joint with intact skin	60 per cent heal with control of infection, oedema, and pain
Infections: Staphylococci or streptococci, thrombotic arterial occlusion and gangrene Anaerobes, necrotizing infection, and gas gangrene	Chiropody and made-to-measure footwear are useful treatment adjuncts

of foot care need to be discussed repeatedly, particularly in patients with evidence of peripheral vascular disease, poor foot hygiene, neuropathy, or neuropathic trophic changes such as calluses, hammer toes, and metatarsal subluxation. Patients over 65 years old are at increased risk, particularly if their vision is impaired. Often they cannot see, feel, or reach their feet.

Clinical examination pointers

1. Establish a rapport. Remember that few people like to be lectured about their life style.
2. Make sure that any suggestions you make to the patient are as reasonable as possible. A list of statistics about amputations and heart disease will merely convince the patients that there is no point in even trying.
3. Measure blood pressure carefully and treat hypertension aggressively.
4. If retinopathy is present, ask yourself whether, in a hectic clinic, you can pick up 100 per cent of patients with mild macula oedema or early new vessel formation. If not, request a second opinion.
5. In the clinic, even if the patient appears well, formally check visual acuity, check fundi through dilated pupils, measure blood pressure carefully, and inspect injection sites. Examine the feet for callus formation and incipient skin problems, check pulses for ischaemia, and reflexes ± vibration or proprioception for neuropathy. A blood sample should be taken for lipids, glucose, and HbA1c, and the urine tested for protein.

Key points

- Smoking doubles the risk of heart disease and stroke in diabetes.
- Hypertension quadruples the risk of heart disease and stroke in diabetes.
- The strongly hereditary nature of type 2 diabetes (NIDDM) is a screening opportunity that should be exploited.
- Insulin resistance, impaired glucose tolerance, or diabetes are strongly associated with acromegaly, Cushing's syndrome, and polycystic ovarian disease.
- Proteinuria in diabetics is not invariably caused by diabetic nephropathy. Up to 20 per cent of cases have other causes of proteinuria.
- Metabolic targets for diabetics are: a fasting glucose of less than 7 mmol/l, a postprandial glucose of less than 11 mmol/l; an HbA1c of less than 6.5 per cent; LDL and HDL cholesterols of less than 5.2 mmol/l and greater than 0.9 mmol/l, respectively; a triglyceride of less than 2.3 mmol/l; body mass index of less than 25 kg/m^2; and a blood pressure of less than 140/90.

'My evening blood sugars are high, but when I increase my insulin, I go hypo during the night'

History

A 53-year-old insulin-dependent diabetic, who was eventually stabilized on M1® insulin via a pen injector twice daily, found that in the evening she consistently ran blood glucose levels of between 15 and 17 mmol/l. She increased the evening insulin from 18 to 20 U, and then to 22 U, but instead of the evening blood glucose levels coming under control, they remained unchanged. Instead, she found herself waking up with symptoms of hypoglycaemia between 3 and 4 a.m. in the mornings.

On closer questioning she explained that she took 36 U of M1® insulin in the morning at about 07.30, and her evening dose at 19.00. Supper was at 19.30 and, being a dutiful diabetic, she measured her blood glucose at about 21.00 before retiring to bed.

Management

M1® insulin is 90 per cent long acting and 10 per cent short acting (M2® is 20 per cent short acting, M3®—the equivalent of Mixtard®—is 30 per cent short acting, and so on). To increase insulin action in the evening, she was therefore advised to leave the evening dose unchanged, but increase the morning dose.

Explanation

By increasing the 7 p.m. M1® insulin dose, much of the desired hypoglycaemic *effect* was unfortunately delivered during the early hours of the morning (6–12 h later), rather than the late evening.

Few drug combinations need to be tailored to patients' specific needs, as the same ratio, and two or three dose schedules, work for almost everyone. The same is true for diabetics, although there will always be patients and clinicians who enjoy the apparent freedom (and risk) of 'cooking up' their own combinations. There are now excellent, stable combinations of short- and longer-acting insulins in ready-loaded cartridges, and the same few combinations work well for almost everybody needing insulin treatment.

'My 17-year-old patient is losing weight and feeling run-down. He has glycosuria and polyuria'

History

As above.

Examination

In this age group there are unlikely to be any complications of diabetes. Nevertheless, checking the presence of ankle reflexes and proprioception or vibration in the feet (to exclude neuropathy), the presence of foot pulses, some of which may be absent in normal people (macrovascular complications), the blood pressure and fundi (retinopathy), sets the scene for later consultations and, by being normal, may defuse the anxiety sometimes engendered by physical examinations.

Management

There are no prizes for making the diagnosis of insulin-dependent diabetes once beta cell function has been destroyed, or for treating his blood sugar *per se*. The honours are reserved for the patient, the patient's family, and his medical advisers who optimize treatment, prevent complications, and ensure that the patient, while respecting the condition, is not ruled by it. Clear, consistent information, explanation, education, and reassurance, all frequently repeated and reinforced, are required.

A modern insulin regimen, three injections of short-acting insulin before each meal, and a longer-acting preparation in the evening, delived by pen injector was started. The latest, 'low pain' lancets for blood glucose analysis by electronic meter were provided.

Explanation

The progression from normal beta cell function to frank diabetes does not occur overnight. As autoimmune islet cell destruction progresses over a period of months, maximum insulin output gradually declines. During this 'honeymoon' period, episodes of increased insulin demand may not be met, and overt diabetes may appear and then disappear.

It should always be borne in mind that the diagnosis of diabetes can be psychologically devastating. It is, after all, a chronic disease with a strong hereditary component that significantly interferes with life style and is often frustrating and uncomfortable to treat. Adolescence is a particularly difficult time to achieve glycaemic control. At puberty, lean body mass doubles over 2–5 years and insulin requirements increase accordingly.

Insulin-dependent diabetes has an incidence of about 1 in 700 per annum. With the excellent range of stable insulin mixtures in cartridges and ultrafine needle technology making injecting more comfortable and quicker than shaving a beard, the four injection/day regimens that mimic intact beta cell function are no longer onerous. A long-acting preparation such as isophane insulin once daily (often in the evening) provides stable 24 hour insulin cover, which is increased at meal times by the injection of small boluses of soluble insulin (usually 4–10 U) 20 min earlier. An injection pen kept in a handbag or jacket pocket will deliver an accurate dose through a skirt or trouser leg and can be returned to a pocket without the other dinner party guests noticing that anything has happened.

'My patient feels faint and "hypo" if she doesn't eat regularly. The symptoms are relieved by eating'

History

The 24-year-old patient claimed that from the age of 16 she had found 'hunger' incapacitating. Unless she ate during the day at intervals of 4 hours or less, she would feel disorientated and faint. She was frightened about what might happen if she found herself unable to eat for longer, but in fact this situation had never arisen. She also felt perfectly well in the morning on waking. Her weight was steady.

Examination

No abnormal findings.

Investigations

None undertaken.

Management

The patient was reassured.

Explanation

The clear implication of the referral letter, and the explicit complaint of the patient is of 'spontaneous hypoglycaemia'. Fortunately, in view of its sinister associations, spontaneous hypoglycaemia at any time is, in reality, a very rare event. Almost invariably, the patient has learned to over-react to the painful and very powerful symptom complex known as hunger. Hypoglycaemia caused by an insulin-secreting tumour of the pancreas (an insulinoma) can be ruled out by having the patient fast for 72 hours in hospital (an extremely uncomfortable endurance test for anyone), checking blood glucose and insulin levels if and when symptoms occur.

Multiple-choice questions

1. The following suggest neuropathic rather than ischaemic ulceration of the foot:
   a. Build up of callus around the ulceration site;
   b. Marked local discomfort;
   c. A cold foot;
   d. Bounding pulses;
   e. Normal proprioception at the great toe.

2. Diabetic retinopathy:
   a. Is usually present at the diagnosis of insulin-dependent diabetes;
   b. Increases in prevalence with increasing duration of disease;
   c. Initially shows a marked improvement after instigation of tight diabetic control;
   d. Results from excessive and uneven retinal arteriolar dilatation;
   e. Is a universal phenomenon in patients with diabetic endstage renal failure.

3. In diabetic ketoacidosis:
   a. Profound dehydration is characteristic;
   b. Hyperglycaemia may mask hypernatraemia;
   c. Pulmonary emboli are a major problem;
   d. Treatment with 5 per cent dextrose may be appropriate in hypernatraemia even if blood sugar remains high;
   e. The fluid deficit is usually 10–15 litres. 5-8 L

4. In diabetes: ↗ Type I
   a. The genetic component of insulin-dependent diabetes is more pronounced than in non-insulin-dependent diabetes; F

b. It usually takes 1 year or less for insulin levels in IDDM to decline from normal to near zero;

c. Impaired glucose tolerance is associated with a risk of microvascular complications similar to that of diabetes itself;

d. In pregnancy, the criteria for diagnosis of gestational diabetes are more strict than those used to diagnose diabetes in non-pregnant subjects;

e. The risk of developing diabetes is increased if the patient has suffered an episode of gestational diabetes.

5. Microalbuminuria:

a. Is urinary albumin excretion sufficient to give one plus (+) of protein on routine dipstick testing;

b. Is a better predictor of vascular disease and premature mortality than cholesterol level, smoking or hypertension;

c. Is stabilized or reduced by intensified insulin treatment;

d. Diagnosis requires analysis of a 24 h collection of urine;

e. Patients may benefit from treatment of blood pressure as low as 120/80 mmHg.

6. In the treatment of diabetes:

a. The total amount of insulin delivered by intravenous infusion over 24 h in a hospital patient is a poor guide to subsequent subcutaneous insulin requirement;

b. In a newly diagnosed insulin-dependent diabetic, insulin should be started as a single daily dose and the frequency of injections increased until control is achieved;

c. When a twice daily insulin regimen is devised, it is usual to give approximately two-thirds of the total daily dose in the evening, and one-third in the morning;

d. A high 7 a.m. blood glucose in a young insulin-dependent diabetic can sometimes be reduced by lowering the evening dose of insulin;

e. Sulphonylurea drugs should be used in preference to metformin in non-insulin-dependent diabetics, as the latter causes lactic acidosis.

Answers

1. The following suggest neuropathic rather than ischaemic ulceration of the foot:

a. Build up of callus around the ulceration site   T

If the skin was ischaemic, it would be unable to mount this kind of proliferative activity.

b. Marked local discomfort   F

Pain and anaesthesia are opposite ends of the sensory spectrum, yet a bizarre mixture of symptoms giving rise to what appears to be 'painful anaesthesia' is common in diabetic neuropathy. However, trauma caused by local anaesthesia seems to play a part in neuropathic ulceration and, in general, these lesions are not as painful as ischaemic ulceration, where nerve endings may still be in the process of dying from ischaemia.

    c. A cold foot   F

This is more characteristic of ischaemia, although both may be present, and both feet cold, depending on the weather.

    d. Bounding pulses   T

    e. Normal proprioception at the great toe   F

2. Diabetic retinopathy
   a. Is usually present at the diagnosis of insulin-dependent diabetes   F
      The incidence is only about 1.5 per cent at this time, but the fundi should always be examined, nevertheless.
   b. Increases in prevalence with increasing duration of disease   T
   c. Initially shows a marked improvement after instigation of tight diabetic control   F
      Initially, over the first year to 18 months, retinopathy progresses more rapidly than it does in control subjects. After this time the benefits become clear, and increase further with time.
   d. Results from excessive and uneven retinal arteriolar dilatation   F
      Capillary shutdown and ischaemia seem to be the most important early events.
   e. Is a universal phenomenon in patients with diabetic endstage renal failure   T
      The incidence of background retinopathy is 100 per cent, and proliferative retinopathy, 75 per cent.

3. In diabetic ketoacidosis:
   a. Profound dehydration is characteristic   T
      There is an osmotic diuresis, compounded by the patient being too ill to drink.
   b. Hyperglycaemia may mask hypernatraemia   T
      For every 3 mmol/l that the glucose exceeds 5 mmol/l, serum sodium is underestimated by 1 mmol/l.
   c. Pulmonary emboli are a major problem   F
      Hyperosmolar coma rather than ketoacidosis is strongly associated with hypercoagulability, and hyperosmolar patients are routinely heparinized at the beginning of treatment.
   d. Treatment with 5 per cent dextrose may be appropriate in hypernatraemia even if blood sugar remains high   T
      High blood sugars are much easier to control (with insulin), than high sodium levels. It is probably safer to do this, than switch to hypotonic sodium solutions.

    e. The fluid deficit is usually 10–15 litres   F

The patient would be seriously awash, if you answered 'true' here. Five to 8 litres is more usual but, clearly, every patient has to be treated individually. Patients should never be treated on 'automatic pilot'. The biochemistry should be repeated at intervals and changes to the regimen made accordingly.

4. In diabetes:

    a. The genetic component of insulin-dependent diabetes is more pronounced than in non-insulin-dependent diabetes   F

Identical twin studies show a concordance rate of about 40 per cent in insulin-dependent diabetes, compared to almost 100 per cent in non-insulin-dependent diabetes. Up to about 15 genes are thought to be involved in determining the susceptibility to IDDM, the most important of which is MHC (HLA-DQ). The environmental agents that precipitate insulin-dependent diabetes are unknown. There is no evidence that a virus is responsible but some data to suggest that exposure to cow's milk before the age of 3 months increases the risk.

    b. It usually takes 1 year or less for insulin levels in IDDM to decline from normal to near zero   F

It actually takes about 3 years for this to happen. The disease is often diagnosed during the last few months of this (honeymoon) period, when the patient may dip in and out of frank diabetes during periods of stress, but be relatively normal at other times. It is during the final, rather than the initial, stages of the process of autoimmune destruction of pancreatic islet beta cells that hyperglycaemia appears, i.e. the patient has *had* IDDM, and as a result suffers from hyperglycaemia, a biochemical problem. Future prevention of IDDM, if possible, will depend on the identification of those at risk, using a panel of antibody tests, followed by long-term immune modulation to suppress or divert the development of anti-islet cell antibodies.

    c. Impaired glucose tolerance is associated with a risk of microvascular complications similar to that of diabetes itself   F

The risk of microvascular complications is normal. The risk of macrovascular complications (stroke, heart attack, etc.) is similar to that of frank diabetes.

    d. In pregnancy, the criteria for diagnosis of gestational diabetes are more strict than those used to diagnose diabetes in non-pregnant subjects   F

The criteria are exactly the same.

    e. The risk of developing diabetes is increased if the patient has suffered an episode of gestational diabetes   T

The chance of development of true diabetes is between 25 and 50 per cent.

5. Microalbuminuria:

    a. Is urinary albumin excretion sufficient to give one plus (+) of protein on routine dipstick testing   F

Standard dipsticks become positive at above 0.5 g of protein/24 h. Microalbuminuria is urinary albumin excretion below this, but above the normal range (1.5–20 μg/min), i.e. 20–200 μg/min.

b. Is a better predictor of vascular disease and premature mortality than cholesterol level, smoking, or hypertension   T

In fact, it is better than all three combined, and is therefore a very important predictor of cardiovascular complications, diabetic nephropathy, and vascular disease. Other long-term complications such as retinopathy and peripheral vascular problems are also associated

c. Is stabilized or reduced by intensified insulin treatment   T

It is useful in predicting those patients in whom a special effort should be made to gain good diabetic control.

d. Diagnosis requires analysis of a 24 h collection of urine   F

In practice, a timed overnight collection (i.e. the patient emptying the bladder at a set time before retiring to bed, and then collecting a urine sample at a set time the following morning) is more practical. An albumin/creatinine ratio of greater than 2 mg/mmol predicts microalbuminuria with a sensitivity and specificity of greater than 95 per cent. Albumin excretion rate should be in the microalbuminuric range in at least two out of three collections within a period of 3 months. Heavy exercise, urinary tract infection, acute illness, and cardiac failure are confounding factors that may produce a false positive test for microalbuminuria. Equally, one in five cases of proteinuria in diabetics are not due to diabetic nephropathy. Reduced complement levels, protein electrophoresis, antinuclear antibodies, renal ultrasound, and sometimes renal biopsy to identify glomerulonephritis, myeloma, systemic lupus erythematosus (SLE), and pyelonephritis may be required.

e. Patients may benefit from treatment of blood pressure as low as 120/80 mmHg   T

At this level or even below, ACE inhibitors have been shown to reduce progression of complications. At least 85 per cent of insulin-dependent diabetics with nephropathy become hypertensive.

6. In the treatment of diabetes:

a. The total amount of insulin delivered by intravenous infusion over 24 h in a hospital patient is a poor guide to subsequent subcutaneous insulin requirement   F

If a newly diagnosed insulin-dependent diabetic has been stabilized using a sliding-scale infusion of soluble insulin, the sum of the amount given per 24 h provides a rough idea of the total amount that they will subsequently need by injection, bearing in mind that the patients' activity level and diet in hospital are atypical, and that an underlying problem may have temporarily increased insulin requirements. For these patients, the insulin can be divided into a bolus of 4–6 units of soluble insulin

20 min before each of the three main meals of the day, with the remainder of the 24 h total (often 0.5–1 U/h) given as a bolus of isophane insulin in the evening. It is wise to give less than the patient is likely to eventually require and gently increase the dose, rather than induce hypoglycaemia at the outset and end up struggling with the effects of counter-regulatory hormone release (i.e. adrenaline, glucagon, growth hormone, etc.) and patient anxiety.

b. In a newly diagnosed insulin-dependent diabetic, insulin should be started as a single daily dose and the frequency of injections increased until control is achieved   F

The modern, versatile regimen is to give three injections of short-acting insulin daily before meals, and provide a continuous low level of insulin throughout the day and night using a single injection of isophane insulin. In a patient who is new to insulin, a reasonable starting point is to give soluble insulin, 4–6 units before meals and an injection of 16 units of isophane insulin in the evening, increasing the latter until the blood glucose on waking is between 4 and 7 mmol/l. In patients who have developed insulin-dependent diabetes following pancreatectomy, the amount of insulin required is often surprisingly low, sometimes as little as 2–6 units/day *in total*.

c. When a twice daily insulin regimen is devised, it is usual to give approximately two-thirds of the total daily dose in the evening, and one-third in the morning   F

In patients who had previously been stabilized on two injections of insulin daily (such as a 30 : 70 mixture of short- and longer-acting insulin (Mixtard® or M3®)) it is usual, at least initially, to give around two-thirds of the total daily dose in the morning and one-third in the afternoon.

d. A high 7 a.m. blood glucose in a young insulin-dependent diabetic can sometimes be reduced by lowering the evening dose of insulin   T

In the past, rebound hyperglycaemia following an episode of hypoglycaemia (the 'Somogyi phenomenon') was thought to be common. Although it is occasionally seen, hyperglycaemia on waking following nocturnal hypoglycaemia is unusual, and virtually confined to insulin-dependent diabetic children. Somogyi described an intensive insulin treatment regimen (before long-acting preparations were available) which included an injection of insulin at 3 a.m. He made no mention of rebound hyperglycaemia. Perhaps the origin of the 'Somogyi phenomenon' was 'the effect seen when the Somogyi treatment regimen was implemented'.

e. Sulphonylurea drugs should be used in preference to metformin in non-insulin-dependent diabetics as the latter causes lactic acidosis   F

In an obese non-insulin-dependent diabetic, metformin is often the drug of choice as it does not increase appetite. Unfortunately, abdominal discomfort occasionally limits treatment and the tablets themselves are rather large (see Fig. 17.2). Lactic acidosis, although a dangerous complication of biguanides, is exceedingly rare. Sulphonylureas are in general more powerful hypoglycaemics than metformin but tend to cause weight gain. Chlorpropamide (100–500 mg/day as a single dose) and glibenclamide (5–15 mg/day as a single dose) are powerful enough to cause hypoglycaemia at therapeutic doses if used without care. Tolbutamide (typically 500 mg three times daily) is a very mild hypoglycaemic. Gliclazide (40–160 mg as a single dose or up to 320 mg in divided doses) and glipizide (2.5–15 mg as a single dose or up to 40 mg in divided doses) are useful intermediate-acting drugs. Sulphonylureas and biguanides can safely be given in combination.

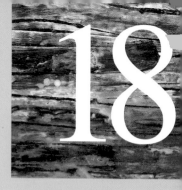

18

Hyperlipidaemia

- Summary

- Introduction

- Fat metabolism

- Risk analysis

- Diet

- Key points

- Case history

- Multiple-choice questions

Summary

Normal function

- Lipids are used principally as a medium of energy storage and regulator of fuel use. They are also required for the synthesis of steroid hormones, bile salts, and cell membranes.
- Adipose tissue is endocrinologically active. It converts pre-androgens to androgens and to the cyclic oestrogen 'oestrone'. The net effect is to increase circulating oestrogens and androgens in obese patients.

Typical pathology

- Inherited abnormalities of lipid handling that predispose to the deposition of cholesterol at sites other than peripheral fat stores, the most important being vascular walls.
- Secondary causes of hyperlipidaemia such as hypothyroidism, diabetes, and alcohol abuse.

'Typical clinical scenario'

- A 64-year-old man, recently discharged from hospital following a myocardial infarction, whose total cholesterol, measured within hours of the onset of chest pain, was 5.8 mmol/l.

Introduction

Coronary heart disease (CHD) accounts for 30 per cent of deaths in men and 25 per cent of deaths in women. There is clear epidemiological evidence of the benefits of treating hyperlipidaemia in the prevention of coronary heart disease (if the risk of death from the same exceeds 1.5 per cent/year), and the more at-risk the patient (i.e. the coexistence of high initial total cholesterol levels, diabetes mellitus, ischaemic heart disease, peripheral vascular disease, left ventricular hypertrophy, and/or hypertension in an old, cigarette-smoking, male patient) the bigger the benefit of intervention.

The management of hyperlipidaemia has, in the past, been complicated by classifications of circulating lipid particles based on irrelevant molecular characteristics such as size, density, and electrophoretic mobility, by the inherent complexity of lipid metabolism itself, and by lipid-lowering drugs with major side-effects and modest beneficial effects. A series of new, powerful, broad-spectrum-lipid-lowering drugs with improved side-effect profiles, together with excellent epidemiological data (at least for the 'statins' (see below)) has greatly simplified the management of these conditions.

Even after a patient has had a coronary artery bypass graft, reduction in cholesterol results in the formation of fewer new atheromatous lesions and regression (albeit minimal) of pre-existing plaques. The apparent association between lipid-lowering drug treatment and suicide, violent death, and cancer appears to have been a statistical artefact of the cholesterol-lowering effect of major illnesses such as tumours and depression.

The history and examination, combined with measurement of blood lipids, will often alert the clinician to the possibility of familial hyperlipidaemia. Common causes of secondary hyperlipidaemia such as renal and hepatic disease, diabetes, alcohol abuse, and hypothyroidism need to be excluded at the outset.

Fat metabolism

Triglycerides are major energy stores, and cholesterol is needed for the synthesis of steroid hormones, bile salts, and cell membranes. Neither are water soluble, so both are carried in special complexes containing phospholipids and proteins (apolipoproteins).

The liver controls the rate at which it synthesizes cholesterol by modifying the activity of 3-hydroxy-3-methylglutaryl CoA (HMG CoA) reductase—the rate-limiting enzyme in the formation of cholesterol from acetyl CoA. The level of cholesterol-containing low density lipoproteins (LDL) particles in the blood is controlled by regulation of hepatic LDL receptor expression and, hence, LDL uptake. High density lipoprotein (HDL) particles take up excess cholesterol from peripheral cells and are *anti*atherogenic. LDL are atherogenic and constitute 70 per cent of circulating cholesterol. Lp(a) ('LP little a') particles are closely related to LDL in structure and associated risks. Fats absorbed from the gut or released from the liver are deposited in fat stores and thus removed from the circulation by the action of the enzyme lipoprotein lipase (LPL). Fibrinogen is an independent risk factor for CHD and stroke. It is increased in diabetes and by smoking, obesity, and vascular disease, and is decreased by exercise and moderate alcohol intake.

Table 18.1
Causes of secondary hyperlipidaemia

Common	Lipid/s increased
Hypothyroidism	Cholesterol
Obesity	Cholesterol and triglycerides
Diabetes	Triglycerides
Alcohol abuse	Triglycerides
Less common	
Renal disease	Cholesterol and triglycerides
Liver disease	Cholesterol
Glucocorticoids	Cholesterol
Thiazides and beta-blockers	Triglycerides

Risk analysis

The dietary intake of saturated fats by a population is directly related to its average blood cholesterol, and, like hypertension and cigarette smoking, blood cholesterol is directly related to the rate of heart attacks.

Meta-analysis shows that a 1 per cent reduction in cholesterol produces a 2 per cent fall in coronary heart disease mortality, and that lipid-lowering drug treatment results in a 4 per cent overall reduction in coronary heart disease events. It follows that if a patient is at very low risk (for example, an otherwise normal young woman with a total cholesterol of 9.5 mmol/l), the benefits of treatment with lipid-lowering drugs will be negligible. However, if the patient has a high absolute risk of a fatal coronary heart disease event of greater than 1.5 per cent annum (which equates with a coronary heart 'event' rate of 4.5 per cent annum), for example, a cholesterol of 5.7 mmol/l in a patient following a myocardial infarction, treatment is likely to be beneficial (Fig. 18.1).

Diet

For many people the processes of buying food, cooking it, and consuming it take up a large and very pleasurable part of life. The habits and prejudices that make up these rituals are often deeply ingrained in our behaviour. Too often, what are by many people considered to be 'real foods' contain the saturated animal fat, hydrogenated oils, and dairy products that make up the bulk of the fats that together constitute 38 per cent of our daily calorie intake (Table 18.4).

The goal is to reduce total fat intake to 30 per cent of our calorie intake, substitute saturated fats with monounsaturated olive oil, polyunsaturated sunflower, soya and safflower oil, and use fish oils where appropriate. The calorie shortfall should be replaced with complex carbohydrates such as jacket potatoes, wholemeal bread, pasta, and whole-grain rice. Soluble fibre in the form of legumes, oatmeal, and fruit may also help to reduce the absorption of fat.

A very vigorous dietary regimen can reduce circulating lipids by over 10 per cent. A more standard lipid-lowering diet is unlikely to reduce lipid levels by more than 2 per cent, and although it should be employed as sole treatment for a short while, it is unfair to criticize the patient for failing to follow dietary advice if no change can be detected in lipid levels after a few weeks. It should be remembered that thin, as well as obese people can be hyperlipidaemic.

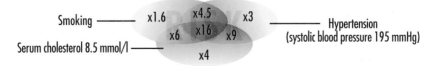

Smoking —— x1.6 x4.5 x3 —— Hypertension (systolic blood pressure 195 mmHg)
x6 x16 x9
Serum cholesterol 8.5 mmol/l —— x4

Fig. 18.1 Relative risks of coronary heart disease.

Table 18.2
Hypercholesterolaemia (and mixed hyperlipidaemia)

When to intervene	What to use	Notes
Cholesterol 5.2–6.5 mmol/l	Diet	A random blood sample is representative, provided it is taken <24 h after a myocardial infarction or > 3 months after surgery or a major illness. Patients with known CHD and cholesterol ≥5.5 mmol/l should be treated with Simvastatin in addition to diet
Cholesterol 6.5–7.8 mmol/l	1. Diet + statin 2. Diet + statin + resin 3. Diet + statin + fibrate	
Consider treatment if diet alone is insufficient and two or more elements of the following description are present: An obese, male, diabetic, cigarette smoker, with a personal and family history of early onset coronary heart disease and peripheral vascular disease, who has been found to have an HDL cholesterol level of <0.9 mmol/l	(consider a trial of sex hormone replacement therapy for postmenopausal women)	Exclude hypothyroidism, renal, and hepatic problems, and treat uncontrolled diabetes mellitus A 3–6 month trial of diet alone is often worthwhile in all types of hyperlipidaemia With statins, muscle enzymes and liver function tests need to be checked every 3 months initially, then every 6 months after 1 year treatment
Cholesterol > 7.8 mmol/l	1. Diet + statin 2. Diet + statin + resin 3. Diet + statin + fibrate	Concurrent use of statins and fibrates is probably quite safe and works better than either alone. A painful but reversible myopathy sometimes occurs

Table 18.3
Hypertriglyceridaemia

When to intervene	What to use	Notes
Triglyceride 2.3–5.6 mmol/l	Diet	Patients need to fast for at least 14 h before the sample is taken
Triglyceride >5.6 mmol/l	1. Diet 2. Diet + fibrate 3. Diet + fibrate + acipimox	Correction of secondary causes, such as uncontrolled diabetes or excessive alcohol intake, is usually all the treatment that is required

Table 18.4
Cholesterol-containing food (mg/100 g)

Eggs	450
Liver	330
Butter	230
Cheese (cheddar)	102
Milk	14
Vegetable oil	0

Key points

- Evidence that treatment of hyperlipidaemia saves lives is unequivocal.
- Groups at high absolute risk of coronary heart disease events, such as diabetics and patients with peripheral vascular or ischaemic heart disease, should be targeted for treatment.
- In isolation, a high cholesterol is a poor predictor of risk: a 75 per cent reduction in an already negligible risk, is not worthwhile.
- Fasting blood samples are required for triglyceride, but not for cholesterol measurement.
- A total cholesterol of over 5.5 mmol/l in a patient who has had a myocardial infarction should be treated with a statin.
- Fibrinogen and Lp(a), like raised cholesterol and low HDL cholesterol, are independent risk factors for ischaemic heart disease.

Table 18.5
Effects of lipid-lowering treatments

Treatment	Effects on			Costs	Mechanism of action and side-effects
	C	TG	HDL		
Lifestyle					
Ignore it	↑	↑	↑	No immediate costs	Depending on the circumstance, this is no longer a tenable course of action. Lowering total cholesterol in individuals with a high absolute risk of coronary heart disease saves lives
Diet	→	→	←	Saves money	20 per cent of men and 30 per cent of women are overweight. Central obesity (beer belly) is a greater risk than peripheral obesity. Although always recommended, attempts to change diet and life-style rarely produce substantial or sustained improvements in lipid levels
Exercise	↑	→	←	Variable	Can produce a feeling of well-being, and increases self-respect. But is also time consuming and associated with musculoskeletal injuries. In practice, exercise without dietary manipulation is a difficult and slow way to lose weight
Alcohol	→	↑	→	Variable	Up to 14 or 21 units of alcohol/week (female/male) age ≥50, has a beneficial effect on coronary heart disease mortality by increasing HDL levels
Smoking	←	↑	→	Saves money	Smoking has minor direct effects on lipids but a major impact on coronary heart disease risk. Patients should be advised to stop smoking if possible. Nicotine patches may be useful

continued below

Treatment	Effects on			Costs	Mechanism of action and side-effects
	C	TG	HDL		
Major lipid-lowering treatment modalities					
Statins	↓	↓	↑	£15–30 per month	Statins inhibit HMG-CoA reductase, and their effects are therefore most marked on cholesterol levels, with an increase in LDL receptor activity and fall in LDL. They are well tolerated but can cause myalgia, rashes, and insomnia. Reversible myopathy may occur when used with fibrates, particularly with the older derivates. Epidemiological evidence for their use in secondary prevention of coronary heart disease events is excellent
Fibrates	↓	↓	↑	£8–30 per month	Fibrates increase LDL receptor and LPL activity and reduce VLDL synthesis and fibrinogen levels. They are well tolerated and effective in most hyperlipidaemic scenarios, but are particularly effective for hyperlipidaemia involving raised triglycerides. Unfortunately, there is little good epidemiological data to support their use in secondary prevention. They should be avoided in hepatic or severe renal disease, or in the presence of gallstones
Less commonly used lipid-lowering treatments					
Acipimox	↓	↓	↑	£25–35 per month	Nicotinic acid derivatives, such as acipimox, limit adipocyte lipolysis and therefore the flow of fatty acid precursors to the liver for triglyceride synthesis. They are potentially dangerous drugs with significant side-effects such as flushing, itching, and diarrhoea. They should be avoided in peptic ulcer disease and used in a specialist setting
Resins	↓	↑↓	↑	£25–50 per month	Resins limit bile acid reabsorption, increase hepatic LDL receptor activity, and increase bile acid synthesis. They cause constipation, bloating, and interfere with the absorption of folic acid, fat-soluble vitamins, and drugs, including fibrates

continued next page

Treatment	Effects on			Costs	Mechanism of action and side-effects
	C	TG	HDL		
Other treatments of less proven benefit					
Vitamin E	↑	↑	↑	£1–2 per month	Antioxidants, such as fat-soluble vitamin E (≥100 U/day) may reduce coronary heart disease events by 40 per cent. There is currently insufficient evidence to advocate the widespread use of these supplements. Confirmatory studies are underway
Garlic	→	→	←	Not available on prescription	Modest beneficial effects of garlic are seen on lipid profiles in patients with non-insulin-dependent diabetes. The German Health Office recommends a daily intake of 4 g of fresh garlic bulb daily: 2–3 g may be enough to reduce C & TG by 10 per cent, but this needs to be confirmed
Oestrogen	→	↑→	←	£3–10 per month	For postmenopausal women with a moderately raised cholesterol, a trial of HRT is useful, as oestrogens raise HDL and lower LDL
α-Blockers	→	→	←	£8–40 per month	Together with ACE inhibitors and calcium antagonists, these are the treatments of choice for hypertension in diabetics

C, cholesterol; HDL, high-density lipoproteins; TG, triglycerides.

'My patient was found to have a high cholesterol at a routine health check. Please advise'

History

A 56-year-old businessman attended a 'well man' screening clinic and was found to have a total cholesterol of 8.2 mmol/l. He smoked 15–20 cigarettes daily, drank 'a pint or two' occasionally after work and often relaxed with a glass of whisky in the evening. He took no regular exercise but believed himself to be generally fit, unlike his 49-year-old brother who had been diagnosed as having angina (pectoris). His father died of a 'heart attack' at 63 years.

Examination

The patient was moderately obese (BMI = 28 kg/m^2) with predominantly central obesity. A bilateral arcus corneus was present, but no xanthomas or xanthelasmata. Heart sounds were normal and his blood pressure was 158/90 mmHg.

Investigations

Full blood count, urea, creatinine, electrolytes, and liver function tests were normal, with the exception of a raised γGT. Random blood glucose was 5.6 mmol/l; free T$_4$, 9.5 pmol/l (normal range 10–23 pmol/l); and TSH 6.8 mU/l (normal range 0.3–6 mu/l). Repeat thyroid function test and lipid analysis showed a FT$_4$ of 10.1 pmol/l, TSH of 7 mu/l, total cholesterol of 7.9 mmol/l, and an HDL cholesterol of 1.2 mmol/l. Triglyceride was 2.4 mmol/l. Thyroid microsomal autoantibodies were positive at 1:120.

Management

The consequences of the patient's life style—diet, exercise, cigarette and alcohol consumption—were discussed with the patient who was encouraged to adopt a calorie-restricted, low-fat diet. In view of the positive thyroid autoantibodies, his chance of developing unequivocal rather than just biochemical hypothyroidism was high, and he was started on thyroxine (100 μg daily). After 3 months, his total cholesterol had fallen to 7 mmol/l and his weight had decreased by 3 kg. Nevertheless, his TSH was still towards the upper end of the normal range (4.2 mU/l) and his thyroxine replacement was increased to 112.5 μg daily (as 100 and 125 μg on alternate days). His weight stabilized at this level and as his cholesterol remained at around 7 mmol/l, a fibrate was added to his tablet regimen.

Multiple-choice questions

1. In coronary heart disease, risk factors include:
   a. Number of years spent smoking;
   b. Diabetes;
   c. A parent dying of heart disease;
   d. Cholelithiasis;
   e. Systolic blood pressure.

2. The following drugs have a beneficial effect on blood lipids:
   a. Moderate ethanol ingestion;
   b. Oestrogens;
   c. Atenolol (beta-adrenergic blocker);
   d. Thiazide diuretics such as bendrofluazide;
   e. Naproxen.

3. The following statements are true:
   a. Once a heart attack has occurred, it is not worth instituting drug treatment to reduce blood lipids;
   b. A serum cholesterol of 8.5 mmol/l or greater quadruples the risk of coronary heart disease;
   c. 10–30 per cent of circulating cholesterol is in the form of LDL;
   d. Low blood lipids are causally related to cancer deaths and suicide;
   e. Although binding resins such as cholestyramine cause unpleasant symptoms, they should be used because they are much less expensive than 'statins' and 'fibrates'.

4. The following are signs of hyperlipidaemia:
   a. Cholelithiasis (gallstones);
   b. Carpal tunnel syndrome;
   c. Tendon xanthomata;
   d. Arcus corneus;
   e. Xanthelasmata.

Answers

1. In coronary heart disease, risk factors include:
   a. Smoking   T
      Smoking is one of a number of factors that contribute to coronary heart disease risk. For each patient, the 'absolute' risk of coronary heart disease events needs to be estimated to determine whether treatment with lipid-lowering drugs is likely to be beneficial. A marked reduction in 'relative' risk of a cardiac event is irrelevant if the risk was already very low.
   b. Diabetes   T
      Diabetes is a major risk factor for coronary artery disease.

c. A parent dying of heart disease   T

This is one of many risk factors for coronary heart disease. Complex equations can be used to estimate risk but are not particularly practical for use in the clinic. For that reason, major risk factors (such as the presence of peripheral vascular disease) take precedence.

d. Cholelithiasis   F

e. Systolic blood pressure   T

The relative risks of the major factors in coronary heart disease risk, and particular the high risks of hypertension and smoking, are neatly quantified by the following equation from the British Regional Heart Study:

(7.5 × number of years spent smoking) + (4.5 × systolic blood pressure (mean of two readings)) + 265 if a man recalls a doctor diagnosis of coronary heart disease + 150 if current angina + 80 if parent died of 'heart trouble' + 150 if diabetic (or impaired glucose tolerance).

A score of 1000 or more defines the top quintile of risk, who would then be offered a serum cholesterol estimation.

2. The following drugs have a beneficial effect on blood lipids:

a. Moderate ethanol ingestion   T

A beneficial effect is evident with the consumption of 2–3 units daily (1–1.5 pints of beer). At higher doses, hypertriglyceridaemia occurs and can remain even after the patient has ceased heavy intake.

b. Oestrogens   T

Traditionally, sex hormone replacement therapy is something that has been contraindicated in hyperlipidaemia. Yet, oestrogens raise HDL and lower LDL—effects that may be in part responsible for the effects of female sex hormone replacement therapy on longevity.

c. Atenolol (beta-adrenergic blocker)   F

Beta-blockers have an adverse effect on blood lipids. However, alpha-blockers, such as prazosin, doxazosin, and terazosin, decrease both cholesterol and triglycerides, while increasing HDL cholesterol.

d. Thiazide diuretics such as bendrofluazide   F

These should be avoided in hyperlipidaemics and also in diabetes, as they tend to have an adverse effect on blood glucose and blood lipids.

e. Naproxen   F

Non-steroidal anti-inflammatory drugs do not have any significant effects on blood lipids.

3. The following statements are true:

a. Once a heart attack has occurred, it is not worth instituting drug treatment to reduce blood lipids   F

The potential benefits will not be as great as they would have been had the treatment been commenced earlier, nevertheless there is increasing evidence that late treatment is worthwhile, and that if lipid levels are lowered, coronary artery lesions are capable of regression.

b. A serum cholesterol of 8.5 mmol/l or greater quadruples the risk of coronary heart disease   T
The relative risk exceeds that of smoking and of a systolic blood pressure in excess of 195 mmHg.

c. 10–30 per cent of circulating cholesterol is in the form of LDL   F
About 70 per cent of cholesterol is in this form.

d. Low blood lipids are causally related to cancer deaths and suicide   F
This spurious but much publicized association is an artefact of the cholesterol-lowering effect of major illnesses such as tumours and depression.

e. Although binding resins such as cholestyramine cause unpleasant symptoms, they should be used because they are much less expensive than 'statins' and 'fibrates'   F
In most cases they are just as expensive.

4. The following are signs of hyperlipidaemia:

a. Cholelithiasis (gallstones)   F
However, the treatment for hyperlipidaemia may predispose to gallstone formation by increasing cholesterol excretion into bile.

b. Carpal tunnel syndrome   F
Very common in acromegaly. Also occurs in hypothyroidism, pregnancy, and rheumatoid arthritis.

c. Tendon xanthomata   T
A major clinical manifestation of familial type II hypercholesterolaemia, and essentially diagnostic of the condition or the heterozygous state.

d. Arcus corneus   T
The sign is very common in the elderly and is of little clinical significance. However, in younger patients it is a very useful sign.

e. Xanthelasmata   T
Again, a sign of hyperlipidaemia, but not much use diagnostically because they are so common in the normal population.

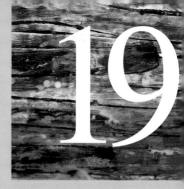

19

Calcium metabolism and bone

- Summary

- Introduction

- Skeletal development

- Remodelling

- Hormones (and inorganic ions) involved in calcium regulation

- Common clinical problems in calcium metabolism

- Calcium emergencies

- Key points

- Case histories

- Multiple-choice questions

Summary

Normal function

- To facilitate skeletal growth and mineral accretion.
- To allow for bone remodelling and repair.
- To maintain extracellular calcium within the narrow limits required for optimal physiological function.

Typical pathology

- Osteoporosis is the single biggest endocrine problem. It affects almost 100 per cent of women by the age of 80 years and their lifetime risk of osteoporotic fracture is close to 40 per cent.
- Hypercalcaemia
  - → Primary hyperparathyroidism. Calcium levels are controlled principally by parathyroid hormone (PTH) and vitamin D, both of which increase circulating calcium.
  - → Hypercalcaemia of malignancy. The elaboration of PTH-related peptide (PTHrp) from solid tumours or 'calcaemic factors' from haematological malignancies accounts for most cases of hypercalcaemia that are not due to primary hyperparathyroidism.
- Hypocalcaemia
  - → Primary hypocalcaemia is rare and results from either inadequate PTH secretion or effect.
  - → Vitamin D deficiency gives rise to rickets in children and osteomalacia in nutritionally and sunlight-deprived adults.

'Typical clinical scenario'

- A 26-year-old amenorrhoeic patient with a low body mass index (more than 10 per cent below ideal weight) who does not want to risk osteoporosis in later life, but does not 'like the thought of' sex hormone replacement therapy or putting on weight either.

Introduction

At first sight, the panoply of hormones and tissues involved in calcium homeo-stasis appears daunting. Fortunately, in most cases, the reasons for abnormal calcium levels are easily evaluated and the causes simple to identify. A single con-dition, osteoporosis, makes calcium metabolism numerically one of the most important of all problems for the endocrinologist. Up to 40 per cent of women suffer one or more osteoporotic fractures and by the age of 80 years, the incidence of oestoporosis in women approaches 100 per cent.

Skeletal development

Depending to some extent on genetic potential, exercise, diet, hormonal status, and calcium intake, total body calcium increases from 25 g at birth to 1200 g in the adult. During this time, an average of 400 mg of calcium is added to the skeleton daily, with most rapid accretion between the ages of 11 and 15 years. Peak bone mass occurs at about 30 years in women (peak spinal mass at 15 years) and is then lost at about 3 per cent decade, accelerating to about 9 per cent per decade (1–2 per cent per year) from the menopause (usually 45–50 years) until the seventy-fifth year. From then on, bone mineral loss slows to about 3 per cent per decade—the rate of loss experienced in men from the peak mass at 40 years (spinal mass peaks at 17 years) throughout adult life. Women have less bone mass/volume than men at all ages, and typically, by the age of 80, 30 per cent of peak bone mass may have been lost. At the present time, although bone quantity can be measured with reasonable accuracy, bone quality (i.e. its fracture resistance) cannot.

Remodelling

Continual remodelling of internal and external bone surfaces allows for accretion (bone formation) and resorption, microfracture repair, and adjustment of the load-bearing properties of the skeleton. Once recruited, osteoclasts actively resorb bone at about 5 μm/day for 10 days, leaving resorption pits or lacunae. Osteoblasts follow in their wake, forming and then mineralizing osteoid.

With every remodelling cycle of bone resorption and formation in adulthood, there is a very slight reduction in bone mass, so that merely increasing the number of 'normal' remodelling cycles tends to reduce overall bone mass. Cancellous bone is most affected by this process, as although it accounts for only 20 per cent of the total bone mass, it represents 80 per cent of the bone surface area (the exact opposite to cortical bone).

Hormones (and inorganic ions) involved in calcium regulation

Parathyroid hormone (PTH)

PTH mobilizes calcium from bone and reduces renal calcium clearance. PTH also increases renal phosphate loss and indirectly increases gut calcium absorption by stimulating formation of 1,25-dihydroxycholecalciferol (1,25(OH)$_2$D). PTH is thought to stimulate osteoclast activity via the osteoblasts.

Vitamin D

The main function of vitamin D is to stimulate calcium absorption from the gut. As vitamin D is a fat-soluble vitamin, it is no surprise that it is found pre-

Parathyroids:
The parathyroid glands secrete PTH in response to a fall in calcium, & are turned off within seconds by an increase in calcium.

Thyroid:
Calcitonin (from 'C' cells) has a minimal effect on calcium regulation, even at high levels.

Skin:
Sunlight on the skin induces vitamin D (cholecalciferol) formation from 7-dehydrocholesterol.

Liver:
The liver hydroxylates cholecalciferol at the 25 position. It also produces plasma proteins which bind about 50% of circulating calcium, and bile, without which fat soluble vitamin D could not be absorbed.

Kidneys:
Renal reabsorption of calcium and clearance of phosphate is stimulated by PTH. The kidneys hydroxylate 25-hydroxycholecalciferol in the 1 position, to produce $1,25(OH)_2D$. Thiazide diuretics also reduce calcium clearance.

Intestines:
Calcium absorption from the gut is regulated by $1,25(OH)_2D$. Phosphate is absorbed in parallel with dietary supply. Therefore plasma phosphate levels are highly unreliable unless patients are fasted & renal function is normal.

Bones:
The skeleton contains more than 98% of total body calcium. PTH stimulates osteoclasts & increases calcium & phosphate loss from bone. As PTH also increases renal phosphate clearance, circulating phosphate falls.

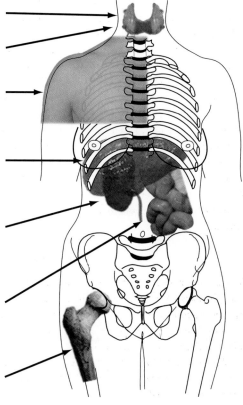

Fig. 19.1 Tissues involved in calcium regulation.

dominantly in fish and dairy products, and is absorbed from the small bowel in the presence of bile. Sunlight on the skin induces vitamin D (cholecalciferol) formation from 7-dehydrocholesterol. Cholecalciferol is hydroxylated at the 25 position in the liver, and further hydroxylated to $1,25(OH)_2D$ by the kidneys.

Calcitonin

Despite its name, endogenous calcitonin is only a minor player in calcium regulation, producing a small increase in renal clearance of calcium and phosphate, and reduction in bone resorption. Its main use in clinical medicine is as a marker of medullary thyroid carcinoma—also derived from thyroid 'C' cells—and in the treatment of painful osteoporotic fractures.

Parathyroid hormone-related peptide (PTHrp) and other 'calcaemic factors'

Many malignancies, irrespective of whether they have metastasized to bone, are associated with hypercalcaemia. This appears to be because they elaborate PTH-related peptide (predominantly a solid tumour product) or 'calcaemic factors', some of which have been identified as cytokines (from haematological malignancies). The physiological function of these peptides in man is unclear. PTHrp is a useful (solid) tumour marker.

Sex hormones

Oestrogens increase serum PTH and 1,25(OH)$_2$D, decrease urinary calcium clearance, and increase retention of whole-body calcium. Androgens have a similar effect but probably act via local conversion to oestrogens.

Glucocorticoids

Pharmacological doses of glucocorticoids are dramatically effective at removing bone. In response to 30 mg of prednisolone daily, bone density falls initially by an astounding 17.5 per cent/year. A tapering dose of prednisolone from 10 mg daily to zero over 3 months, *permanently* reduces overall bone density by about 5 per cent, and even at 7.5 mg daily (or 15 mg every other day), increased bone loss is inevitable. However, release of 'calcaemic factors' from some haematological malignancies can be inhibited by glucocorticoids.

Thyroid hormones

Thyroid hormones stimulate bone resorption and increase circulating calcium levels. This suppresses PTH production and increases renal calcium loss.

Fluoride

High-dose fluoride treatment dramatically increases spinal bone mineral density, but fracture rates remain unchanged. Complications such as abdominal pain and plantar fasciitis limited treatment in early high-dose trials. The use of lower doses in controlled-release preparations (40 mg sodium monofluoride) may find a therapeutic niche in the future.

Bisphosphonates

Bisphosphonates are analogues of pyrophosphate, the substrate of bone crystal formation. They are potent inhibitors of bone turnover that have revolutionized the treatment of Paget's disease of bone (see p. 313). They are also increasingly used in the treatment of osteoporosis and hypercalcaemia.

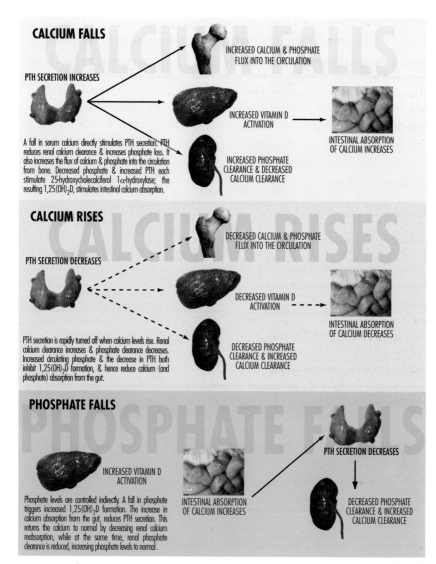

CALCIUM FALLS

PTH SECRETION INCREASES

INCREASED CALCIUM & PHOSPHATE
FLUX INTO THE CIRCULATION

INCREASED VITAMIN D
ACTIVATION

INCREASED PHOSPHATE
CLEARANCE & DECREASED
CALCIUM CLEARANCE

INTESTINAL ABSORPTION
OF CALCIUM INCREASES

A fall in serum calcium directly stimulates PTH secretion. PTH reduces renal calcium clearance & increases phosphate loss. It also increases the flux of calcium & phosphate into the circulation from bone. Decreased phosphate & increased PTH each stimulate 25-hydroxycholecalciferol 1α-hydroxylase; the resulting 1,25(OH)$_2$D, stimulates intestinal calcium absorption.

CALCIUM RISES

PTH SECRETION DECREASES

DECREASED CALCIUM & PHOSPHATE
FLUX INTO THE CIRCULATION

DECREASED VITAMIN D
ACTIVATION

DECREASED PHOSPHATE
CLEARANCE & INCREASED
CALCIUM CLEARANCE

INTESTINAL ABSORPTION
OF CALCIUM DECREASES

PTH secretion is rapidly turned off when calcium levels rise. Renal calcium clearance increases & phosphate clearance decreases. Increased circulating phosphate & the decrease in PTH both inhibit 1,25(OH)$_2$D formation, & hence reduce calcium (and phosphate) absorption from the gut.

PHOSPHATE FALLS

INCREASED VITAMIN D
ACTIVATION

PTH SECRETION DECREASES

INTESTINAL ABSORPTION
OF CALCIUM INCREASES

DECREASED PHOSPHATE
CLEARANCE & INCREASED
CALCIUM CLEARANCE

Phosphate levels are controlled indirectly. A fall in phosphate triggers increased 1,25(OH)$_2$D formation. The increase in calcium absorption from the gut, reduces PTH secretion. This returns the calcium to normal by decreasing renal calcium reabsorption, while at the same time, renal phosphate clearance is reduced, increasing phosphate levels to normal.

Fig. 19.2 Control of serum calcium and phosphate levels.

Common clinical problems in calcium metabolism

Hyperparathyroidism

Primary

The prevalence of primary hyperparathyroidism is 0.1 per cent, making it one of the most common endocrine conditions. At least 80 per cent of cases are caused by a

Table 19.1
Serum calcium, phosphate, and alkaline phosphatase levels in a variety of disorders of calcium metabolism

	Calcium	Phosphate	Alkaline phosphatase
Osteoporosis	N	N	N
Osteomalacea	N or low	Low	N or raised
Primary hyperparathyroidism	Raised	N or low	Raised
Secondary hyperparathyroidism	N or low	N or raised	Raised
Tertiary hyperparathyroidism	Raised	Variable	Raised
Hypoparathyroidism	Low	Raised	Normal
Paget's disease of bone	N unless immobilized	N	Often markedly raised

Phosphate levels are influenced by diet and are therefore often diagnostically unhelpful.

Table 19.2
Calcium measurement

Different laboratories use a variety of methods to measure either total or ionized calcium in serum. Neuromuscular excitability and feedback regulation of PTH secretion is mediated by ionized calcium, but the measurement of calcium ions is complicated by the effect of changes in sample pH (as pH increases, ionized calcium decreases). Total calcium, corrected for serum albumin (e.g. add 0.0225 mmol/l to the calcium concentration for every 1 g albumin below 42 g/l) is therefore usually measured

single adenoma, and most of the rest, by multiple adenomas or hyperplasia of all four glands. Parathyroid carcinomas occur in up to 3 per cent of cases, and the multiple endocrine neoplasia syndromes are involved in a very small proportion of cases.

Treatment

As raised calcium levels in primary hyperparathyroidism tend to be stable, surgery, particularly in elderly patients, is often reserved for those with symptoms, such as weakness, dehydration, or renal impairment. Debate continues about the adverse effects on bone mineral content of prolonged periods of even mild hyperparathyroidism.

Table 19.3
Hyper- and hypocalcaemia: symptoms and signs

Hypercalcaemia	Hypocalcaemia
Pathogenesis	Pathogenesis
Major causes	Major causes
Primary hyperparathyroidism	Osteomalacia
Malignancy	Hypoparathyroidism (iatrogenic)
	Laboratory artefact
Minor causes	
Vitamin D intoxication	Minor causes
Sarcoidosis	Pseudohypoparathyroidism
Hyperthyroidism	'Hungry bones' following surgery for
Addison's disease	primary hyperparathyroidism
Symptoms	Symptoms
Usually none unless $Ca^{2+} \geqslant 3$	Ionized calcium determines membrane
Polyuria and polydipsia	excitability, and as this falls in
Fatigue and depression	hypocalcaemia or alkalosis, increased
Muscular aches and pains	neuromuscular excitability leads to:
Constipation	
Headaches	Cramps
Nausea and vomiting	Fits
	Cardiac arrhythmias
	Signs
	Chvostek's sign—twitching of the facial muscles when the branches of the facial nerve are gently percussed as they cross the mandible
	Trousseau's sign—tonic spasm of the forearm muscles when a cuff occludes vascular supply

Secondary

Secondary hyperparathyroidism is compensatory hypersecretion of PTH in response to hypocalcaemia. This occurs typically in chronic renal failure and is the province of nephrologists, rather than endocrinologists. Reduced renal clearance of phosphate decreases $1,25(OH)_2D$ production, intestinal calcium absorption is reduced, and PTH levels increase. There may also be peripheral (uraemia-induced) resistance to PTH and direct impairment of renal $1,25(OH)_2D$ synthesis.

Treatment

Plasma phosphate and calcium levels are controlled, and osteomalacia corrected with vitamin D supplements. In general, management consists of oral calcium supplements (such as calcium carbonate) and calcitriol (1,25(OH)$_2$D) or alpha-calcidol (1α-hydroxycholecalciferol) to facilitate calcium absorption from the gut. These are powerful vitamin D metabolites, and their use requires careful monitoring. Renal transplantation usually corrects or greatly improves the condition.

Tertiary

The development of autonomous PTH secretion in secondary hyperparathyroidism is called tertiary hyperparathyroidism. It is most often associated with the end stage of long-standing renal disease and is rarely seen in the endocrine clinic.

Treatment

Subtotal parathyroidectomy may be required in this condition, in addition to the management options outlined above.

Hypoparathyroidism

The association of hypocalcaemia (usually in the range of 1.2–1.5 mmol/l) and hyperphosphataemia in a patient with normal renal function strongly suggests hypoparathyroidism. Iatrogenic hypoparathyroidism following thyroidectomy and autoimmune destruction of the parathyroid glands are the most common causes.

Treatment

Treatment consists of long-term use of oral calcium and calcitriol (1,25(OH)$_2$D) or alphacalcidol (1α-hydroxycholecalciferol) to facilitate calcium absorption from the gut. In acute hypocalcaemia, for example, following surgically induced hypoparathyroidism, intravenous calcium supplements (20 ml of 10 per cent calcium gluconate over 10 min) may be required.

Pseudohypoparathyroidism

Pseudohypoparathyroidism is the condition in which functional receptors for PTH are absent, or biologically inactive PTH is produced. The biochemical picture is similar to that of hypoparathyroidism (low calcium and high phosphate), but with a markedly raised PTH. When the typical phenotype of pseudo-hypoparathyroidism (short, obese, and round-faced with short fingers, dental defects, and predisposition to *Candida* infections) occurs in normocalcaemic family members of patients with pseudohypoparathyroidism, the condition is referred to as pseudopseudohypoparathyroidism.

The action of PTH on the kidneys is accompanied by a marked increase in urinary cyclic AMP excretion. The absence of a urinary cyclic AMP response to PTH is used to distinguish pseudohypoparathyroidism from hypoparathyroidism in hypocalcaemic patients.

Table 19.4
Features of osteomalacia and rickets

Clinical	Radiological	Biochemical
Frequent	Osteomalacia	Frequent
Diffuse bone pain	Pseudofractures—Looser's	Serum calcium normal
Tenderness, often	zones	or low
pre-tibial	Decreased radiological	Serum 25(OH)D low
Apparent muscular	density	Serum alkaline
weakness	Abnormal trabecular	phosphatase normal or
	pattern	raised
Less frequent	Rickets	Less frequent
Neuromuscular	Thickened, cupped, and	Serum phosphate low
excitability	hazy metaphyseal border	(variable)
Fractures	Bone deformity	Mild acidosis
Bone deformity		

Treatment

Vitamin D (usually 1α-hydroxycholecalciferol (alfacalcidol) or 1,25(OH)$_2$D (calcitriol)) and calcium supplements are used to keep plasma calcium in the low normal range—enough to stop neuromuscular excitability but not enough to predispose to nephrolithiasis.

Osteomalacia (and rickets)

A vitamin D-deficient diet and insufficient exposure to solar ultraviolet radiation, still common in underprivileged communities, leads to defective bone mineralization. If this occurs during development, it is known as rickets. If it occurs after the epiphyseal plates have closed, it is called osteomalacia. Rarely, osteomalacia is caused by vitamin D resistance. More often, it accompanies malabsorption in conditions such as coeliac disease.

Osteoporosis

The World Health Organization defines osteoporosis as a decrease in bone mass by more than 2.5 standard deviations from the normal peak bone density in youth. Unlike 'complicated osteoporosis', in which a fracture has already occurred, it cannot be diagnosed radiologically, although any radiograph of a female octogenarian who has not received oestrogens will show osteoporosis, as the incidence of the condition at that age is 100 per cent. In real terms, fracture rates double when bone density is 1 SD below the young normal mean, and increase eightfold at 2 SD. There are no biochemical markers for osteoporosis.

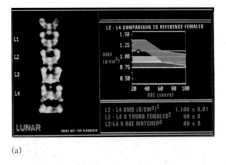

(a)

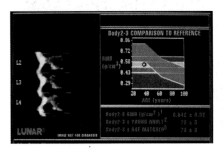

(b)

Fig. 19.3 Dual energy X-ray absorptiometry (DEXA) bone mineral density scan output (courtesy of Aura Scientific Ltd). The areas of interest, mean changes in bone mineral mass with age, and the patient's bone mineral density at each site can be clearly seen.

Prevention of osteoporosis

1. Make every effort to limit the dose and duration of glucocorticoid treatment.
2. Treat secondary hypogonadism if menses are irregular or absent.
3. Prevent secondary hyperparathyroidism by assuring a calcium intake of 1500 mg/day.
4. Maintain vitamin D levels near the top of the normal range.

Treatment for osteoporosis

1. Until recently, accepted use of oestrogens was to begin replacement treatment (sex hormone replacement therapy) within 10 years of the menopause, preferably within 6 years, and continue for 10 years or until the age of 65 if there is no family history of breast cancer. This indication is being revised as new data about breast cancer risk and new, more powerful bisphosphonate drugs become available.
2. Cyclical etidronate, 400 mg daily for 14 days every 3 months for 3 years, has been shown to be effective. Pamidronate, or other more powerful bisphosphonates such as alendronate, may be used increasingly in the future.

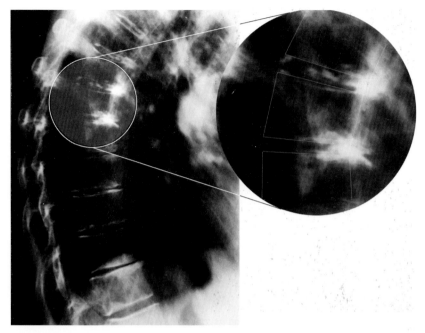

Fig. 19.4 Typical appearance of multiple spinal wedge fractures leading to kyphosis in an elderly female.

3. Women of 70 years or over should receive 400–800 U of vitamin D$_3$ (chole-calciferol) daily. This is conveniently given as one or two 'calcium and vitamin D' tablets daily. There are no side-effects, the cost is minimal, and even in patients over 80 years old, the incidence of hip fractures is reduced.
4. Dietary sodium restriction, thiazide diuretics to reduce urinary calcium loss, calcitonin, and fluoride treatments are also used in some carefully selected circumstances.
5. A series of exercises to improve spinal muscle strength. The patient is asked to do gentle push-ups against a wall, pinch the shoulder blades together, stretch a rubber band between the hands and, if the patient is able to get down on all fours (and get up again), extend each leg in turn (donkey kicks). Each exercises is repeated 10 times, two or three times daily.

Calcium emergencies

Calcium levels are usually tightly controlled between 2.12 and 2.62 mmol/l. Levels of 3 mmol/l do not often cause symptoms, but above about 3.25 mmol/l renal impairment and ectopic calcification may occur, particularly if phosphate levels are high. Levels over 3.5 mmol/l require urgent treatment and as the calcium reaches 4 mmol/l, coma and cardiac arrest can occur.

Table 19.5
Physical and biochemical measures of bone density, formation, and resorption

Bone density	Measures of formation (osteoblast activity)	Measures of resorption (osteoclast activity)
DEXA scan. Dual energy X-ray absorptiometry at the femoral neck and lumber spine is the most accurate method	Alkaline phosphatase (bone isoenzyme)	Pyridinium cross links (urinary excretion)
Calcaneal ultrasound, the speed of ultrasound transmission through the ankle is not yet as accurate	Osteocalcin (excretion rate in 24 h urine collection)	Hydroxyproline (urinary excretion)

Emergency treatment of hypercalcaemia

Until the underlying condition is diagnosed and definitive therapy instituted, the steps described in Table 19.7 are merely 'holding treatments'. The reduction in calcium is unlikely to last for long and the response to treatment the second time around is unlikely to be as good. As the prognosis is often poor, always consider the patients' comfort as well as their biochemistry. Blood samples for biochemical analysis, particularly PTH estimation, must be taken before treatment is commenced as subsequent measurements are likely to be unreliable.

Paget's disease of bone

Table 19.6
Paget's disease of bone

Definition	A chronic skeletal condition characterized by one or more foci of abnormally rapid and disorganized bone remodelling (up to 20 times normal)
Diagnosis	Findings on radiography are very characteristic. During bone remodelling, hydroxyproline is released from the collagen matrix. High levels of hydroxyproline are usually detected in urine
Pathogenesis	Still unknown. At present, attention is focused on the effects of a chronic viral infection
Prevalence	Varies widely, but about 1 per cent of people over 40 have radiological evidence of the condition
Presentation	Usually as an incidental finding on radiography or as a result of investigation of an unexplained, isolated elevation of alkaline phosphatase
	Less commonly, patients present with lumbar back pain, bone pain, or bone deformity
Complications	Complications are very rare. They include pathological (chalk stick) fracture, hypercalcaemia if the patient is immobilized, compression of structures surrounded by bone, such as the eighth nerve, high-output cardiac failure, and sarcomas
Treatment	Treatment is usually unnecessary. Simple analgesics such as aspirin are useful. Bisphosphonates, particularly pamidronate, dramatically reduce bone turnover and induce remissions lasting months or years. These drugs have swept glucocorticoids and calcitonin into the therapeutic small print

Table 19.7
Emergency treatment of hypercalcaemia

Hypercalcaemia is compounded by polyuria and dehydration. Rehydration is the initial treatment. Give at least 3 litres of saline over the first 24 h if possible, and continue at 2 litres or more per day until the patient is fully rehydrated. The calcium will fall by 0.1–0.3 mmol/l

Glucocorticoids rarely help except in haematological malignancies. Nevertheless, as most cases of extreme hypercalcaemia are caused by malignant disease, prednisolone 40 mg/day can be given

After 24–48 h consider using a bisphosphonate such as pamidronate 15–30 mg in 500 ml/0.9 per cent saline over 4 h (or 60–90 mg when the calcium is over 4 mmol/l). Calcium falls over a few days. Repeat doses may be required

Calcitonin, 100 units subcutaneously, three times daily after a test dose, works more quickly than the bisphosphonates, but does not normalize calcium

If calcium is dangerously high (>4.5 mM) and cardiovascular complications are present, there may be a case for rapid removal of calcium from the circulation using 50–100 mM of 0.1 M neutral phosphate buffer over 4–6 h, or EDTA infusion

Mithramycin (plicamycin) is used at 25 μg.kg.day in 1 l of 0.9 per cent saline over 4 h. It is an extremely toxic drug

Key points

- Skeletal integrity, neuromuscular excitability, and intracellular signalling are all calcium dependent.
- Hypercalcaemia is usually the result of primary hyperparathyroidism.
- The elaboration of 'calcaemic factors' from haematological malignancies, or PTH-related peptide (PTHrp) from solid tumours, accounts for most of the remaining cases of hypercalcaemia.
- Spontaneous hypocalcaemia sufficient to cause tetany is unusual and results from either inadequate PTH secretion, or inadequate PTH effect.
- Vitamin D deficiency gives rise to osteomalacia in nutritionally and sunlight-deprived communities.
- Osteoporotic fractures occur at some time in 40 per cent of the population.
- A tapering dose of prednisolone from 10 mg daily to zero over 3 months, permanently reduces overall bone density by about 5 per cent.
- To see if micro-fractures are the source of pain in a limb, run a finger down the leg and tape a paper clip to the painful area. If the pain corresponds to a lesion on a subsequent radiograph, the two are related.

'A routine check showed my patient to have a raised calcium. Please advise'

History

This 68-year-old man had previously been fit and well, but for the last few months had felt rather run down. He denied any change in his bowel habit or in the frequency of passing urine. A routine blood test as part of a workup for tiredness had been carried out, and led to the referral.

Examination

Unremarkable. Blood pressure 164/90 mmHg.

Investigations

Calcium 3 mmol/l (normal range 2.25–2.7 mmol/l); phosphate, 1.2 mmol/l (normal range 1–1.5 mmol/l); alkaline phosphatase, 150 U/l (normal range 20–120 u/l); urea, 7.3 mmol/l (normal range 3–7 mmol/l); creatinine, 143 μmol/l (normal range < 120 μmol/l). FBC and ESR normal. A parathyroid hormone estimation was 13 mmol/l (normal range 0.9–5.4 pmol/l).

Management

The diagnosis is primary hyperparathyroidism. As his renal function is good and he has no symptoms from the raised calcium, no action was taken other than to arrange follow up.

Explanation

In primary hyperparathyroidism calcium levels are elevated but still regulated appropriately, suggesting that the 'calcium sensing' mechanism has been re-set. The benefits of reducing calcium are often so minimal that surgical parathyroidectomy is not warranted. A potentially exciting advance is the development of new calcium-receptor blockers (distinct from calcium-*channel* blockers) that will 'fool the parathyroids into thinking that ambient calcium levels are higher than they actually are', and reduce parathyroid hormone secretion.

'My elderly patient has back pain and is losing height'

History

A 74-year-old lady suddenly developed back pain 5 weeks ago. It was very severe initially, but has eased a little since then. Two similar episodes of back pain had occurred during the past couple of years and, in each case, the symptoms largely resolved over a period of 8 weeks. Between attacks she was well, although after standing for a few minutes—doing housework or washing up—a dull ache developed between her shoulder blades and forced her to sit down. She believes that she has lost about 3″ (7.6 cm) in height over the past 5 years.

She had had a cholecystectomy and an appendectomy in the past, and her menopause occurred at 50 years of age.

Examination

There was marked kyphosis and pain on palpation at T8–9. Otherwise, no significant abnormalities were detected.

Investigations

A lateral radiograph of her spine confirmed the diagnosis of 'established osteoporosis' with a number of wedge fractures (Fig. 19.4). There was no evidence of Paget's disease and no lytic lesions. A full blood count was normal.

Management

The problem was explained to the patient using the following analogy: the back is like a flagpole held up with muscular guyropes. If the flagpole is shortened by fractures, the guyropes become lax and need to be tightened to maintain posture. Between fractures, the discomfort comes from muscle strain rather than from the bones themselves.

She was given a series of exercises to improve the muscle strength in her back and, in addition, was started on cyclical etidronate (400 mg daily for 2 weeks every 3 months) and two tablets of calcium and vitamin D (400 IU each) daily, long term.

Explanation

The normal full blood count and absence of lytic lesions on radiography excluded myeloma. The lifetime risk of osteoporotic fracture is 40 per cent. Of these 80–90 per cent are vertebral and 40–50 per cent in the hip. For every SD the bone mineral density (BMD) is below the mean, the risk doubles. The usefulness of oestrogens in a 74-year-old is doubtful. Below 70 years, in a patient without a close family history of breast cancer, oestrogens would still be used, starting at a low dose of 0.3 μg Premarin® once every 2–3 days, gradually increasing if tolerated to a full replacement at 0.625 μg, with Provera® (medroxyprogesterone acetate) 5 mg daily for 5 days every 2–3 months.

'My patient has malaise and pains in the arms and legs'

History

A 63-year-old Indian female who spoke very little English despite having lived in the country for 12 years, was referred with general malaise and 'pain in the arms and legs'. Through an interpreter, it was clear that she had initially put her 18 months of symptoms down to overwork. Nevertheless the pain in her legs had progressively worsened and it was becoming difficult for her to look after her husband and four children. Her diet consisted of mostly vegetarian, Indian cuisine and apart from shopping at the local grocers she rarely went out.

Examination

On examination she was moderately obese but essentially well. There were no areas of localized discomfort on palpation of her limbs, and no arthralgia. She was able to stand from squatting, but clearly found it painful to do so.

Investigations

Calcium was 2.1 mmol/l (normal range 2.1–2.6 mmol/l); phosphate, 0.9 mmol/l (normal range 0.8–1.4 mmol/l); and alkaline phosphatase, 137 U/l (normal range 20–120 u/l). Chest radiography and radiography of her pelvis and hips were normal.

Management

The history suggests that she spent most of the time indoors with very little exposure to the sun. A diagnosis of probable osteomalacia was made and she was treated with calcium and vitamin D tablets (400 IU/tablet). Her symptoms resolved completely over a period of 12 weeks, and the alkaline phosphatase returned to normal.

Explanation

In many extended Indian households, there are one or two middle-aged or elderly women who rarely venture beyond the confines of the home. When they do, they expose very little skin to the sun and the small amount of vitamin D in their diet (unless they consume large amounts of dairy products) compounds the problem. A common complaint is 'too much pain' or 'total body pain'. A therapeutic trial of calcium and vitamin D, even in the absence of biochemical support of the diagnosis, is inexpensive, safe, and often successful.

Multiple-choice questions

1. Bone mineral loss is accelerated by:
   a. Increased PTH;
   b. Increased T_4;
   c. Immobilization;
   d. Oestrogen or testosterone withdrawal;
   e. Glucocorticoid treatment.

2. In general therapeutics:
   a. Treatment with 15 mg of prednisolone every other day, rather than 7.5 mg daily, spares bone mineral;
   b. High-dose fluoride increases bone density and reduces fracture rates;
   c. Hypercalcaemia of malignancy is diagnostic of bone metastases;
   d. Bisphosphonates are first-line treatment for primary hyperparathyroidism;
   e. Daily exercise (such as aerobics) is beneficial for bone density.

3. Hypercalcaemia is a common feature of:
   a. Prolonged treatment with thiazide diuretics;
   b. Hyperthyroidism;
   c. Sarcoidosis;
   d. Ingestion of antacids;
   e. Paget's disease.

4. Bisphosphonates:
   a. Are well absorbed orally;
   b. Maintain their effect for as long as they remain in the skeleton;
   c. Increase the ability of osteoblasts to stimulate osteoclasts;
   d. Are rapidly cleared through hepatic metabolism;
   e. Are useful for hypercalcaemia of malignancy.

5. Primary hyperparathyroidism:
   a. Is one of the most common causes of hypercalcaemia;
   b. Is typically associated with hyperphosphataemia;
   c. Is typically associated with a raised urinary hydroxyproline;
   d. Usually results in a progressive and inexorable rise in serum calcium levels;
   e. Is associated with thirst, polyuria, and constipation.

6. The following groups are at increased risk of osteoporosis:
   a. Women who have had a simple hysterectomy;
   b. Smokers;
   c. Patients with treated hypothyroidism;
   d. Asthmatics taking beclomethasone dipropionate by inhaler;
   e. Cosmonauts.

Answers

1. Bone mineral loss is accelerated by:
   a. Increased PTH   T

   PTH increases within seconds of a reduction in plasma calcium level, and restores the situation by reducing renal calcium clearance, by increasing hepatic activation of vitamin D, and by increasing the calcium and phosphate flux out of bone.

   b. Increased T_4 T

   Thyroxine-induced osteoporosis may be caused by excessive thyroxine replacement in patients with hypothyroidism but is more usually the result of a prolonged period of unrecognized or inadequately treated thyrotoxicosis before treatment rendered the patient hypothyroid and replacement therapy was commenced.

   c. Immobilization   T

   This may well be one of the limiting problems in space travel. Bone integrity depends on weight bearing. Isometric muscle exercises help, but have to be pretty vigorous.

   d. Oestrogen or testosterone withdrawal   T

   Oestrogen (generated by aromatization) is the key bone mineral-preserving sex steroid in women and possibly in men, too. Because of this, an early menopause is associated with an increased risk of osteoporosis in later life.

   e. Glucocorticoid treatment   T

Glucocorticoids induce dramatic bone mineral loss. There is a good theoretical case but no data as yet to treat patients who are about to receive high-dose glucocorticoids (for a flare up of inflammatory bowel disease, asthma, or thyroid eye disease, for example) with bisphosphonates.

2. In general therapeutics:
   a. Treatment with 15 mg of prednisolone every other day, rather than 7.5 mg daily, spares bone mineral   F

There might be benefits as far as adrenocortical atrophy is concerned, but alas, not with bone mineral loss.

   b. High-dose fluoride increases bone density and reduces fracture rates   F

At high doses, 75 mg/day, bone density increases dramatically, but fracture rates tend to remain unchanged. The main changes are in the spine, so low-dose treatment might be considered in osteoporosis where the femoral neck density is relatively normal, but lumbar spine density is reduced.

   c. Hypercalcaemia of malignancy is diagnostic of bone metastases   F

Although in breast cancer, hypercalcaemia is usually associated with bone metastases, in many other malignancies hypercalcaemia is secondary to the production of calcium-releasing humoral factors.

   d. Bisphosphonates are first-line treatment for primary hyperparathyroidism   F

If treatment is needed, first-line therapy, at present, is surgery.

   e. Daily exercise (such as aerobics) is beneficial for bone density   T

While the pupils in the aerobics class may benefit from 'the burn' one or twice a week, the amount of exercise the teacher is having may be enough to render her amenorrhoeic. Oestrogen deficiency can then lead to dramatic osteoporosis despite the exercise, and many of these 'ultra-fit' people are shocked when their bone mineral density equates to that of a 70-year-old.

3. Hypercalcaemia is a common feature of:
   a. Prolonged treatment with thiazide diuretics   F

Hypercalcaemia may occur, but changes are mild, rare in the long term, and not usually clinically significant. By reducing urinary calcium loss, thiazide diuretics are potentially useful in the prevention of osteoporosis.

   b. Hyperthyroidism   F

It occurs in, at the most, 2–20 per cent of uncontrolled thyrotoxics.

   c. Sarcoidosis   F

Fewer than 1 in 5 cases of sarcoidosis are complicated by hypercalcaemia. It is thought to result from excessive vitamin D activation (by hydroxylation). The hypercalcaemia of vitamin D intoxication, unlike that of hyperparathyroidism or malignancy, is amenable to a reduction in dietary calcium intake, as the primary action of vitamin D is to enhance intestinal calcium absorption.

    d. Ingestion of antacids   F

Proton pump inhibitors and H_2 antagonists, some of which are available over the counter (i.e. without prescription), have greatly reduced the frequency of this complication of excessive antacid ingestion.

    e. Paget's disease   F

Only if patients are immobilized, and the disease is active and fairly extensive.

4. Bisphosphonates:

    a. Are well absorbed orally   F

Unfortunately, the absorption of etidronate is at best 1–3 per cent of the oral dose. Even coffee blocks absorption, so patients have to fast for 4 h before taking a dose last thing at night.

    b. Maintain their effect for as long as they remain in the skeleton   F

Although they are not metabolized, and remain in the bone long term, their activity wanes.

    c. Increase the ability of osteoblasts to stimulate osteoclasts   F

If anything, the opposite is true. There is, however, some evidence that bisphosphonates may inhibit osteoblast activity. Inhibition of bone mineralization has been a cause for concern with etidronate, but seems to be much less of a problem with the more potent bisphosphonates now available. With long-term use of alendronate, for example, osteoid seam width (unmineralized bone) does not appear to increase.

    d. Are rapidly cleared through hepatic metabolism   F

They remain in the skeleton for long periods.

    e. Are useful for hypercalcaemia of malignancy   T

However, if no other action is taken to deal with the tumour, the respite is often short lived, particularly with solid tumours.

5. Primary hyperparathyroidism:

    a. Is one of the most common causes of hypercalcaemia   T

The routine measurement of calcium as part of biochemical screening in hospital was largely responsible for the appreciation of the true incidence of this condition and its generally benign clinical course.

    b. Is typically associated with hyperphosphataemia   F

Plasma phosphate levels are not particularly reliable. If anything, however, phosphate is usually reduced. Renal resistance to vitamin D and defects in phosphate metabolism give rise to a series of rare conditions (such as vitamin D resistant rickets) that are characterized, amongst other biochemical characteristics, by hypophosphataemia.

    c. Is typically associated with a raised urinary hydroxyproline   F

Hydroxyproline, an amino acid, is a breakdown product of collagen that is not immediately re-used during bone synthesis. Released during resorption of the organic phase of bone, a raised urinary hydroxyproline is a typical finding in Paget's disease of bone.

    d. Usually results in a progressive and inexorable rise in serum calcium
levels   F

This would be unusual. The raised calcium level tends to be fairly static, as if the calcium-sensing mechanism of the parathyroid glands has been re-set.

    e. Is associated with thirst, polyuria, and constipation   T

These are symptoms associated with marked hypercalcaemia, which can be caused by hyperparathyroidism.

6. The following groups are at increased risk of osteoporosis:

    a. Women who have had a simple hysterectomy   T

After a simple hysterectomy, in which the ovaries are left *in situ*, about 25 per cent of women suffer premature ovarian failure within the subsequent 2 or 3 years. The reason for this is currently obscure—it might be related to interference with ovarian blood supply or perhaps a non-causal association between medical conditions currently treated with hysterectomy and ovarian failure. Nevertheless, women who have had their uterus removed are at risk of premature ovarian failure.

    b. Smokers   T

Smoking has anti-oestrogenic effects. Perimenopausal women who smoke may find that regular periods return for a time if they give up cigarettes.

    c. Patients with treated hypothyroidism   F

Thyrotoxicosis is associated with accelerated bone mineral loss, not hypothyroidism. There is some evidence that even after treatment, bone mineral density does not recover completely.

    d. Asthmatics taking beclomethasone dipropionate by inhaler   F

There is no convincing evidence that inhaled glucocorticoids at the doses generally used to treat bronchial asthma have significant effects on bone mineral, although they can be absorbed in amounts sufficient to suppress endogenous steroid secretion.

    e. Cosmonauts   T

Weightlessness produces dramatic bone mineral loss, much of which is not recoverable. The problem of 'skeletal off-loading' is not only a major limiting factor in long-term occupation of microgravity environments and space travel, but a major problem for patient who are bed bound for any length of time. To prevent this, muscle contractions with generated forces in excess of 12 Watts are required.

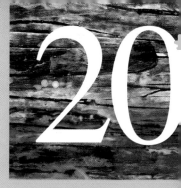

Water and salt

- Summary
- Introduction
- Diabetes insipidus
- SIADH
- Water deprivation test
- Hyperaldosteronism
- Key points
- Case history
- Multiple-choice questions

Summary

Normal function

- To maintain serum osmolality and electrolyte levels within the optimal range for normal physiological functioning.

Typical pathology

- Hypernatraemia (most major, acute problems of salt and water metabolism are seen in accident and emergency rather than in the clinic)
  - → Poorly controlled diabetes. Hyperglycaemia-induced osmotic diuresis compounded by decreased conscious level and failure to respond appropriately to thirst. The problem is sometimes obscured by hyperglycaemia (a blood glucose of 35 mmol/l results in an underestimation of serum sodium by 10 mmol/l) and made worse by injudicious rehydration with large amounts of 0.9 per cent saline.
- Hyponatraemia
  - → Overuse of diuretics, particularly combinations of amiloride and thiazides.
  - → SIADH (syndrome of inappropriate antidiuretic hormone secretion). Much less common than iatrogenic hyponatraemia, and usually self-limiting.

'Typical clinical scenario'

- A 62-year-old lady with central diabetes insipidus following subfrontal surgery for a craniopharyngioma. The patient is taking DDAVP (a synthetic analogue of vasopressin with enhanced half-life and reduced pressor effects) by nasal aerosol as well as thyroxine, hydrocortisone, and sex hormone replacement. She adjusts the dose to control symptoms of polyuria, polydipsia, and thirst, and omits a dose once a week to prevent water intoxication. The onset of thirst, with continued polyuria, indicates ongoing need for treatment.

Introduction

Under normal conditions serum osmolality is kept within remarkably tight limits. A 3 per cent increase in plasma osmolality (from 280 mOsm/l to 290 mOsm/l) is enough for the central osmoreceptors to switch regulation of free water clearance from maximum diuresis to maximum antidiuresis (Fig. 20.1).

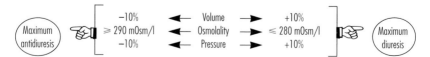

Fig. 20.1 Principal haemodynamic factors affecting diuresis.

Vasopressin acts on renal 'V2' receptors which increase water reabsorption from the distal tubule and collecting duct, and concentrate the urine. At high vasopressin levels, for example in severe hypotension or when pharmacological doses are used to control bleeding oesophageal varices, vascular 'V1' receptors are also stimulated, causing vasoconstriction.

A 5–10 per cent decrease in blood pressure, or a decrease in effective circulating volume by 10 per cent is sensed by peripheral baroreceptors. Increased osmolality and decreased blood volume and pressure result in enhanced posterior pituitary vasopressin release, reduced free water clearance and, at about 290 mOsm/l, by the onset of thirst.

The 'thirst centre' straddles the midline at the front of the hypothalamus (Fig. 20.2). The sensation of thirst in response to osmotic stimuli is so powerful that significant hypertonicity does not develop in conscious individuals given free access to water even when vasopressin is completely absent.

Diabetes insipidus

In diabetes insipidus there is insufficient vasopressin to concentrate the urine. In almost all cases seen in the endocrine clinic, the problem is 'central', i.e. the urine

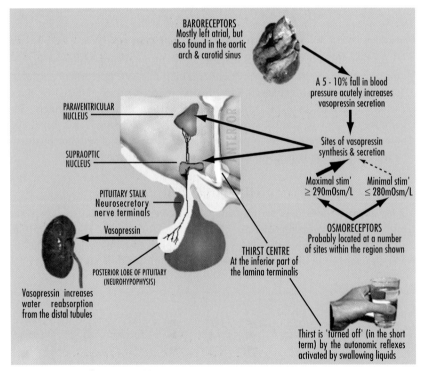

Fig. 20.2 Control of serum osmolality.

Table 20.1
Atrial natriuretic peptide (ANP)

ANP is one of a number of peptides (including brain natriuretic peptide) released from the cardiac atria (and ventricles) in response to atrial distension, sodium load, or increased catecholamines. ANP relaxes smooth muscle and directly inhibits both aldosterone secretion from the zona glomerulosa of the adrenal cortex and vasopressin release from the posterior pituitary. Consequently, immediately after injection of ANP into healthy volunteers, blood pressure falls and within 30 min sodium excretion and urine volume increase.

remains inappropriately dilute in the presence of raised plasma osmolality, and the condition can be corrected by giving exogenous vasopressin or a vasopressin analogue.

Nephrogenic diabetes insipidus, in which vasopressin levels are high, but ineffective, is typically found in childhood or in postobstructive nephropathy, and is the cause of the polyuria seen in hypokalaemia and hypercalcaemia.

Treatment

Therapeutically the long-acting analogue of vasopressin, desmopressin (DDAVP), is used either as a spray, as a propellant-driven aerosol, or in tablet form. DDAVP

Table 20.2
Causes of central diabetes insipidus

Relatively common

Transcranial, subfrontal surgery:
   usually carried out for craniopharyngiomas or pituitary
   macroadenomas; in some cases the condition eventually resolves

Transphenoidal pituitary surgery:
   diabetes insipidus is much less common with this approach as the hypothalamus
   itself is not directly accessible to the surgeon, and the pituitary tumour itself
   usually shields the posterior pituitary from the surgeon's advances
   Post-traumatic

Rare

Idiopathic (presumably autoimmune)
Granulomatous diseases—histiocytosis, sarcoidosis
Pregnancy: in pregnancy patients tend to have lower vasopressin reserves

Table 20.3
Causes of hyper- and hyponatraemia

Hypernatraemia	Hyponatraemia
Common	**Common**
Inability to drink for whatever reason (e.g. coma, confusion or cerebrovascular accident)	Iatrogenic — infusions of dextrose or dextrose/saline
	Diuretics, particularly amiloride in elderly people
Osmotic diuresis (i.e. hyperglycaemia)	Cardiac, renal, or hepatic failure
Rare	**Rare**
Diabetes insipidus	Syndrome of inappropriate vasopressin release (SIADH)
Burns (i.e. increased insensible loss)	Excessive water or beer intake
	Pseudohyponatraemia in hypertriglyceridaemia
	Untreated Addison's disease

liquid for injection is also available, but its use is rarely necessary in conscious patients. The dose of vasopressin is adjusted by the patient to control symptoms of polyuria, polydipsia, and particularly thirst. Patients are sometimes asked to omit a dose at intervals of a week or two to see, first, whether the underlying condition has resolved and, secondly, to prevent water intoxication. The onset of thirst, with continued polyuria, indicates ongoing need for treatment.

The presence of a number of discrete sites of vasopressin synthesis in each hemisphere explains why diabetes insipidus is usually caused by diffuse trauma or infiltration, rather than, for example, a single neoplastic lesion. The proximity of the thirst centre to the paraventricular and supraoptic nuclei accounts for the unusual but hazardous association of impaired thirst sensation with diabetes insipidus. Trauma, surgery for suprasellar lesions such as craniopharyngiomas, and infiltrative lesions can also impair thirst sensation in isolation.

SIADH

The syndrome of inappropriate antidiuretic hormone release (SIADH) is sustained vasopressin release or apparent action on the kidneys without appropriate osmotic or hypovolaemic stimuli. Total body salt levels are normal, but in a volume expanded state. Patients are typically drowsy and confused. Convulsions may also occur.

Table 20.4
Causes and treatment of SIADH

Causes	Treatment
Idiopathic (the most frequent 'diagnosis')	The condition usually resolves spontaneously after a few days
Lung infections	Fluid restrict
Tumours	Drugs that produce reversible nephrogenic
Central nervous system disorders	diabetes insipidus (i.e. demeclocycline)
Hypothyroidism	
Drugs (particularly phenothiazines)	

In most cases of SIADH, the condition resolves spontaneously while the cause is being investigated. Water deprivation is the most effective and elegant way to redress the biochemical disturbance, and is usually sufficient. If hypertonic solutions are used, it is critically important that they are given very cautiously (maximum rate of correction of 0.5–1 mmol/l.h) to minimize the risk of the brain-stem catastrophe 'central pontine myelinolysis'. Correction beyond a sodium of 125–130 mmol/l is unnecessary.

Water deprivation test

In practice, the precipitating cause of diabetes insipidus is usually apparent and the correct diagnosis clear from the history of unremitting thirst, polyuria, and nocturia. A single plasma osmolality can be useful to confirm the diagnosis, and a formal water deprivation test is often unnecessary.

The water deprivation test is the classical test to establish the presence of diabetes insipidus. Unless hysterical polydipsia (excessive drinking) has been so excessive and prolonged that the concentration gradient in the renal medulla has been 'washed out' (leading to reversible nephrogenic diabetes insipidus), a carefully carried out water deprivation test readily solves the usual clinical conundrum, which is to distinguish central diabetes insipidus from hysterical polydipsia (Table 20.5). Although the dangers of depriving patients with diabetes insipidus of water should be borne in mind throughout the test, if the patient is asked to restrict his or her fluid intake modestly from the previous afternoon, conclusive changes are often achieved more rapidly. Weight loss does not usually exceed 1 kg during the test. If it exceeds 2 kg, or if the condition of the patient deteriorates, the test (which was probably unnecessary in the first place) should be abandoned.

Table 20.5
Features that help to distinguish diabetes insipidus from hysterical polydipsia

Diabetes insipidus	Hysterical polydipsia
History of head trauma or tumour	History of psychiatric/behavioural disorders
Sudden onset	24 h urine volume >18 l
Unrelenting polyuria	History of episodic polyuria
Random osmolality >290 mOsm/l	Random plasma osmolality less than 285 mOsm/l

Hyperaldosteronism

Primary hyperaldosteronism is most often caused by a solitary adrenal adenoma (Conn's syndrome: see p. 91).

Table 20.6
Secondary hyperaldosteronism

Causes	Pathogenesis
Reduced circulating volume	This is a physiological response in patients with, for example, congestive cardiac failure, nephrotic syndrome, or hepatic cirrhosis
Diminished cardiac output	Again, a physiological response in heart failure
Hepatic cirrhosis	Reduced hepatic metabolism of aldosterone is often blamed, but a number of factors, including diminished blood volume, are implicated
Renin-secreting tumours	A rare cause of secondary hyperaldosteronism
Renal artery stenosis	Significant renovascular stenosis occurs in approximately 1 per cent of hypertensive patients

Key points

- In most cases, diabetes insipidus can be diagnosed from the history alone.
- If a water deprivation test is required to differentiate diabetes insipidus from hysterical polydipsia, ensure that the patient is weighed before *and* after passing urine.
- SIADH is usually self-limiting.

'My patient complains of uncontrollable thirst. Does she have diabetes insipidus?'

History

A 48-year-old female presented with thirst and polyuria. The letter from her GP made it clear that diabetes mellitus and renal glycosuria had been unequivocally excluded, and that although the patient had had a past history of multiple psychological and psychiatric problems, the symptoms were so dramatic that she was sure her patient had developed diabetes insipidus. The patient herself claimed that the symptoms had come on quite suddenly 3 months previously. She could scarcely contain her thirst by drinking large amounts of water, fruit juices, tea, and coffee, and had to make frequent trips to pass copious volumes of dilute urine during the day. She was woken up once, or occasionally twice, each night by the call to pass urine, usually within a couple of hours of retiring to bed.

Examination

The patient provided an animated description of her symptoms and showed no signs of depression or mental illness. Her visual fields were full to confrontation.

Investigations

Urea, calcium, Na^+, and K^+ were within normal limits. As the GP had specifically requested that diabetes insipidus be excluded, a water deprivation test was carried out. The initial serum osmolality of 280 mOsm/l remained essentially unchanged during the test, while urine osmolality rapidly increased.

Table 20.7
Results of water deprivation test

Time (hours after start)	08.00	09.00	10.00	11.00	12.00	13.00
Urine output (ml/h)	—	180	220	60	30	20
Urine osmolality (mOsm/l)	—	50	50	234	688	1020
Weight after voiding (kg)	65.2	65.1	65	64.6	64.6	64.5

Management

The diagnosis is hysterical polydipsia. The patient was reassured, leaving her GP to address the true problem—the psychological state of the patient.

Explanation

The initial increase in urine volume is the result of the patient drinking a large amount of fluid before presenting for the test 'to tide her over the trauma of being water deprived'. After the resulting transient diuresis had passed, however, there was a rapid decline in urine volume and increase in urine osmolality, as expected.

Given the history of past mental problems and the lack of profound diuresis throughout the night, the diagnosis was almost certain without resorting to a water deprivation test. The single call to pass urine each night, within 2 or 3 hours of retiring, represents the tail end of a normal diuresis caused by drinking excessively (i.e. exactly the same pattern as that demonstrated by the water deprivation test). It is sometimes worth excluding conditions that cause a dry mouth, as the patient may be responding to this with frequent sips of water that accumulate to a considerable fluid load.

Multiple-choice questions

1. Vasopressin secretion is induced by the following:
   a. A rise in blood pressure;
   b. A fall in effective blood volume;
   c. A decrease in blood osmolality;
   d. Nausea;
   e. Pituitary stalk transection.

2. Causes of diabetes insipidus include:
   a. Treatment with demeclocycline;
   b. Pituitary surgery;
   c. Stroke;
   d. Histiocytosis X (Langerhans cell histiocytosis);
   e. Head trauma.

3. SIADH (syndrome of inappropriate ADH (vasopressin) secretion) is characterized by:
   a. Increased plasma sodium ion concentration;
   b. Reduced plasma osmolality;
   c. Inappropriate diuresis;
   d. Drowsiness or fits;
   e. Decreased plasma urea concentration.

4. In a water deprivation test:
   a. An initial decrease in urine osmolality at the first time point after time zero suggests that the patient has had a large amount to drink immediately before the test;
   b. A mismatch between the volume of urine passed and decrease in weight at one or more time points suggests that the patient has had a surreptitious drink while in the toilet;
   c. A rapid decrease in urine volume and increase in urine osmolality indicates normality;
   d. Persistent passage of large amounts of dilute urine with a matching decrease in body weight confirms the diagnosis of diabetes insipidus;
   e. The patient is allowed to eat dry food.

Answers

1. Vasopressin secretion is induced by the following:
   a. A rise in blood pressure   F
   A 5–10 per cent *decrease* in blood pressure stimulates vasopressin release.
   b. A fall in effective blood volume   T
   A 10 per cent decrease in blood volume stimulates vasopressin release.
   c. A decrease in blood osmolality   F
   An *increase* in blood osmolality by only 3 per cent (from 280 to 290 mOsm/l) induces vasopressin release, turning maximum diuresis to maximum antidiuresis.
   d. Nausea   T
   Nausea is a powerful stimulus of vasopressin secretion.
   e. Pituitary stalk transection   F
   This cuts off the flow of vasopressin to the posterior pituitary, and is likely to reduce vasopressin output.

2. Causes of diabetes insipidus include:
   a. Treatment with demeclocycline   T
   This is used to induce mild, reversible nephrogenic diabetes insipidus.
   b. Pituitary surgery   T
   The most common cause. It is much more common after transcranial, sub-frontal surgery.
   c. Stroke   F
   SIADH is more likely than diabetes insipidus to follow a cerebrovascular accident.
   d. Histiocytosis X (Langerhans cell histiocytosis)   T
   Diabetes insipidus is the most common endocrine manifestation of this condition, in which the hypothalamus is diffusely affected. Bone and visceral involvement may also be found.
   e. Head trauma   T
   Anything that can produce widespread damage to the hypothalamus or disrupt the pituitary stalk can produce diabetes insipidus.

3. SIADH (syndrome of inappropriate ADH (vasopressin) secretion) is characterized by:
   a. Increased plasma sodium ion concentration   F
   b. Reduced plasma osmolality   T
   c. Inappropriate diuresis   F
   The opposite is true.
   d. Drowsiness or fits   T
   These symptoms and signs can certainly occur, and may be the first sign of a problem.
   e. Decreased plasma urea concentration   T

4. In a water deprivation test:
   a. An initial decrease in urine osmolality at the first time point after time zero suggests that the patient has had a large amount to drink immediately before the test   T
   This often indicates that the patient is particularly anxious about the test, and tends to suggest hysterical polydypsia rather than diabetes insipidus.
   b. A mismatch between the volume of urine passed and decrease in weight at one or more time points suggests that the patient has had a surreptitious drink while in the toilet   T
   The diagnosis of diabetes insipidus is usually clear without resort to a water deprivation test. When a water deprivation test is warranted, the history is usually unclear and the patients may be pursuing another agenda that is furthered by maintaining the impression of a bona fide cause of their symptoms.

c. A rapid decrease in urine volume and increase in urine osmolality
    indicates normality   T
d. Persistent passage of large amounts of dilute urine with a matching
    decrease in body weight, confirms the diagnosis of diabetes insipidus   T
    It also suggests that the test should be terminated.
e. The patient is allowed to eat dry food   F

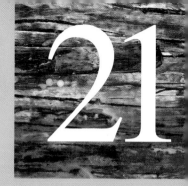

Endocrine hypertension

- Summary

- Introduction

- Key points

- Case history

- Multiple-choice questions

Summary

Normal function

- Appropriate perfusion of body tissues irrespective of posture or activity.

Typical pathology

- Idiopathic hypertension, with no identifiable endocrine cause. Primary endocrine hypertension is rare but, because hypertension occurs in 20 per cent of the adult population, the coexistence of hypertension and endocrine disease is common. Endocrinologists are usually asked for an opinion when hypertensive patients (on or off treatment) are noted to be hypokalaemic.
- 'Classical, rather than typical pathology'
  - → Conn's syndrome. Aldosterone-secreting adrenal cortical adenoma (see p. 91).
  - → Phaeochromocytoma. The majority arise from cells of the adrenal medulla, with 10 per cent or less arising from the sympathetic chain or elsewhere (see p. 87).
  - → Cushing's syndrome. Hypercortisolaemia from pituitary or ectopic production of ACTH, or excessive adrenal production of cortisol (see p. 55).
  - → Acromegaly (see p. 38).

'Typical clinical scenario'

- A 65-year-old hypertensive with hypokalaemia that resolved once K^+-wasting diuretics were discontinued.

Introduction

Endocrine causes are responsible for only a very small fraction of cases of hypertension. Nevertheless, as hypertension is a common, treatable problem that causes major morbidity and mortality, it is worthwhile excluding secondary causes, particularly if the patient is unusually young, unresponsive to normal antihypertensive agents, or has unprovoked hypokalaemia. Even if the hypertension does not fully resolve, it may become easier to manage after appropriate treatment.

Table 21.1
Causes of hypertension

	Incidence
Essential hypertension, chronic renal and renovascular disease	≥ 99%
The contraceptive pill	≤ 0.2%
Hypercalcaemia	≤ 0.1%
Cushing's syndrome	≤ 0.1%
Conn's syndrome	≤ 0.1%
Phaeochromocytoma	≤ 0.1%
Acromegaly	≤ 0.1%
Hypothyroidism	≤ 0.1%

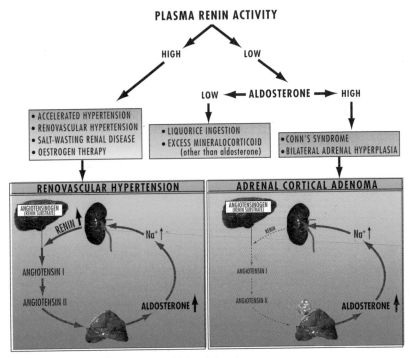

Fig. 21.1 Investigation of hypertension with hypokalaemia.

Key points

- Almost all hypertension associated with a specific underlying diagnosis is related to renal or renovascular disease.
- About one-third of acromegalics, and most patients with Cushing's disease, are hypertensive.

'My patient has hypertension and hypokalaemia that is proving difficult to control. Am I missing an endocrine problem?'

History

A 48-year-old schoolteacher was referred to clinic with a 6 year history of poorly controlled hypertension. The problem had been identified during a consultation for migrainous headaches. He smoked 20 cigarettes daily and claimed to be otherwise well. A variety of antihypertensives had been tried, the latest combination being a single daily dose of bendrofluazide 5 mg, atenolol 100 mg, and amlodipine 10 mg. On this regimen, his blood pressure was 174/96 mmHg. Whenever his electrolytes had been tested, the potassium was noted to be between 2.8 and 3.5 mmol/l. Attempts to replace it with supplements were unsuccessful, and mild hypokalaemia persisted even after the thiazide diuretic was stopped.

Examination

On examination, the only abnormalities were early retinal artery changes in keeping with chronic hypertension, and a blood pressure of 188/94 mmHg after 5 min recumbency.

Investigations

Na$^+$ was 142 mmol/l (normal range 133–153 mmol/l); urea, 4.7 mmol/l (normal range 3–7 mmol/l); K$^+$, 2.9 mmol/l (normal range 3.7–5.2 mmol/l). Plasma renin activity was less than 0.2 pmol/ml.h (normal range 0.5–3.1 pmol/ml.h: random, i.e. not after overnight recumbency, which would tend to minimize levels); aldosterone, 790 pmol/l (ambulant normal range 200–900 pmol/l).

After antihypertensives were stopped and potassium and sodium intake was liberalized (with effervescent potassium and sodium) for 3 weeks, plasma renin activity was less than 0.2 pmol/ml.h; aldosterone, 690 pmol/l; and K^+, 3.2 mmol/l. An abdominal MR scan showed a single lesion 1.2 cm in diameter on the right adrenal cortex.

Management

He was treated with spironolactone 100 mg daily until surgery. An aldosterone-secreting adenoma was excised from his right adrenal cortex.

Explanation

Under normal circumstances, high plasma sodium directly reduces renin production, and in turn, angiotensin I, angiotensin II and aldosterone should fall. In addition, low plasma potassium should directly reduce aldosterone secretion. In this patient, aldosterone remained well up in the normal range despite high sodium and low potassium levels, suggesting autonomous aldosterone secretion by the adrenal cortex. This was confirmed by the suppressed plasma renin activity.

Had the MRI been less clear cut, other tests such as venous sampling of the adrenal outflow (95 per cent sensitivity) or adrenal iodoscintigraphy (70 per cent sensitivity) might have been required. In addition to spironolactone, amiloride, which amongst other effects blocks the Na^+ channels that aldosterone opens up, can be very useful.

Multiple-choice questions

1. The following endocrine conditions are associated with hypertension:
   a. Acromegaly;
   b. Macroprolactinoma;
   c. Cushing's syndrome;
   d. Conn's syndrome;
   e. Carcinoid syndrome.

2. The following are associated with hypertension:
   a. The combined oral contraceptive pill;
   b. Liquorice ingestion;

    c. Intracorporeal (the penile corpora) injection of papaverine in a patient with a venous leak;

    d. Use of desmopressin aerosol for diabetes insipidus;

    e. Congenital adrenal hyperplasia.

3. In hypertensive patients:

    a. A potassium of greater than 4.0 in a patient off treatment excludes Conn's syndrome;

    b. Hyperparathyroidism may be implicated in the condition;

    c. Hypothyroidism may be implicated in the condition;

    d. Sex hormone replacement therapy should be avoided;

    e. The dose of thyroxine used in thyroid hormone replacement therapy should be kept as low as possible.

Answers

1. The following endocrine conditions are associated with hypertension:

    a. Acromegaly   T

        There are a number of explanations why this occurs in acromegaly, including an increase in plasma volume and total sodium, defective fluid secretion in view of volume expansion but normal atrial natriuretic peptide, inappropriate renin–angiotensin system activation, or a direct action of GH or IGF-I at the kidneys, causing sodium retention.

    b. Macroprolactinoma   F

Hypertension is not associated with macro- or microprolactinomas.

    c. Cushing's syndrome   T

        Hypertension is also more common in obese patients. However, in cushing's disease there is osteopenia, a tendency to bruise easily and marked proximal myopathy. The absence of any one of these three symptoms or signs is against the diagnosis of Cushing's disease.

    d. Conn's syndrome   T

        A combination of high aldosterone, low renin, hypokalaemia, and moderate hypertension is characteristic. Bartter's syndrome is a rare condition characterized by normotensive hypokalaemia, due to a defect in tubular chloride or potassium transport. It usually presents in childhood as hypokalaemia with raised aldosterone and renin. Hypertension is occasionally present.

    e. Carcinoid syndrome   F

Carcinoid syndrome is not associated with hypertension.

2. The following are associated with hypertension:

    a. The combined oral contraceptive pill   T

        The incidence of hypertension in women taking oestrogen-containing contraceptives is 5 per cent, more than twice the proportion of age-matched controls.

b. Liquorice ingestion   T

Unexpectedly, glucocorticoids (e.g. cortisol) and mineralocorticoids such as aldosterone have equal affinity at the renal mineralocorticoid type 1 receptor. The enzyme 11β-hydroxysteroid dehydrogenase prevents gluco-corticoids working in this way and 'protects' the receptor from gluco-corticoids. One of the active ingredients of liquorice, glycyrrhizic acid, reversibly blocks the enzyme and produces an effect similar to Conn's syndrome, with potassium loss and sodium retention.

c. Intracorporeal (the penile corpora) injection of papaverine in a patient with a venous leak   F

Papaverine is a vasodilator. It is more likely that the patient will become hypotensive rather than hypertensive.

d. Use of desmopressin aerosol for diabetes insipidus   F

Pharmacological doses of vasopressin are required to produce hyper-tension, and desmopressin is specific for the renal 'V2' rather than the vascular 'V1' receptors.

e. Congenital adrenal hyperplasia   T

It can be, although it is unusual for hypertension to be a problem.

3. In hypertensive patients:

a. A potassium of greater than 4.0 in a patient off treatment excludes Conn's syndrome   T

Conn's characteristically produces a potassium at or below the lower limit of the normal range.

b. Hyperparathyroidism may be implicated in the condition   T

The mechanism is unknown.

c. Hypothyroidism may be implicated in the condition   T

The mechanism is unknown and the causal association is probably very rare.

d. Sex hormone replacement therapy should be avoided   F

If the hypertension is controlled, there is no reason for excluding the patient from this treatment. In fact, as hypertension is a risk factor for cardiovascular disease and hormone replacement therapy protects against this, there is an added incentive to treat.

e. The dose of thyroxine used in thyroid hormone replacement therapy should be kept as low as possible   F

There should be no change in treatment. The right dose is the amount that returns the TSH to within the normal range.

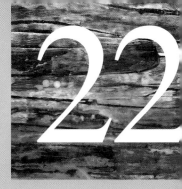

Endocrine neoplasia

- Summary
- Introduction
- Phaeochromocytomas
- Tumours giving rise to hypercalcaemia
- Multiple endocrine neoplasia syndromes
- Key points
- Case histories
- Multiple-choice questions

Summary

Normal function

- Any gene can aspire to be an oncogene (a gene responsible for the induction of tumours) if the protein that it codes for directly or indirectly tells a cell that it is time to divide. These 'proto-(or potential)-oncogenes' are normally regulated by 'anti-oncogenes' or tumour suppressor genes that mediate the opposite signal. Inactivation of anti-oncogenes or transformation of proto-oncogenes into oncogenes by mutation, results in tumour formation. For the great majority of endocrine tumours, specific oncogenes have yet to be identified.

Typical pathology

- Adenoma formation (relatively common)
  - → Parathyroid adenomas. Primary hyperparathyroidism has a prevalence as high as 0.1 per cent.
  - → Pituitary tumours. Endocrinologically inactive adenomas and pro-lactinomas are the most common subtypes.
- Carcinoma formation (relatively rare)
  - → Thyroid carcinomas are the most common of all endocrine malignancies. Even so, they account for only 1 per cent of deaths from malignant disease. Subtypes are papillary, follicular, medullary, and anaplastic. Of these, papillary carcinomas are the most common, and are the most benign.
  - → Carcinoid tumours—so-called because of their malignant-looking histology but relatively benign behaviour. Production of 5-hydroxy-tryptamine (serotonin) and other bioactive peptides produce the clinical syndrome once hepatic metastases (which circumvent hepatic first-pass metabolism by draining directly into the systemic circulation) are present.
  - → Phaeochromocytoma—usually due to adrenaline-or noradrenaline-secreting tumours of the adrenal medulla. Prediction of malignant or benign behaviour from histological examination is notoriously difficult. Approximately 10 per cent metastasize.
- Non-endocrine malignancies that respond to endocrine treatment (very common)
  - → Carcinoma of the breast is responsible for 20 per cent of all female cancer deaths. Many are oestrogen-dependent.
  - → Carcinoma of the prostate is the second most common malignancy in men. They are androgen-dependent tumours. The removal of endogenous androgens can dramatically affect disease progression.

'Typical clinical scenario'

- A 55-year-old woman with episodic abdominal cramps, loose stools, and facial flushing from the carcinoid syndrome.

Introduction

The production or metabolism of hormones or their precursors at low levels is a characteristic of many normal tissues. In malignancy the ability to produce these factors is often retained, and as tumour mass increases, a variety of paracrine, autocrine, and distal effects as diverse as neuropathy, dermatomyositis, anorexia, and fever can occur.

Hormone-*responsive* non-endocrine tumours, such as prostatic and breast cancers, are amongst the most common of all tumours. However, the production of clinically significant amounts of classical endocrine hormones is rare. Typical examples are the production of ACTH or ACTH-like peptides by small-cell lung carcinomas and chorionic gonadotrophin (hCG) by trophoblastic (placental) tumours or germ-cell neoplasms of the ovary and testis. Others, such as erythro-poietin from renal or hepatic tumours and vasopressin from small-cell lung carcinomas, can lead to polycythaemia or SIADH (see p. 328), respectively.

Hypercalcaemia is one of the most common endocrine problems of neoplasia. Solid tumours can produce parathyroid hormone-related protein (PTHrp) and haematological malignancies may produce a variety of 'calcaemic' factors that mobilize bone mineral. Rarely, malignancies can enhance vitamin D hydroxy-lation, secrete PTH or, in the presence of multiple bone metastases, directly increase bone resorption.

A number of other peptides, such as prostatic-specific antigen, α-fetoprotein (from hepatocellular and testicular tumours), and calcitonin (from medullary thyroid carcinomas) have insignificant physiological effects but are useful tumour markers.

Phaeochromocytomas

Phaeochromocytomas (p. 87) can be difficult to diagnose as urinary cate-cholamines may not be raised between attacks. In addition, symptoms may be difficult to distinguish from those produced by psychiatric disease. The classical headache of phaeochromocytoma is a throbbing pain throughout the head—as if held in a vice—with a distinct crescendo, decrescendo over a period of minutes to hours, sometimes with palpitations and sweating (diaphoresis). Between attacks, the patient often feels perfectly well. In non-malignant phaeochromocytoma, the 5 year survival is greater than 95 per cent, and the recurrence rate after surgery is less than 10 per cent (see Fig. 4.2).

Tumours giving rise to hypercalcaemia

Many solid tumours can give rise to hypercalcaemia and, in the majority, the pro-duction of parathyroid hormone-related peptide (PTHrp) is responsible. PTHrp is found in many endocrine tissues, with particularly high levels in lactating mammary gland and breast milk. The normal physiological function of the peptide is obscure, but as it is present in more than 90 per cent of squamous

Table 22.1
Tumours of the principal endocrine organs

Type	Notes
Thyroid	Although the most common endocrine carcinomas, they account for fewer than 1% of all invasive tumours. Most cases occur between the ages of 25 and 65 years. About 75% of people with thyroid cancer die from other conditions
Parathyroid	The prevalence of hyperparathyroidism is as high as 1:1000. Parathyroid carcinomas account for < 3% of cases of primary hyperparathyroidism. They are associated with very high calcium levels
Pituitary	Account for 10–15% of intracranial tumours coming to surgery. Approximately 30% are prolactinomas, 25% endocrinologically inactive, 15% somatotroph, and 10% corticotroph
Pancreatic	Gastrinomas
	Most common islet cell tumour. Gives rise to the Zollinger–Ellison syndrome of peptic ulceration, diarrhoea, and oesophagitis. One-third are associated with MEN 1
	Diagnosis
	Fasting gastrin usually >171 pmol/l
	Gastrin secretion increases by more than 114 pmol/l after 3 h of infusing 4 mg elemental calcium/kg.h
	Treatment
	Surgical excision. Proton pump inhibitors and H_2 antagonists are very useful. Somatostatin analogues and partial gastrectomy may also be useful

continued next page

Type	Notes
Pancreatic	**Insulinomas**
	Second most common islet cell tumour
	Diagnosis
	Demonstrate fasting hypoglycaemia with elevated insulin levels. 'C' peptide (the amino acid chain cleaved from pro-insulin to give rise to the mature peptide) should also be elevated
	Treatment
	Surgical, but diazoxide and streptozotocin can be useful in unresectable disease
	Glucagonomas
	Extremely rare
	Diagnosis
	Hyperglycaemia accompanied by necrolytic, migratory erythema, diarrhoea, anorexia, and wasting
	Treatment
	Surgical resection or somatostatin analogues can be used
	VIP-Omas
	Vasoactive intestinal polypeptide produced in excess can give rise to the watery diarrhoea syndrome
	Treatment
	Somatotatin analogues are useful

continued below

Type	Notes
Ovarian	Ovarian tumours rarely present with endocrine manifestations. However, a variety of ovarian neoplasms, such as those derived from sex cord or stromal cells, can secrete androgens and produce an abrupt onset of hirsutism and virilization. Other ovarian hormones may also be produced in excess
Testicular	These account for 1% of male cancer deaths and are the second most common malignancy in men aged between 20 and 35 years. Tumours commonly affect both testes simultaneously or in turn, are five to ten times more common in undescended testes and are usually derived from germ cells. Most present to surgeons, but rarely, oestrogen secretion may cause the rapid onset of painful gynaecomastia in adults, or, if androgens are produced in childhood, precocious puberty
Adrenal	Cortex
	Adrenal cortical tumours can produce cortisol, aldosterone, or androgens, leading to Cushing's syndrome, Conn's syndrome, or virilization. Rarely, oestrogens are produced, leading to feminization.
	Medulla
	Adrenaline and/or noradrenaline-secreting adrenal medullary tumours (phaeochromocytomas) account for 0.1% of cases of hypertension. In two-thirds of cases, the hypertension is sustained rather than paroxysmal. In 10%, it is absent altogether

Table 22.2
Carcinoid tumours

Definition	Carcinoid tumours are slow-growing tumours derived from neural crest cells that usually arise within the lower gastrointestinal tract or lung. They are histologically 'carcinoma-like', but follow a more benign clinical course – hence 'carcinoid'
Diagnosis	The urine content of 5-hydroxyindoleacetic acid (5-HIAA) over 24–72 h is usually elevated
Incidence	Found in the small intestine in 1:150 autopsies and identified in 1:300 appendicectomy specimens
Age and sex	They can occur at any age, but the mean age is 50. The incidence in males and females is similar
Symptoms	Do not occur unless the secretions of bioactive peptides, 5-hydroxytry pamine (serotonin) and sometimes bradykinin and histamine, circumvent hepatic first-pass metabolism. Hepatic metastases are usually present before episodes of facial flushing lasting a minute or two to hours, sweating, abdominal pain, colic, nausea, vomiting, diarrhoea, dizziness, and hypotension occur
Signs	Endomyocardial fibrosis of the right heart leading to a pulmonary stenotic murmur, an abdominal mass from an enlarging primary tumour and/or hepatomegaly and facial flushing, form a classical symptom triad that occurs infrequently during the late stages of the condition
Treatment	Traditional chemotherapy is of very little use. Somatostatin analogues are often tried in an attempt to reduce peptide secretion, along with the anti-histamines with anti-serotonin activity (such as cyproheptadine) to block the peripheral effects of vasoactive peptides. Nicotinic acid supplements are used to prevent pellagra, as consumption of this vitamin by the tumour can be excessive

tumours and 50 per cent of breast tumours in hypercalcaemic patients, it is a useful marker of 'solid tumours' (the exception being acute T-cell leukaemia).

The presence of hypercalcaemia does not necessarily imply direct bony involvement with metastases.

Multiple endocrine neoplasia syndromes

The multiple endocrine neoplasia (MEN) syndromes are rare. Like many endocrine conditions, their clinical significance is considerably outweighed by the

Table 22.3
Common non-endocrine tumours that are amenable to hormonal manipulation

	Carcinoma of the prostate	Carcinoma of the breast
Epidemiology	Second only to lung cancer in terms of male cancer deaths	Breast cancer is responsible for 20% of all female deaths from cancer
Hormone Dependence	These are androgen-dependent tumours. Their growth is inhibited by depriving them of androgens.	Many breast cancers are oestrogen-dependent, and their growth is inhibited by depriving them of oestrogens.
Rationale for treatment	Prostatic cancer shows the best response to endocrine therapy of all hormone-sensitive cancers:- • GnRH superagonists block pituitary LH production. • Finasteride blocks 5α-reductase within prostatic cells from converting circulating pre-androgens (mostly from the adrenals) to dihydrotestosterone. • Flutamide is an androgen receptor blocker	In pre-menopausal women, the ovaries are the main source of oestrogens. Ovarian androgens are converted to oestrogens by aromatase under the influence of FSH and LH. In post-menopausal women, the ovaries do not contain aromatase, but androgens from the ovaries and adrenals continue to form a substrate for peripheral aromatase (which is twice as active in this age group).

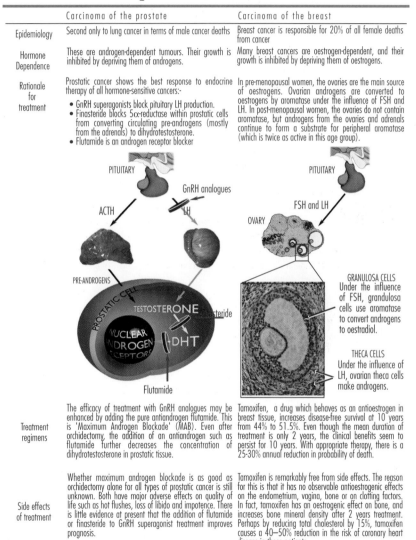

PITUITARY

GnRH analogues

ACTH   LH

PITUITARY

FSH and LH

OVARY

PRE-ANDROGENS

PROSTATIC CELL

TESTOSTERONE

finasteride

NUCLEAR ANDROGEN RECEPTOR

DHT

Flutamide

GRANULOSA CELLS
Under the influence of FSH, granulosa cells use aromatase to convert androgens to oestradiol.

THECA CELLS
Under the influence of LH, ovarian theca cells make androgens.

	Carcinoma of the prostate	Carcinoma of the breast
Treatment regimens	The efficacy of treatment with GnRH analogues may be enhanced by adding the pure antiandrogen flutamide. This is 'Maximum Androgen Blockade' (MAB). Even after orchidectomy, the addition of an antiandrogen such as flutamide further decreases the concentration of dihydrotestosterone in prostatic tissue.	Tamoxifen, a drug which behaves as an antioestrogen in breast tissue, increases disease-free survival at 10 years from 44% to 51.5%. Even though the mean duration of treatment is only 2 years, the clinical benefits seem to persist for 10 years. With appropriate therapy, there is a 25-30% annual reduction in probability of death.
Side effects of treatment	Whether maximum androgen blockade is as good as orchidectomy alone for all types of prostatic cancer is still unknown. Both have major adverse effects on quality of life such as hot flushes, loss of libido and impotence. There is little evidence at present that the addition of flutamide or finasteride to GnRH superagonist treatment improves prognosis.	Tamoxifen is remarkably free from side effects. The reason for this is that it has no observable antioestrogenic effects on the endometrium, vagina, bone or on clotting factors. In fact, tamoxifen has an oestrogenic effect on bone, and increases bone mineral density after 2 years treatment. Perhaps by reducing total cholesterol by 15%, tamoxifen causes a 40–50% reduction in the risk of coronary heart disease in these patients.
Future treatment	A primary prevention study using finasteride, a 5α reductase inhibitor (that blocks the production of dihydrotestosterone from testosterone) is in progress.	Direct aromatase inhibitors such as 4-hydroxyandrostenedione may also have a role in the future in adjuvant therapy in primary breast cancer.

Table 22.4
Multiple endocrine neoplasia syndromes

	Type 1 Wermer's syndrome	Type 2a Sipple's syndrome	Type 2b (sometimes type 3)
Clinical syndrome	Parathyroid hyperplasia Pituitary tumours Pancreatic tumours Lipomas	Medullary thyroid carcinoma Phaeochromocytoma 50% Parathyroid hyperplasia 10–20%	Medullary thyroid carcinoma Marfanoid habitus Mucosal neuromas Phaeochromocytomas Colonic polypi Parathyroid hyperplasia
Chromosomal localization	Type 1 maps to a locus on the long arm of chromosome 11, near the centromere	Both type 2a and 2b appear to be associated with the activation of the *RET* proto-oncogene on the long arm of chromosome 10, near the centromere	
Diagnosis	The identification of closely linked nucleic acid markers is making carrier status predictable. The 100% penetrance by the age of 40 equates carrier status with disease	The polymerase chain reaction (PCR) can be used to identify the presence of the *RET* oncogene before any hormonal tests become positive. As the penetrance is very high, this is sufficient evidence to make the diagnosis and to advise total thyroid ablation in those affected	
Notes	In MEN 1, 50% of parathyroid tumours recur within 10 years of surgery Hyperparathyroidism may increase gastrin levels when it occurs concurrently with Zollinger–Ellison syndrome 35% of patients with functional pancreatic adenomas have insulinomas	Phaeochromocytomas are screened for and removed before thyroid surgery is contemplated Although it is not used at present, radioiodine treatment may in future be used instead of surgery for thyroid ablation	Mucosal neuromas are found on the distal portion of the tongue, as well as the lips and subconjunctiva Medullary thyroid carcinoma is more aggressive in 2a than 2b with metastases reported in babies less than 1 year old Hyperparathyroidism is rare

scientific interest with which they are associated. Nevertheless, it should be remembered that the expression of the multiple endocrine neoplasia syndromes is life threatening, and blights the lives of generation after generation of the families involved.

Multiple endocrine neoplasia are divided into three distinct syndromes (Table 22.4), all of which are dominantly inherited and share the same characteristic of tumours of multiple endocrine organs that progress histologically from hyperplasia, through adenoma, to carcinoma. Thus tumours are often multicentric. For example, hyperparathyroidism, when it occurs, tends to be associated with hyperplasia of all four glands, rather than a single adenoma.

Key points

- Tumours of endocrine tissue are rare, but hormone-responsive non-endocrine tumours are common.
- Thyroid tumours are the most common endocrine malignancy.
- Hypercalcaemia is one of the most common endocrine problems of neoplasia.
- The syndromes of multiple endocrine neoplasia are dominantly inherited.

'My patient has malignant carcinoid syndrome. Please advise'

History

A 63-year-old female had been admitted under the surgeons with abdominal pain 6 months previously. At laparotomy, a small bowel stricture with local lymphadenopathy and a hepatic mass, assumed to be a secondary deposit, was revealed. A 30 cm length of small bowel was resected and continuity restored. Histologically the tumour was identified as a small bowel carcinoid with local nodal metastases. Postoperatively the patient was asymptomatic, but increasingly, she noticed episodes of abdominal cramps and loose stools, and on two occasions had facial flushing lasting almost 2 hours.

Examination

The only abnormality on examination was a 4 cm liver edge. Heart sounds and blood pressure were normal.

Investigations

Her urinary 5-hydroxyindoleacetic acid (5HIAA) was 320 μmol/24 h (normal range 0–35 μmol/24 h), compared to a postoperative level of 180 μmol. Biochemistry was otherwise normal. Hepatic ultrasound confirmed the presence of a large cyst, but also demonstrated a number of other cysts, the largest being 3 cm in diameter.

Management

The patient was symptomatically improved on cyproheptadine 4 mg three times a day and multivitamin tablets. A long-acting somatostatin analogue made her feel worse and was withdrawn after a short clinical trial. Hepatic lobectomy or selective embolization was dismissed in view of the number of cysts present.

Explanation

Carcinoid tumours are often very slow growing. Although they are generally not susceptible to radiotherapy, there are many anecdotes of patients with proven hepatic metastases from carcinoid tumours living reasonably comfortably for many years. In some patients, symptoms due to the release of 5HIAA and other small bioactive peptides produced by the tumour can be limited by somatostatin analogues or antihistamines with 5HT antagonist activity, such as cyproheptadine. As metabolically active carcinoids tend to consume nicotinamide, vitamin supplements can be useful to prevent the development of pellagra, particularly if abdominal discomfort has led to anorexia.

'My patient complains of excessive sweating. Is there an endocrine cause'

History

A 67-year-old female complained of excessive sweating going back almost 5 years, and emphasizes the fact by dabbing her brow with a tissue throughout the consultation. The sweating was continual rather than paroxysmal, and although she explained that it was present day and night, she did not have to change the bed linen in the morning. Her menopause was at the age of 52 and her only past medical history was of two pulmonary valvotomies for pulmonary stenosis of unknown cause. She denied headaches or palpitations. Her bowel habit was normal.

Current treatment was sex hormone replacement therapy with tibolone (Livial®), which had not altered her symptoms in any way.

Examination

She was clinically euthyroid, obese (BMI = 31 kg/m^2), plethoric (i.e. flushed), and had a supine blood pressure of 218/104 mmHg (with a large cuff). A soft ejection systolic murmur of pulmonary stenosis was audible in the pulmonary area, but no abdominal masses were palpable. Her skin was moist, but the sweating did not appear excessive.

Investigations

Two 24 h urine collections (into a bottle containing 25 ml of 6 M HCl), assayed for 5HIAA, metanephrines, and nor-metanephrines were normal. Thyroid function tests, FSH, LH, and a full blood count were also unremarkable.

Management

The patient was reassured that a sinister underlying cause of sweating was most unlikely. A weight reducing diet was tentatively suggested, and the patient was also given some antiperspirant solution to rub on the parts worst affected.

Explanation

There are a number of endocrinological causes of sweating, including hot flushes of oestrogen withdrawal, thyrotoxicosis, pheochromocytoma, carcinoid syndrome, and acromegaly. The incidence of phaeochromocytoma in patients presenting with hypertension is very low, and this patient's long history without episodic or paroxysmal symptoms made an underlying endocrinopathy unlikely. The patient's propensity to sweat would certainly be reduced if the patient managed to lose weight, but this rarely proves a feasible option.

Tibolone is a sex hormone replacement used particularly to ameliorate hot flushes, that combines oestrogenic and progestogenic activity with mild androgenic effects.

Aluminium salts are the active ingredients of over-the-counter anti-perspirants and of solutions such as Anhydrol Forte® and Driclor®.

Multiple-choice questions

1. Characteristic features of phaeochromocytoma include:
   a. Severe headaches lasting for days with extreme fatigue between attacks;
   b. Symptoms that can be confused with anxiety attacks;
   c. Paroxysms of headache and sweating induced by movements such as straining or lifting;
   d. Sweating (diaphoresis);
   e. Palpitations.

2. In carcinoid tumours:
   a. The presence of symptoms of flushing and diarrhoea suggests that the tumour is more than 5 cm in diameter;
   b. Right heart murmurs are often heard;
   c. Can be confirmed by finding high levels of VMA or metanephrines in the urine;
   d. Conventional chemotherapy and radiotherapy are useful;
   e. Women are affected twice as often as men.

3. Features of MEN 1 (multiple endocrine neoplasia type 1) include:
   a. Autosomal recessive inheritance;
   b. Parathyroid hyperplasia;
   c. Phaeochromocytoma;
   d. Pancreatic tumours;
   e. Medullary thyroid carcinoma.

4. Hormone-responsive tumours:
   a. Tamoxifen, an anti-oestrogen used in breast tumours, produces osteoporosis;
   b. Prostatic cancer shows a poor response to endocrine treatment;
   c. Breast cancer is responsible for 1 in 5 of all female deaths from cancer;
   d. Prostatic cancer is the second most common cause of cancer-related death in men;
   e. In postmenopausal women, the ovaries no longer make significant amounts of oestrogen, and tamoxifen is therefore ineffective in breast tumour therapy.

5. In endocrine neoplasia:
   a. Symptoms of systemic mastocytosis can be confused with carcinoid syndrome;
   b. The *RET* oncogene is associated with MEN 1;
   c. Production of PTHrp (parathyroid hormone-related peptide) is typical of haematological malignancies;
   d. Hypercalcaemia equates with metastatic involvement of bone;
   e. Patients with carcinoid tumours are predisposed to pellagra (nicotinic acid deficiency).

Answers

1. Characteristic features of phaeochromocytoma include:
   a. Severe headaches lasting for days with extreme fatigue between attacks   F
   It is more usual for the patient to feel well between attacks, and for the headaches to last for a shorter time.
   b. Symptoms that can be confused with anxiety attacks   T
   Paroxysmal episodes suggesting fits, hyperventilation, or panic attacks are well described.
   c. Paroxysms of headache and sweating induced by movements such as straining or lifting   T
   This is a fairly unusual feature of a rare tumour, but can be useful in distinguishing psychiatric symptoms from phaeochromocytoma, as mental stress does not produce paroxysms in the latter.
   d. Sweating (diaphoresis)   T
   Almost three-quarters of all patients complain of excessive sweating.
   e. Palpitations   T
   Up to 60 per cent of patients complain of palpitations.

2. In carcinoid tumours:
   a. The presence of symptoms of flushing and diarrhoea suggests that the tumour is more than 5 cm in diameter   F
   Not necessarily. Rather than indicating a particular tumour size, symptoms suggests that hepatic metastases are present. These are very often small but multiple.
   b. Right heart murmurs are often heard   F
   This is a classical but unusual sign that is sometimes heard late on in the course of the disease.
   c. Can be confirmed by finding high levels of VMA or metanephrines in the urine   F
   These are the breakdown products of catecholamines rather than 5-HT, and would suggest phaeochromocytoma. 5HIAA is found in the urine of patients with carcinoid. Many carcinoid tumours also produce ACTH or ACTH-like peptides, but rarely in amounts sufficient to cause Cushing's syndrome. Nevertheless, about 20 per cent of cases of ectopic ACTH production result from hormone secretion from bronchial, thymic, or pancreatic carcinoid tumours.
   d. Conventional chemotherapy and radiotherapy are useful   F
   Unfortunately not. Somatostatin analogues are the latest modality to be tried. The results of clinical trials are still awaited, but it seems likely that even if symptoms are reduced, life expectancy will not be increased.
   e. Women are affected twice as often as men   F
   The sex incidence is equal.

3. Features of MEN 1 (multiple endocrine neoplasia type 1) include:
    a. Autosomal recessive inheritance   F
       All of the MEN syndromes are dominant.
    b. Parathyroid hyperplasia   T
       This is found in all three types, but is most common in type 1.
    c. Phaeochromocytoma   F
       This would suggest MEN 2a or 2b.
    d. Pancreatic tumours   T
       Gastrinomas (Zollinger–Ellison syndrome) and insulinomas occur.
    e. Medullary thyroid carcinoma   F
       This condition is strongly associated with type 2a and 2b. There is also a
       related but distinct syndrome of isolated medullary thyroid carcinoma.

4. Hormone-responsive tumours:
    a. Tamoxifen, an anti-oestrogen used in breast tumours, produces osteo-
       porosis   F
       Although the drug acts as an anti-oestrogen at the breast, it does not
       have anti-oestrogenic properties at other sites, such as the vagina,
       endometrium, or bone.
    b. Prostatic cancer shows a poor response to endocrine treatment   F
       Prostatic cancer shows one of the best responses to endocrine treatment of
       all hormone-sensitive cancers. GnRH agonists block pituitary LH pro-
       duction and block testosterone production by the testes. However, there is
       still ACTH drive to the adrenals that continues to produce pre-androgens
       that can be converted to androgens by prostatic tumour cells.
    c. Breast cancer is responsible for 1 in 5 of all female deaths from cancer   T
    d. Prostatic cancer is the second most common cause of cancer-related death
       in men   T
       Lung cancer is the most common.
    e. In postmenopausal women, the ovaries no longer make significant
       amounts of oestrogen, and tamoxifen is therefore ineffective in breast
       tumour therapy   F
       Although the ovaries do not contain aromatase (to convert androgens to
       oestrogens), they do continue to secrete androgens, which, with adrenal
       androgens, are converted to oestrogen peripherally. Tamoxifen remains
       useful.

5. In endocrine neoplasia:
    a. Symptoms of systemic mastocytosis can be confused with carcinoid
       syndrome   T
       Mastocytosis is a rare, systemic disease characterized by mast cell pro-
       liferation, and produces symptoms resulting from paroxysmal release of
       peptide mediators of inflammation from these cells. Flushing is often a
       prominent feature, accompanied by tachycardia, vasodilatation, nausea,
       vomiting, and diarrhoea. A characteristic, but not invariable feature, is

the presence of a pigmented, erythematous or acneiform rash that becomes urticarial on stroking (urticaria pigmentosa). Occasionally, episodes are precipitated by aspirin. Blood histamine levels during an acute flushing episode are useful, or 24 h urinary histamine or histamine metabolite levels (methylhistamine and methylimidazolacetic acid) can be measured.

b. The *RET* oncogene is associated with MEN 1   F

It is associated with MEN 2a and MEN 2b. This is an important finding as its identification in very young children is now used to identify unequivocally individuals who will develop the disease. A prophylactic total thyroidectomy, removes the 'C cell' substrate for medullary thyroid carcinoma development.

c. Production of PTHrp (parathyroid hormone-related peptide) is typical of haematological malignancies   F

PTHRP is a marker of solid tumours. Haematological malignancies produce other factors (currently ill-defined) that give rise to hypercalcaemia.

d. Hypercalcaemia equates with metastatic involvement of bone   F

Hypercalcaemia in patients with breast cancer is almost always related to bone metastases. However, in many other tumours the association between hypercalcaemia and bone metastases is poor.

e. Patients with carcinoid tumours are predisposed to pellagra (nicotinic acid deficiency)   T

Serotonin (5HT) synthesis requires tryptophan. Carcinoid tumours consume much more than the usual 1 per cent of body tryptophan that is usually turned over for this purpose. The resulting niacin (nicotinic acid) deficiency may lead to pellagra, characterized by dermatitis, dementia, and diarrhoea.

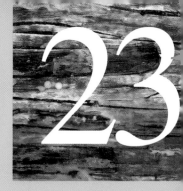

23

Endocrine prophylaxis

- Introduction
- Key points

Introduction

Within the boundaries imposed by health economics and politics, the endocrinology clinic offers enormous potential for effective prophylaxis of common and dangerous diseases. Too often, the chances are squandered.

Key points

- Oestrogen replacement is still first-line therapy for postmenopausal osteoporosis. It should be introduced at low dose to minimize unpleasant side-effects.
- First-degree relatives of patients with NIDDM have a 33 per cent risk of developing the same.
- The complications of diabetes and gestational diabetes are, at least to some extent, preventable.

Table 23.1
Potential prophylactic opportunities

Target population	Potential intervention and benefits
Perimenopausal or postmenopausal women	Sex hormone replacement therapy for 5 years halves the risks of osteoporotic fractures and halves the incidence of subsequent cardiovascular events. The uptake of HRT in postmenopausal women is between 2.3 and 12% only
Women up to 34 years old (whether they smoke or not)	The death rate from the contraceptive pill is lower than the pregnancy (birth)-associated death rate in women who do not want fertility but are having unprotected intercourse
Obese people with a family history of ischaemic heart disease, and patients with known ischaemic heart disease	Treatment of hyperlipidaemia, particularly in high-risk patients, reduces the incidence of cardiovascular events, or further cardiovascular events if one has already occurred.
All pregnant women	The incidence of gestational diabetes is 5%, and the infant mortality if the condition remains untreated is 7%. All women should be screened for gestational diabetes at booking and at the beginning of the third trimester
Pregnant women who have previously given birth to a child with congenital adrenal hyperplasia	Low-dose oral dexamethasone is started from week 9 of gestation until chorionic villus sampling can be carried out at 9–11 weeks. If the result of this, or of amniocentesis at 15–18 weeks shows an affected female, treatment is continued to term. By suppressing fetal ACTH, virilization will be reduced or prevented
Men aged 55 or older	Finasteride (a 5α-reductase inhibitor, that blocks the conversion of testosterone to dihydrotestosterone) prophylaxis against the development of prostatic cancer is currently being tested in a large double-blind study in the USA

continued below

Target population	Potential intervention and benefits
Patients with multiple endocrine neoplasia type 2a (MEN 2a, Sipple's syndrome)	The identification of the *RET* oncogene in this condition now allows affected individuals to be identified in childhood and offered total thyroidectomy to prevent the development of medullary thyroid carcinoma
Patients with insulin-dependent diabetes	There is now unequivocal evidence that good diabetic control minimizes complications and should be strived for
First-degree relatives of patients with non-insulin-dependent diabetes	About one-third of siblings and offspring of patients with NIDDM have either diabetes or impaired glucose tolerance. The concordance for identical twins is almost 100%—double that in insulin-dependent diabetes. They should be screened
Patients taking glucocorticoids long term, such as bad asthmatics and people with rheumatoid arthritis	Particularly in female patients, treatment to increase calcium intake and keep vitamin D levels near the top of the normal range should be encouraged (i.e. calcium and vitamin D tablets). Bisphosphonate treatment should be considered
The whole population	Evidence that a reduction in salt and fat content of foods is useful in preventing hypertension and heart disease is very good. The food industry (a powerful lobby akin to the tobacco industry) only promotes changes that enhance sales. The fat removed to make 'healthy' skimmed milk, is ploughed into other foods such as soup, to make them creamy. Moves to reduce our fat and salt intakes should be encouraged.

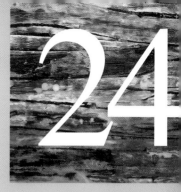

24

Endocrine function tests

- Summary
- Frequently used tests
- Less commonly used tests
- Tests used by endocrinologists in paediatric clinics

Summary

The number of dynamic function tests used routinely to assist in the diagnosis and management of endocrine disease has decreased as the range and sensitivity of peripheral hormone assays has improved. With the exception of the glucose tolerance test, the Synacthen test—used particularly to diagnose secondary adrenal cortical failure due to hypopituitarism—is perhaps the most widely used. The insulin stress test is uncomfortable for the patient and hypoglycaemia makes it a potentially dangerous way of diagnosing adrenocortical insufficiency. It has been largely superceded in this capacity by the short Synacthen test, but is still sometimes used to identify GH-deficient adults (see p. 232).

Second- and third-generation TSH assays and accurate assays for free thyroid hormones have together rendered the TRH test (TSH-releasing hormone) almost obsolete in the diagnosis of thyrotoxicosis. However, a paradoxical GH-secretory response to TRH is occasionally used to confirm the diagnosis of acromegaly.

The water deprivation test is still used to differentiate diabetes insipidus from hysterical polydipsia. If the diagnosis of diabetes mellitus is in doubt, a blood glucose 2 h after a 75 g dose of oral glucose is now all that is required.

Actual values vary between laboratories.

Table 24.1
Dexamethasone suppression test

Indications	Method	Interpretation
To exclude Cushing's syndrome (hypercortisolaemia of whatever cause)	Give the patient a 1 mg tablet of dexamethasone to take at home at 11 p.m. the evening before a single blood test for cortisol estimation at 9 a.m.	A cortisol below 138 nmol/l excludes the diagnosis; a level of <50 nmol/l is usual
If the overnight dexamethasone suppression test is abnormal (the sleeping midnight cortisol is ≥138 nmol/l), a single >50 nmol/l, or if 24 h urinary cortisol excretion is elevated (>275 nmol/24 h), go on to formal dexamethasone suppression testing	The patient is admitted to hospital and a blood sample taken at 11 p.m. on the day of admission for cortisol and ACTH. This is repeated at 8 a.m. daily for the next 4 days with sequential 24 h urine collections (8 a.m. to 8 a.m.) for free cortisol. Oral dexamethasone (0.5 mg) is given 6 hourly for the first 2 days, and increased to 4 mg qds for the last 2 days	Normally the cortisol is suppressed to <138 nmol/l and urinary free cortisol to <70 nmol/day. Once increased cortisol secretion has been confirmed, any consistent suppression or urinary cortisol by oral dexamethasone, no matter how small, suggests pituitary disease, and complete failure of suppression suggests primary adrenal disease or ectopic production. In practice, circulating cortisol is usually suppressed to < 50 nmol/l by a single dose of 1 mg dexamethasone, and, if not, is certainly suppressed by 2 mg/day

qds, four times a day.

Table 24.2
Glucose tolerance test

Indications	Method	Interpretation
To diagnose DM when fasting or random levels are inconclusive It is rarely necessary to do this except in pregnancy	Give 75 g glucose (388 ml Lucozade) Take blood for glucose (± GH) at time zero, and at 30 min intervals for 2 h	≤7.8 mmol/l is normal; > 7.8 and ≤ 11.1 mmol/l = impaired glucose tolerance; and > 11.1 mmol/l = diabetes (see p. 257)
To confirm the diagnosis of acromegaly	For the diagnosis of diabetes mellitus, a blood sample for glucose at 2 h is all that is required	Normally, GH is suppressed to < 2 mU/l. In acromegaly, GH remains unchanged, or increases 2 h after 75 g glucose orally

Table 24.3
Provera (medroxyprogesterone) withdrawal test

Indications	Method	Interpretation
To determine whether the endometrium has been exposed to oestrogens	Give 5 mg of provera® daily for 5 days	If this is followed by a menstrual period, the endometrium must have been in a proliferated state

Table 24.4
Short synacthen test

Indications	Method	Interpretation
Suspected primary hypoadrenalcorticalism	Make sure the patients stop their hydrocortisone replacement 24–36 h before the test	Lack of ACTH results in rapid adrenal cortical atrophy (with the exception of the aldosterone-producing zona glomerulosa), and a single bolus of Synacthen® (synthetic-ACTH-en) is insufficient to elicit a cortisol response
Suspected hypopituitarism	Give 250 μg of Synacthen® as a single im bolus and measure cortisol at 0, 30, and 60 min	Circulating cortisol should rise to ≥495 nmol/l, and usually does so by 1 h
		There are no indications for the long Synacthen test, as ACTH levels distinguish primary from secondary adrenal failure

Table 24.5
Corticotrophin-releasing hormone (CRH) test

Indications	Method	Interpretation
Used in patients with documented hypercortisolaemia, particularly as an adjunct to inferior petrosal sinus sampling It is *not* used as an ACTH secretogogue to test for hypopituitarism	Give 100 μg iv and take blood for ACTH and cortisol at 10, 15, 20, 30, and 60 min	An increase in petrosal ACTH occurs in Cushing's disease, but not ectopic ACTH secretion Unstimulated ACTH levels alone are very useful for separating Cushing's disease, adrenal tumours and ectopic ACTH almost completely. A pituitary MR scan is often even better

Table 24.6
Insulin stress test for GH deficiency

Indications	Method	Interpretation
One of the (not very good) tests of GH deficiency in adulthood Little used now as a test of hypopituitarism	Inject 0.1–0.15 U/kg iv at time zero Test BM stick glucose every 15 min to ensure that blood glucose falls to less than 2.2 mmol/l during the test Take blood for GH at 15 min intervals for 1 h If the patient collapses during the test (i.e. becomes markedly hypoglycaemic and needs resuscitation with glucose), the results are still valid	Still very poorly validated, but GH levels of <15 mU/l are low, 17–20 are borderline, and over 20 are taken as normal In deficiency, GH usually remains ≤5 mU/l, with <10 mU/l taken as mild and <3 mU/l, severe deficiency Note that the chances of GH deficiency if two or three other anterior pituitary hormones are deficient, are 80% and almost 100% respectively

Table 24.7
Pentagastrin test for medullary thyroid carcinoma

Indications	Method	Interpretation
To diagnose medullary carcinoma of the thyroid in patients with euthyroid goitre	Give 0.5 μg/kg pentagastrin IV Take blood for calcitonin 3, 5, and 10 min later	>300 ng/l or a threefold increase in calcitonin is a positive test

Table 24.8
Synacthen test for congenital adrenal hyperplasia

Indications	Method	Interpretation
Patients with marked hirsutism, equivocal basal 17-hydroxyprogesterone, and raised testosterone	Give 250 μg Synacthen® between 8 a.m. and 9 a.m. during the follicular phase of the cycle. Measure 17-hydroxyprogesterone at 50 min	A positive result is a level of >45.4 nM. In 3β-dehydrogenase deficiency, DHEA is also elevated

Table 24.9
Thyrotrophin-releasing hormone (TRH) test

Indications	Method	Interpretation
Used mostly to confirm the diagnosis of acromegaly—in which paradoxical GH secretion occurs.	Inject 200 μg TRH as rapid iv bolus—tell patient to expect curious side-effects such as transient discomfort at the back of the throat, or strange taste, with marked but fleeting nausea	A paradoxical GH secretory response suggests acromegaly
It is occasionally used to confirm the diagnosis of thyrotoxicosis if the TSH is persistently suppressed, but both the FT_4 and FT_3 remain well within the normal range	Take samples for GH (or TSH ± PRL) at 0, 20, or 30 min and 60 min	In primary thyrotoxicosis, the TSH-secretory response to TRH is suppressed
It is no longer used to test for hypopituitarism		

Table 24.11
Arginine stimulation of GH reserves

Indications	Method	Interpretation
Not used to identify GH deficiency in adults, but occasionally used in children	Give 0.5 g/kg arginine iv to a maximum of 40 g and measure GH levels at 15 min intervals	A GH of < 9 mU/l strongly suggests GH deficiency, although the deficiency may be partial
This test should only be undertaken by paediatric endocrinologists with a special interest in growth		

Table 24.10
Water deprivation test

Indications	Method	Interpretation
To distinguish diabetes insipidus from polydipsia. It can also help to distinguish cranial from nephrogenic DI, although the former, if untreated, can so reduce the concentration gradient in the renal medulla that nephrogenic DI occurs as a complication. This is an unusual conundrum in practice The patient must not drink or smoke during the test	In practice you get a 'head start' if you ask the patient not to drink overnight and to restrict their fluid intake on the morning of the test, if it does not make them too uncomfortable. Weigh the patient with an empty bladder at 8 a.m., then collect total voided urine hourly from 8 a.m. (record the volume and save a sample for osmolality) and weigh the patient *before and after* each visit to the toilet Take blood samples every 2 h for osmolality. A dose of DDAVP is usually given at the end of the test	In diabetes insipidus, the urine volume and osmolality change very little. If the patient has drunk a huge amount of water to 'tide them over the test', the urine osmolality often decreases in the second ± third sample, and the volume increases. DDAVP should result in a reduction in urine volume in the next hour and an increase in osmolality

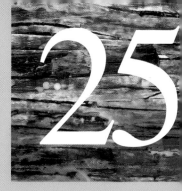

25

Examination hints

- What does the examiner want?

- Who fails?

- The attitude to have

What does the examiner want?

Very few examiners take delight in seeing an overanxious student sweating and writhing under pressure. For most, the only pleasure derived from exams is when they see their students confidently and competently gliding through, and are able to think to themselves 'I wouldn't mind having any of them look after my patients ... or after me, for that matter.'

Given a little personal effort, almost everybody who gets into medical school in the first place is gifted enough to become an excellent doctor. By failing students, clinical teachers recognize that they are failing themselves, and if examining people the first time is bad, having to organize further exams—drag another series of long and short cases back to hospital and set aside time to re-agonize over the outcome—is worse. So every effort is made to help the student pass.

Table 25.1
Viva voce hints

Prepare for the exam by setting yourself questions and answering them out loud

Ask your personal tutor, your lecturers, or junior medical staff to give you a trial viva, to practise answering 'on the fly'

When you answer a question in a viva, speak up and speak clearly: it is no time to allow shyness or nervousness to wreck your careful preparation

Do not give the impression of boredom or arrogance. There is nothing more offensive

Induce the examiners to ask you the questions you want to be asked. For example, if you have polished up your knowledge about diabetes and are answering a question about splenectomy, you final words might be '... the risks of overwhelming infection might be even higher in *diabetes*

Do not accidentally induce the examiners to ask you questions about a subject you know little about. If you are answering a question about diabetic ketoacidosis (about which you know a great deal) and the first complication you mention is 'Respiratory distress syndrome', do not be surprised if the examiner stops you and asks you all about RDS

Do not give protracted answers. You cannot score points if the examiners cannot ask enough questions.

Do not forget the obvious. If you are asked what tests you might request in a diabetic annual review, do not start with retinal angiograms, autonomic function tests, and Doppler flow studies, without first mentioning blood glucose, HbA1c, creatinine, urea and electrolytes, urine stick test for protein, and so on

Table 25.2
Written exam hints

Read the rubrics. If is says 'give the 4 most common causes of hypercalcaemia' give 4, not 24

You must be careful to answer the question that has been asked. If the question says 'describe the *management* of hypercalcaemia', do not give the *clinical signs* of hypercalcaemia

Answer *all* of the questions. If by mistake you have only left yourself 60 seconds to answer the last one, at least write *something*. If nothing at all has been written, nothing at all will be scored – and that is the only time the examiner will feel himself beyond criticism for giving a low mark

Do not hide behind shear volume of prose in essays. It will annoy the examiner

Short answers are SHORT ANSWERS. The examiner is likely to have a set marking scheme and will be looking for key words or concepts

Write legibly. You may be very proud of your stylish scrawl, but it is not in your best interests to irritate the marker

Headings and subheadings are very useful to organize your thoughts and allow you to demonstrate that organization to the examiner. The examiner will find it easier to mark, and that can only help

Do not forget the obvious. If you are asked to write about the symptoms and signs of Addison's disease and you write 600 words on hypercalcaemia (a mild and unusual association) but forget to mention nausea, anorexia, weight loss, and postural hypotension, you will diminish your score

Lastly, if at the end of the day, you think that the marks you were given do not truly reflect your ability, *do not become despondent*. It may be worth asking for the mark to be reviewed if you feel strongly that you have been misjudged

---

However, the examiners are aware that (to use a 'driving test' analogy) you have to share the road with those who pass the test, and doctors who are clearly oblivious of their ignorance are the most worrying for patients and the profession alike.

The job of the examiners is to assess each student to see whether they are competent to be let loose on the population at large. That decision is usually obvious within the first few minutes of the start of the clinical exam. After that, the examiner has little to do unless the student is rather good or rather bad, in which case the examiner will push harder. It should be borne in mind that although a rapidly regurgitated list of 20 causes of 'syndrome x' may be impressive, students (and subsequently doctors) who have no idea which two or three conditions account for almost all of the cases that they will see during their career are often worse than useless.

Table 25.3
Multiple-choice question

Hints

The MCQ format is a powerful way to test knowledge. Because it is so objective it is also in very widespread use, often exploiting banks of questions that have been extensively tested in battle

Do not waste time claiming that 'I just can't do MCQ exams'. It is not a productive attitude to work with

Do not resent marking systems that deduct marks for wrong answers. It is important to know when you don't know

False confidence in medical practice is a killer

Although there is no magic formula for easing the amount of work (and being a medical undergraduate is very hard work), try to identify *aides-mémoire* that are effective for you. For example, memorize a complete pictorial tableau of the disease (i.e. the patient who had all the features) or make up a mnemonic. However ridiculous the association, if it works for you, it works

Work *before* an exam, not afterwards for the re-sits. Do not waste time trying to make sure that other people think you did not have to do any work to pass

If you work hard to master a subject, you will find that the tendency to come out an MCQ exam claiming that 'The questions were so ambiguous!' is greatly reduced

Who fails?

Exams are failed by the ignorant and the arrogant, neither of whom know when they do not know. Although it may not seem so at the time, there are few genuine 'upsets' in undergraduate clinical exams. In most cases people who 'unexpectedly fail' have been fooling themselves and others about their knowledge and ability. If it looks as if you are percussing the chest or testing tendon reflexes for the first time, the examiners will know. When patients acting as long and short cases have been asked what *they* thought of individual medical students after the clinical exams, their opinions concur remarkably well with those of the examiners.

The attitude to have

You have to be honest with yourself. Students who have worked throughout the course do not fail. Again, it is critical in undergraduate and postgraduate medicine to know when you do not know, and it helps to do something about it before an exam. If you have worked hard in the course, and hard for the exam, make sure the examiners know how good you are. Don't let them get you down.

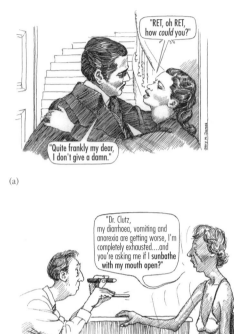

(a)

(b)

Fig. 25.1 Examples of *aides-mémoire*. (a) Many oncogenes, transcription factors, and second messengers are reduced to acronyms that are easy to confuse. *'RET'*, the oncogene associated with MEN 2a and 2b, sounds like 'Rhett' (a.k.a. Rhett Butler), the hero of the film *Gone with the Wind*. Scarlett, protesting, has the lip thickening and goitre associated with the condition. (b) A scene depicting the classical symptoms and signs of Addison's disease. Weight loss, lassitude, anorexia, nausea, and vomiting are the most typical symptoms of primary adrenal failure (Addison's disease). The lack of cortisol feedback inhibition leads to high levels of pituitary ACTH being released and, if the condition develops slowly enough, marked pigmentation of skin and mucous membranes results. This affects particularly the creases on the hands, friction areas, new scars, and the mucous membranes—a fact that has clearly escaped Dr Clutz.

Also, remember that the patients you are clerking or examining are real people, who are often uncomfortable. Establish a rapport with them as you would anyone else, and they will not want to see you fail either (which can be very useful!).

Index

acarbox *see* α-glucoidase inhibitors
ACE *see* angiotensin converting enzyme
acidosis 101, 263, 265
acne 86, 95, 109
acromegaly 37, 38, 203, 343
ACTH 17, 84, 87, 374
   see adrenocorticotrophic hormone
AD *see* androstenedione
Addison's disease 89, 91, 96
  crisis 89, 92
  diagnosis 90, 384
  symptoms and signs 89, 90, 384
  treatment 92
adenohypophysis *see* pituitary
adenoma
  see under specific endocrine organs
adenomatosis, multiple endocrine 354
adenylyl cyclase 7
ADH *see* vasopressin
adrenal cortex
  diseases 87
  physiology 86
adrenal glands 83
  tumours 91, 93, 168
adrenal medulla
  diseases 87
adrenarche 214
adrenocortical insufficiency
  see Addison's disease
α-Glucosidase inhibitors 261
adrenocorticotrophic hormones 17, 84,
    87, 374
aggression 18, 132, 189
alcoholism 141, 192
  hyperlipidaemia and 292
  impotence and 203, 208
aldosterone 85, 86
  metabolism 87
  plasma levels 93
  secretion 87
aldosteronism
  primary *see* Conn's syndrome
  secondary 330
5α-reductase 353
alkaline phosphatase 306, 309, 312
amiodarone 80
anabolic steroids, synthetic 193, 196

androgens
  effects 166, 189
androstenedione 85, 86
angiotensin 87
angiotensin converting enzyme
  inhibitors 102, 272, 281, 294
anorexia nervosa 228, 247
anosmia *see* Kallmann's syndrome 130,
    187, 192
anti-androgens 123, 140, 141, 157, 170,
    172
antidiuretic hormone *see* vasopressin
antiperspirants 357
anxiety, attacks of 51, 88, 201, 204
apolipoproteins 288
apoplexy, pituitary 32
appetite 22, 242, 245
  in hyperthyroidism 61
appetite-suppressing drugs 248
arginine stimulation test, *see* growth
    hormone deficiency, tests of
aromatase 353
arteries, peripheral, obstruction 272
asthma 217, 223, 227
atenolol 196, 297
atheroma, diabetes and 272
atrial natriuretic peptide 327
autoantibodies
  thyroid 70
  adrenal 89
autocrine effects 6, 10
autoimmune disease 10, 59, 89
azoospermia 187, 196

Bartter's syndrome 100, 343
basal temperature 3, 108, 110
beriberi 243
bicarbonate, in ketoacidosis 264
biguanides 260
bisphosphonates 304, 313
bitemporal hemianopia
  see vision
blindness, in diabetes 255, 257
blood glucose level 257, 265
  estimation of 260

BMI *see* body mass index
body mass index 246, 258
body temperature 3, 108, 110
bone 299
    accretion 302
    age 189, 218, 222, 228, 233
    density measurement 312
    hyperparathyroidism 305
breasts 114, 175
    carcinoma, hormone treatment 353
    development during puberty and 178
    lactation and 177
    pain and *see* mastalgia 180, 191
bromocriptine 33, 36, 149
    in acromegaly 38
    in lactation suppression 179
    in prolactinomas 38
bulimia 247

cabergoline 33
CAH *see* congenital adrenal hyperplasia
calcaemic factors 301, 304
calcitonin 303
    in calcium metabolism 59, 303
    in thyroid carcinoma 72
calcium 299
    bone accretion and 302
    emergencies 313, 314
    metabolism 302
    plasma levels 306
    gluconate, in hypocalcaemia 308
    vitamin D tablets and 311
cAMP
cancer, hormonal treatment 353, 360
carbimazole 66
carbohydrate 258, 261, 289
carcinoid syndrome 244, 347, 352
carcinoma
    hormonal treatment of 353
    pancreas 349, 354
    lung 55, 352
    thyroid 70
carpal tunnel syndrome
    acromegaly and 37, 298
cataracts 267
catecholamines 85, 87, 99

C cells 303
    thyroid and 59, 99
CCK-PZ *see* cholecystokinin-pancreozymin
centile charts 229, 233
cerebellar haemangioblastomatosis 101
cervical mucus 110, 115
Charcot's joints 272
chiasm, optic, pituitary tumours and 27, 33, 34
cholecalciferol *see* vitamin D
cholecystokinin-pancreozymin 242
cholesterol 94, 288
    containing foods 291
chorionic gonadotrophin 11, 137
chorionic villi 146
chromosomes 116, 190, 217, 233
Chvostek's sign 307
circadian rhythms 4, 31
clomiphene citrate
    in infertility 137, 140
coeliac disease 214, 223, 227, 228, 309
coma
    diabetic 256
    hyperosmolar 265, 279
    hypoglycaemic 265
    ketotic 263, 279
    lactic acidotic 265
    myxoedema 71
congenital adrenal hyperplasia 10, 94, 148, 218
conjunctivitis 63
Conn's syndrome 91, 100, 340, 344
contraceptives 155
    adverse reactions 158
    contraindications 158, 162
    postcoital 159
    side-effects 139, 159
corpus luteum 107
corticosteroids
    actions 86
    synthesis 85
corticotroph 29
corticotrophin-releasing hormone test 375
craniopharyngioma 18, 217, 245, 327
CRH test *see* corticotrophin-releasing hormone test

Cushing's syndrome 39, 93, 341
  diagnosis 39, 375
  obesity and 38, 245
  osteoporosis and
  treatment 33
cyproheptadine 352
cyproterone acetate *see* anti-androgens
cytokines 3

D₃ *see* vitamin D
danazol 180
DDAVP 43, 45, 329
dehydroepiandrosterone 86, 87, 166, 173
dehydroepiandrosterone sulphate 86, 87,
    166, 173
De Quervain's thyroiditis 74
  see thyroiditis
demeclocycline 329, 334
depression 135, 214, 288
desmopressin 43, 45, 329
dexamethasone suppression test 372
DEXA 310, 312
DHEA 86, 87, 166, 173
  see dehydroepiandrosterone
DHEAS 86, 87, 166, 173
  see dehydroepiandrosterone
diabetes insipidus 16, 327
  causes 327, 328
  water deprivation test and 378
diabetes mellitus 253
  advice to patients 258
  complications 255, 263
  definition 255
  diagnosis 257
  diet 258
  eyes in *see* retinopathy 266, 267
  feet in 272
  gestational 147, 153, 262
  heredity 280
  hyperosmolar, non-ketotic coma 265,
    279
  incidence 256
  ketones and 263, 279
  life expectancy in 256, 257
  pregnancy and 262
  retinopathy 266, 267, 279

surgery and 262
  treatment 258
diarrhoea
  carcinoid and 352, 356
  diabetes and 271
  pancreatic tumours and 350
  thyrotoxicosis and 61
diazoxide 350
diet
  diabetes and 258
  lipid lowering 289, 292
  weight reducing 248
dietary
  thermogenesis and 251
1,25-dihydroxycholecalciferol 302
dihydrotestosterone 6, 106, 190, 353
diplopia 63
dopamine 16, 17, 27, 45
  D₂ agonist drugs 28, 33, 36
drugs
  in breast milk 147
  transplacental passage 67, 147
dysmenorrhoea 124
dyspareunia 20, 105, 110

electrolysis 169
empty sellar syndrome 40, 49
endocrine system 3
endometrium 107, 109
epilepsy 32, 307
  prolactin levels after a fit 51
erectile dysfunction 191, 199
erections *see* erectile dysfunction
ergocalciferol *see* vitamin D
erythropoietin 348
ethinyloestradiol 123, 128, 158, 170
eunuchoïdism 189
excessive height 233
exams 379
exercise
  amenorrhoea and 121, 122, 265
  fibrinogen and 288
  lactic acidosis and 265
  microalbuminuria and 281
  obesity and 250
  osteoporosis and 311, 322

exophthalmometer 64
external-beam radiotherapy *see*
      radiotherapy 35
exophthalmos 62, 63
eyelids, retraction in thyroid disease 62

fat 166, 173
   metabolism and 288
feet, diabetic 272
feminization 170, 351
fertility 133
fetus, diabetes and 262
fibrates 293
fibrinogen 288
finasteride 173, 353
fine-needle aspiration biopsy 62
fludrocortisone 86, 91
fluoride 294, 311
flutamide *see* anti-androgens 173, 353
fluvastatin *see* statins
FNAB *see* fine-needle aspiration biopsy
      75, 77
follicle stimulating hormone 17, 21, 31,
      42
food 239
   psychology of 241
fornix 18
frame size *see* obesity 246
FSH *see* follicle stimulating hormone

galactorrhoea 36, 177, 179
   amenorrhoea and 183
gastrin 242
gastrinoma 349
   see also Zollinger–Ellison syndrome
genitalia
   ambiguous 95
GH *see* growth hormone
gigantism 233, 238
globulin
   thyroid binding 65, 77, 79
   sex hormone binding (SHBG) 114,
      166, 168
glucagon 245, 263, 266
   hypoglycaemia treatment of 266

glucagonoma 350
glucocorticoid
   effects of 55, 86, 304, 314
   and replacement therapy 45, 92, 97
glucose
   tolerance test (GTT) 257, 373
   in acromegaly 373
α-glucosidase inhibitor 261
glycosuria 257
glycosylated haemoglobin 260
GnRH *see* gonadotrophin-releasing
      hormone
goitre
   types 64, 70
gonadotrophins *see* follicle stimulating
      hormone and luteinizing hormone
   chorionic, human 11, 137
gonadotroph 29, 214
gonadotrophin-releasing hormone
   superagonists 125, 131
gonads, dysgenesis 130
goserelin *see* gonadotrophin-releasing
      hormone superagonists
Graffian follicles *see* ovarian follicles
granulomas 18, 327
granulosa cells, of ovarian follicles 353
Graves' disease 10, 52
   pre-tibial myxoedema and 61
growth 225
growth hormone
   deficiency
      characteristics of 227, 229, 231
      tests of 44, 232, 377
   excess 233
   see acromegaly
   series (mean blood level) 38
GTT *see* glucose tolerance test
guar gum 261
gubernaculum 187
gut and calcium absorption 303, 305
gynaecomastia 177, 191, 193, 351

haemorrhage
   postpartum 31, 150
   retinal 267, 269
hair, normal 166

follicles 114
hamartomas 218
Hand–Schüller–Christian disease 327, 334
Hashimoto's thyroiditis 69
HbAlc see glycosylated haemoglobin
HDL see high density lipoproteins
heart disease 62, 247, 367
    in carcinoid 352
    in diabetes 256
    in hyperlipidaemia 289
    in hyperthyroidism 71
height, measurement of 230
5-HIAA see 5-hydroxyindoleacetic acid
high density lipoproteins 288, 292
hippocampus 18
hirsutism 163
    idiopathic 167
    treatment of 169
histamine 361
histiocytosis X see
        Hand–Schüller–Christian disease
HMG CoA reductase 288
homocystinuria 234
hormone replacement therapy
    sex hormones 126
    thyroid hormones 41, 71, 79
    adrenal hormones 41, 92
hormones
    circulating 4
    gastrointestinal 242
    receptors 5
hot flushes 105, 110, 126, 353
HRT see hormone replacement therapy
hunger 241, 276
hungry bones 307
hydrocortisone replacement 41, 148
4-hydroxy androstenedione 353
25-hydroxycholecalciferol 303
5-hydroxyindoleacetic acid
    carcinoid and 352
3β-hydroxylase deficiency 95
11β-hydroxylase deficiency 95
hydroxyproline 312
17-hydroxyprogesterone 95, 96, 100, 376

11-hydroxysteroid dehydrogenase 100, 344
5-hydroxytryptamine (5HT) 347
hyperaldosteronism
    primary see Conn's syndrome
    secondary 330
hypercalcaemia 301, 305, 306, 307, 311, 327
    bone secondaries and 320
    differential diagnosis 307, 320
    treatment 313
hypercholesterolaemia 69, 288
    see hyperlipidaemia 285
hyperkalaemia 89, 92
hyperlipidaemia 285
    treatment of 290, 291, 292
hypernatraemia 271, 325, 328
hyperparathyroidism
    primary 301, 305, 321, 347, 349, 354
    secondary 306, 307
    tertiary 306, 308
hyperphagia 18, 22
hypertension 337
    endocrine causes of 340, 351
hyperthyroidism 59
    toxic adenoma and 64
    botulinum toxin 63
    diagnosis 61
    eye disease and 62, 63
    pathology and aetiology 60
    sex ratio 62
    surgery 66
    treatment 65, 66
hypertriglyceridaemia 291, 292
hypoadrenalism 89
    see Addison's disease
hypocalcaemia 306, 307, 308
    differential diagnosis of 301, 307
    symptoms and signs 307
hypoglycaemia 265
    after insulin 255, 265, 266
    spontaneous 277, 354
    treatment 266
hypogonadism 16, 121, 189, 191, 217
hypogonadotrophic hypogonadism see
        hypogonadism
hypokalaemia 55, 91, 101, 327, 341, 343

hyponatraemia 92, 96, 325, 328
hypoparathyroidism 307, 308
  pseudohypoparathyroidism 233, 308
  pseudopseudohypoparathyroidism 308
hypophysectomy 33, 34, 46
hypopituitarism 40, 233
hypos
  feeling of 265, 266, 274
hypothalamus
  anatomy 18
  hormones secreted by the 17
  symptoms of underactivity of 15, 16,
    31, 41, 69
hypothyroidism
  aetiology 70
  after radioiodine treatment 66
  clinical features 69, 71, 217
  obesity and 250
  tendon reflexes and 69, 71
hysterical polydipsia *see* polydipsia

IDDM *see* insulin dependent diabetes
  mellitus
IGF-I 38, 54, 131, 227, 236, 343
immunocytochemistry 29
impaired glucose tolerance
  risks of 257
impotence 199
  management 203, 204
infertility 133
  female, investigation and treatment
    28, 107, 110, 137, 140, 141
  male, investigation and treatment 28,
    136, 138
inhibin 107, 173, 188
insulin 255, 258
  in insulin dependent diabetes mellitus
    280
  in ketoacidosis 264
  lispro 259
  long acting 259
  pen injection devices 259
  sliding scale 261
insulin-like growth factor I 38, 54, 131,
  227, 236, 343
insulin-like growth factor II 227
insulinoma 245, 350, 354

insulin stress test 376
intermediate lobe of the pituitary 51
iodine
  food sources 60
  in hyperthyroidism 68, 79
  radioactive 66
  trapping 60
ipodate, sodium 68
ischaemic heart disease
  hyperlipidaemia and 287, 289
  risk factors 289

jaw wiring, obesity and 251
jejunoileal bypass 251

Kallmann's syndrome 16, 129, 187, 217
karyotype 217, 220
ketoacidosis 263, 279
  treatment of 264
ketones 263, 264
Klinefelter's syndrome 115, 189, 217,
  223, 237
kyphosis, osteoporosis and 311

lactation
  mechanism 177
  suppression *see* galactorrhoea
lactic acidosis 265, 283
lactogen, placental 147
lactotroph *see* mammotroph 29, 31, 149
lamina terminalis 18, 326
Laron dwarfism 10
laser treatment
  for diabetic retinopathy 267, 270
  for hirsutism 169
LDL *see* low density lipoproteins 288
leptin 245
leukaemia, calcaemic factors and 301,
  304
Leydig cells 10
  function 173, 188
LH *see* luteinizing hormone
LHRH *see* gonadotrophin-releasing
  hormone
libido 191

also see erective dysfunction

lid lag *see* thyroid, eye disease and

lipids

diabetes and 258, 287

lipoprotein lipase 288

liquorice and mineralocorticoid effects

344

lithium 70, 80

Looser's zones 309

low density lipoproteins 288

Lp(a) 288

LPL *see* lipoprotein lipase 288

Lugol's iodine 79

luteinizing hormone 31, 107, 137, 188

lymphocytic hypophysitis 149

MAB *see* maximum androgen blockade

353

macrovascular complications of

diabetes 256, 272, 273

malnutrition, osteoporosis and 233

mammotroph cell 29, 31, 149

Marfan's syndrome 234

mastalgia 115, 180, 191

mastocytosis 360

maximum androgen blockade 353

McCune Albright 222

median eminence 19, 54

medroxyprogesterone acetate (Provera®)

111, 123, 373

melanocyte-stimulating hormone 29, 54

melatonin 215

MEN *see* multiple endocrine neoplasia

menarche 120

menopause 120, 125

effects 126

hormone replacement therapy 126

premature 112, 121

menorrhagia 125, 157

menstrual cycle 117

disorders 105, 120

menstruation 119

dysfunctional 125

mechanism 120

metanephrines 89, 357

also see phaeochromocytoma

methimazole 80

metyrapone, in adrenal cortex, tests 33,

90

MIBG 89

microalbuminuria 267, 278, 280

microaneurysms 267, 270

microprolactinomas

diagnosis 33, 36

treatment of 36

microvascular complications, of diabetes

266

migraine 109, 157, 158

MIH *see* Müllerian inhibiting hormone

187, 188

milk let down 153

mineralocorticoids 86, 90, 344

MSH *see* melanocyte-stimulating hormone

29, 54

Müllarian inhibiting hormone 187, 188

multiple endocrine neoplasia syndromes

101, 251, 352, 354

myasthenia gravis 62

myxoedema

coma 71

pre-tibial 61, 62, 68

Nelson's syndrome 34

nephropathy, diabetic 267

neurohypophysis *see* pituitary, posterior

neuropathy, diabetic 271

autonomic 271

impotence and 199, 271

peripheral 271, 278

nicotinic acid

derivatives 293

supplements 352

NIDDM *see* non-insulin-dependent

diabetes

non-insulin-dependent diabetes mellitus

253

norethisterone 126, 158, 160

normetanephrines 89

also see phaeochromocytoma

obesity 246

aetiology 245

classification 246

obesity (*cont.*):
  consequences of 132, 287
  Cushing's syndrome and 245
  management 248
  mechanical and surgical procedures
    251
ob/ob mouse 252
oestradiol 17, 107
oestrogens
  effects and side-effects 111, 115
  osteoporosis and 114, 304
  therapy with 115, 158
oestrone 166, 173
17OH-P *see* 17-hydroxyprogesterone
oil of evening primrose 125, 180
oligomenorrhoea 137
oncogene 347
ophthalmoplegia, thyroid disease and 63
orchidometer 190
orchitis 189, 192
osmolality 326
  calculation to determine 265
  control of plasma 325, 326
osmoreceptors 326
osteoblasts 302, 312, 321
osteoclasts 302, 312, 321
osteomalacia 243, 301, 309
osteoporosis 237, 247, 301, 309
  definition 309
  ovarian dysfunction and 322
  treatment of 310
ovarian hyperstimulation syndrome 137
ovaries 103, 166
  development 105
  functional assessment 110
  tumours 167, 351
overeating, obesity and 245
ovulation
  tests for 137
oxytocin 17, 178, 179
  functions 153
  secretion 153
  therapeutics, use in 179

Paget's disease, of bone 313
  diagnosis 306, 313
  pathogenesis 313

treatment options 313
pamidronate 314, 321
  also see bisphosphonates
pancreas
  hormone secretion 242
  tumours 349, 350
panhypopituitarism 15, 44, 54, 150
paracrine effects 5
parathyroid glands 303
  carcinoma 306, 349
  hormone actions 302, 305
  overactivity *see* hyperparathyroidism
  underactivity 308
  see hypoparathyroidism
parathyroid hormone-related peptide
    304, 348
parturition and lactation 178
  also see oxytocin
PCO *see* polycystic ovarian disease
PCOD *see* polycystic ovarian disease
pellagra 244, 352
pentagastrin test for medullary thyroid
    carcinoma 376
pergolide 36
phaeochromocytoma 87, 88, 89, 100,
    348, 354
  diagnosis 89
  symptoms 89
phenothiazines 130
phenylethanolamine *n*-methyl transferase
    99, 101
phosphatase, alkaline, osteomalacia and
    306
phosphate, plasma levels of 306
pigmentation 31, 85, 92
pilosebaceous unit 166
pineal gland 34, 53, 215
pituicytes, of neural lobe 29
pituitary 25
  anatomy 28
  anterior 29
    functional assessment 41
    hormones 31
    infarction *see* Sheehan's syndrome
  overactivity 27, 29
  posterior 17
  also see oxytocin and vasopressin
  tumours 29

underactivity 40
placenta
  function 146
  hormones produced by 146, 147, 178
PMT *see* premenstrual syndrome
PNMT *see*
  phenylethanolamine *N*-methyl transferase
polycystic ovary disease 121, 122
  diagnosis 122, 124
  treatment 123, 124, 138
polycythaemia 251, 348
polydipsia 307, 331, 334
polyuria 275, 307, 314
postpartum thyroiditis 65
  see thyroiditis, postpartum
potassium
  see hypokalaemia and hyperkalaemia
pre-androgens *see* DHEA, AD, DHEAS
prednisolone 74, 80, 99, 314
pregnancy 143
  adrenal hormones and 148
  diabetes insipidus and 327
  diabetes and 145, 262
  diagnosis 11, 147
  drugs and 54, 154
  hyperthyroidism and 65
  thyroid hormones and 147
premenstrual syndrome 124, 127, 132
priapism 203
PRL *see* prolactin
progesterone
  as contraceptive 108, 162
  effects and side-effects 108, 109, 162
  plasma levels after ovulation 111
prolactin 17, 31
  erectile dysfunction and 203
  galactorrhoea and 179
prolactinomas 36, 135
prophylaxis 363
propranolol 66, 80, 152
proptosis 63
propylthiouracil 67, 68, 152
prostate 106, 353
  carcinoma, treatment 353
  hypertrophy
    prophylactic treatment 366

Provera test 373
  see also medroxyprogesterone acetate
pseudohypoparathyroidism 308
pseudopseudohypoparathyroidism 308
PTH *see* parathyroid hormone
PTHrp *see* parathyroid hormone-related peptide
puberty 211, 214
  delayed 215, 217
  female, timing of 216
  male, timing of 216
  precocious 218, 219
pyridinium cross links 212

quinagolide 36

radioiodine
  in hyperthyroidism 66
radiotherapy
  gonadal 192
  pituitary 35
5α-reductase 353
  action of 366
renal threshold for glucose 257
renin 93
  angiotensin system 87, 340
  normal values 93
Restandol 52
  also see testosterone replacement
RET oncogene *see* MEN 2a and 2b 354, 384
retinopathy, diabetic 266, 267
rickets 243, 301, 309
Riedel's thyroiditis 75

sarcoidosis 307, 320, 327
satiety 241
scurvy 243
second messengers 6
secretin 242
sella turcica 28
semen, analysis of 136, 190, 197
serotonin *see* 5-hydroxytryptamine
Sertoli cells 173, 188

sex
  differentiation 106
  phylogenetic reasons for 119
Sheehan's syndrome 149
short stature 227, 237
SHRT *see* hormone replacement therapy
    sex hormones
SIADH *see* syndrome of inappropriate
    ADH secretion 328, 329
sick euthyroid syndrome 79
Sipple's syndrome,
  see multiple endocrine neoplasia
    syndromes 354
skin
  pigmentation, Addison's disease and
    31, 85, 92
  vitamin D synthesis 303
sliding scale, insulin 261
smoking
  antioestrogenic effects 125, 322
  macrovascular risks and 287
  pregnancy and 237
somatomammotrophin 147
somatostatin 242
  physiology 5
  therapeutic uses 38, 352
somatotroph 29, 31
somatotrophin *see* growth hormone
Somogyi effect 282
somnolence 18
sperm analysis 136, 190
spermatogenesis 136
spermatogonia 136, 188
spironolactone, in aldosteronism 93,
    342
  as antiandrogen 115, 172, 196, 208
statins 293
stature
  excessive 225, 233
  short 218, 228, 233
  Turner's syndrome and 233
storm *see* thyroid 65
streptozotocin 350
stress 15, 19
struma ovarii 60
suckling 153, 177
sulphonylureas 251, 260
sunlight 303, 318

surgery
  for obesity 251
  hypophysectomy 33, 34
  parathyroidectomy 306
  preparations for
    diabetics 262
    hyperthyroidism 79
  subfrontal 33
  thyroidectomy 66
  transphenoidal 33
Sustanon 45, 52, 193
  see testosterone replacement
sweating 348, 357
synacthen test
  for adrenal insufficiency 374
  for congenital adrenal hyperplasia 376
syncytiotrophoblast 146
syndrome of inappropriate ADH secretion
    328, 329

tamoxifen 180, 193, 353
tall stature 233
temperature, of body 3, 108, 110
tendons, reflex slow 69, 71
testes 185
  agenesis 196
  anatomy 187, 188
  descent 187, 192
  function 188, 190, 196
  Müllerian inhibiting hormone 187,
    188
  tumours 192, 351
testosterone
  absorption 52
  conversion to dihydrotestosterone 52,
    115, 173
  exogenous, effects of 140
  local concentrations 188
  ovarian secretion 166
  patches 52
  replacement 45
tetany 307
Theca cells of the ovary 106, 107, 173,
    353
thelarche 214, 218
thermogenesis 251
thirst 326, 329

thyroid
  anatomy 60
  autoantibodies 70
  calcitonin secretion and 303
  carcinoma 70
    anaplastic 72, 73
    follicular 72, 73
    medullary 72, 73, 354
    papillary 72, 73
  eye disease and 62
  scanning 74
  stimulating hormone 17, 29, 31
  storm 65
    treatment 68
thyroiditis
  de Quervain's 74
  Hashimoto's *see* Hashimoto's thyroiditis
    69
  postpartum 65, 145, 147, 152
  pyogenic 75
  Riedel's thyroditis 75
thyrotoxicosis *see* hyperthyroidism
thyrotroph cell 29, 31
thyrotrophin
  see thyroid stimulating hormone
thyrotrophin releasing hormone
  test 377
thyroxine
  free T_4 60
  free T_3 60
  plasma levels 76
  replacement in hypopituitarism 45
tibolone 357
tiredness 76, 96, 150
TRH test 377
triglycerides 288, 291
tri-iodothyronine (T_3) 54, 60, 80
trophoblast 146
Trousseau's sign 307
TSH *see* thyrotrophin
tumours 345
  hormone secreting 347
  hormone sensitive 347, 353

trophoblastic 60, 348
Turner's syndrome 106, 114, 116, 130,
    213, 220, 233
twins 367

ulcers
  ischaemic 272
  neuropathic, diabetes and 272
  peptic 349
  urinary cyclic AMP 308
urogenital ridge 114

vanillylmandelic acid 89, 359
vasoactive intestinal polypeptide (VIP)
    242
vasopressin 15, 16, 17, 29
  deficiency 326–330
  replacement 327
  syndrome of inappropriate secretion
    328, 329
VIPoma 350
virilization 86, 95
vision
  field defects 32
  tests of 30, 32
vitamin D 243, 301, 302, 319
VMA *see* vanillylmandelic acid
von Hippel–Lindau disease 101

water deprivation test 329, 378
  watery diarrhoea syndrome *see* VIP
Wermer's syndrome *see* multiple endocrine
    neoplasia syndromes 354

xerophthalmia 243

Zollinger–Ellison syndrome 349, 354
Zona glomerulosa 374